Tumors and Cysts of the Jaws

Atlas
of
Tumor Pathology

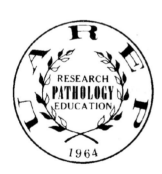

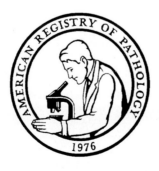

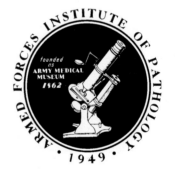

ATLAS OF TUMOR PATHOLOGY

Third Series
Fascicle 29

TUMORS AND CYSTS OF THE JAWS

by

JAMES J. SCIUBBA, D.M.D., Ph.D.
Otolaryngology-Head and Neck Surgery
Director, Division of Dental and Oral Medicine
Johns Hopkins Medical Center
Baltimore, Maryland

JOHN E. FANTASIA, D.D.S.
Associate Professor of Oral Biology and Pathology
School of Dental Medicine
S. U. N. Y. at Stony Brook
Chief, Oral and Maxillofacial Pathology
Long Island Jewish Medical Center
New Hyde Park, New York

LEONARD B. KAHN, M.B.B.Ch., M.Med.Path, F.R.C.Path.
Professor of Pathology and Pathology Chairman
Albert Einstein College of Medicine
Long Island Jewish Medical Center
New Hyde Park, New York

Published by the
ARMED FORCES INSTITUTE OF PATHOLOGY
Washington, D.C.

Under the Auspices of
UNIVERSITIES ASSOCIATED FOR RESEARCH AND EDUCATION IN PATHOLOGY, INC.
Bethesda, Maryland
2001

Accepted for Publication
1999

Available from the American Registry of Pathology
Armed Forces Institute of Pathology
Washington, D.C. 20306-6000
www.afip.org
ISSN 0160-6344
ISBN 1-881041-62-X

ATLAS OF TUMOR PATHOLOGY

EDITOR
JUAN ROSAI, M.D.
Department of Pathology
Memorial Sloan-Kettering Cancer Center
New York, New York 10021-6007

ASSOCIATE EDITOR
LESLIE H. SOBIN, M.D.
Armed Forces Institute of Pathology
Washington, D.C. 20306-6000

EDITORS' NOTE

The Atlas of Tumor Pathology has a long and distinguished history. It was first conceived at a Cancer Research Meeting held in St. Louis in September 1947 as an attempt to standardize the nomenclature of neoplastic diseases. The first series was sponsored by the National Academy of Sciences-National Research Council. The organization of this Sisyphean effort was entrusted to the Subcommittee on Oncology of the Committee on Pathology, and Dr. Arthur Purdy Stout was the first editor-in-chief. Many of the illustrations were provided by the Medical Illustration Service of the Armed Forces Institute of Pathology, the type was set by the Government Printing Office, and the final printing was done at the Armed Forces Institute of Pathology (hence the colloquial appellation "AFIP Fascicles"). The American Registry of Pathology purchased the Fascicles from the Government Printing Office and sold them virtually at cost. Over a period of 20 years, approximately 15,000 copies each of nearly 40 Fascicles were produced. The worldwide impact that these publications have had over the years has largely surpassed the original goal. They quickly became among the most influential publications on tumor pathology ever written, primarily because of their overall high quality but also because their low cost made them easily accessible to pathologists and other students of oncology the world over.

Upon completion of the first series, the National Academy of Sciences-National Research Council handed further pursuit of the project over to the newly created Universities Associated for Research and Education in Pathology (UAREP). A second series was started, generously supported by grants from the AFIP, the National Cancer Institute, and the American Cancer Society. Dr. Harlan I. Firminger became the editor-in-chief and was succeeded by Dr. William H. Hartmann. The second series Fascicles were produced as bound volumes instead of loose leaflets. They featured a more comprehensive coverage of the subjects, to the extent that the Fascicles could no longer be regarded as "atlases" but rather as monographs describing and illustrating in detail the tumors and tumor-like conditions of the various organs and systems.

Once the second series was completed, with a success that matched that of the first, UAREP and AFIP decided to embark on a third series. A new editor-in-chief and an associate editor were selected, and a distinguished editorial board was appointed. The mandate for the third series remains the same as for the previous ones, i.e., to oversee the production of an eminently practical publication with surgical pathologists as its primary audience, but also aimed at other workers in oncology. The main purposes of this series are to promote a consistent, unified, and biologically sound nomenclature; to guide the surgical pathologist in the diagnosis of the various tumors and tumor-like lesions; and to provide relevant histogenetic, pathogenetic, and clinicopathologic information on these entities. Just as the second series included data obtained from ultrastructural (and, in the more recent Fascicles, immunohistochemical) examination, the third series will, in addition, incorporate pertinent information obtained with the newer molecular biology techniques. As in the past, a continuous attempt will be made to correlate, whenever possible, the nomenclature used in the Fascicles with that proposed by the World Health Organization's International Histological Classification of Tumors. The format of the third series has been changed in order to incorporate additional items and to ensure a consistency of style throughout. Close cooperation between the various authors and their respective liaisons from the editorial board will be emphasized to minimize unnecessary repetition and discrepancies in the text and illustrations.

To its everlasting credit, the participation and commitment of the AFIP to this venture is even more substantial and encompassing than in previous series. It now extends to virtually all scientific, technical, and financial aspects of the production.

The task confronting the organizations and individuals involved in the third series is even more daunting than in the preceding efforts because of the ever-increasing complexity of the matter at hand. It is hoped that this combined effort—of which, needless to say, that represented by the authors is first and foremost—will result in a series worthy of its two illustrious predecessors and will be a suitable introduction to the tumor pathology of the twenty-first century.

Juan Rosai, M.D.
Leslie H. Sobin, M.D.

ACKNOWLEDGEMENTS

The presentation of cysts and tumors of the jaws within this text represents the efforts of individuals who have worked in concert, often times overlapping writing assignments and topics. We have remained as faithful to the World Health Organization classifications of odontogenic pathology as possible. In the area of nonodontogenic jawbone pathology and nonodontogenic fibro-osseous lesions, Dr. Leonard Kahn prepared a comprehensive review of the more common conditions while Dr. James Sciubba contributed several of the miscellaneous entities within these sections. Dr. John Fantasia compiled the information and case material concerning odontogenic cysts while Dr. Sciubba prepared the chapters on classification and development of jaw tumors and odontogenic tumors.

Each author provided feedback, cross checking, and editorial commentary to the others throughout the preparation of drafts and final proofs. The reviewers who evaluated our final draft were instrumental in helping clarify several areas in a constructive and appropriate fashion, thus allowing production of a final text that has the necessary breadth and level of detail to make accessing the information straightforward and useful.

The vast majority of the illustrations were obtained from case material within the files of the Departments of Pathology and Dental Medicine at the Long Island Jewish Medical Center. Early recognition of the need to store and catalog such material in a careful and painstaking way by Dr. Leon Eisenbud and the New York Bone Club must be acknowledged. The authors have continued this careful method of case collecting for other endeavors such as this. Other mentors and colleagues who have inspired and molded us over the years are likewise represented within this volume. They include Drs. Lauren Ackerman, Juan Rosai, Charles Waldron, John Waterhouse, and John Batsakis. Our residents and colleagues, interacting with us on a daily basis, sustain the influence of our mentors. Secretarial and organizational support were provided by Ms. Vivian Yip, Barbara Stoja, and Carol Ann Marsigliano.

To our wives, Dolores, Lydia, and Louise, we offer our thanks for their infinite patience and for allowing us to be diverted from family responsibilities during this project.

James J. Sciubba, D.M.D, Ph.D.
John E. Fantasia, D.D.S.
Leonard B. Kahn, M.D.

Permission to use copyrighted illustrations has been granted by:

Medical Association of South Africa:
S Afr Med J 1975;49:2041–5. For figures 8-114, 8-117, 8-118, 8-120, and 8-121.

Mosby:
Oral Surg Oral Med Oral Pathol 1993;76:378–80. For figure 4-19.
Oral Surg Oral Med Oral Pathol 1992;74:319–25. For figure 8-151.
Oral Surg Oral Med Oral Pathol 1985;59:441–5. For figure 4-7.
Oral Surg Oral Med Oral Pathol 1978;46:386–95. For figures 8-89, 8-90, 8-91, and 8-93.

Contents

✧✧✧

TUMORS AND CYSTS OF THE JAWS

1
DEVELOPMENT OF THE TEETH AND JAWS

The pathology of both benign and malignant tumor types within the jaws owes much of its uniqueness to the presence of teeth and associated tissues and structures. The specific nature of the pathologic process tends to be related to the development of these structures and the interaction of epithelial and mesenchymal elements. Additionally, there are many opportunities for pathologic processes to develop, since there are 52 odontogenic structures in the enamel organ which begin their formation at approximately 6 weeks of embryonic life and terminate in the midportion of the third decade. As noted in earlier editions of this series, formative and undifferentiated embryonic structures within the jaw bones persist longer than anywhere else in the skeletal system, hence the pathologist must be aware of the potential opportunities for aberrant development and related pathology.

The jaws are replete with vestiges of odontogenesis, namely, epithelial remnants or rests in the absence of mesenchymal precursors or anlages. Many jaw lesions including cysts and tumors can in fact arise from such embryonally derived remnants. A brief review of the formation of the teeth and jaw is therefore appropriate.

ODONTOGENESIS

Tooth formation depends on the interaction of ectodermally derived oral epithelium and the neural crest ectomesenchyme within the maxillary and mandibular processes. The stomodeum is lined by oral epithelium which contributes the enamel-forming component of the tooth, while the ectomesenchyme of neural crest origin contributes to the formation of both dentin and cementum via reciprocal inductive interaction between the epithelium of the enamel organ and the ectomesenchyme of the dental papilla. Such coordination permits a sequential and orderly process of tooth development.

The Role of the Neural Crest

Soon after development of the neural tube by invagination of the overlying ectoderm, pleuripotential neuroepithelial cells (neural crest cells) begin migrating from the dorsum of the midline of the neural tube. Cranially directed neural crest cells produce bands of migrating ectomesenchymal cells which invade the developing branchial arches. Certain subsets of cranially directed neural crest cells give rise to chondrocytes, osteoblasts, periodontal ligament fibroblasts, cementoblasts, and odontoblasts. Other cells of neural crest origin form the cranial ganglia and most of the peripheral nervous system within the head and neck region. This differentiation, in its final form, is regulated by interactions of those cells with extrinsic factors such as growth factors in the local micro-environment. Important among these factors are nerve growth factor and other members of the neurotrophin family. Abnormalities in neural crest formation can lead to significant developmental defects including anodontia and micrognathia. The ectomesenchymal cells of the neural crest interact in a series of reciprocal inductive steps with early oral epithelium to form the early tooth organs or tooth buds.

The earliest indication of tooth bud development occurs at approximately 6 weeks of gestation with the downgrowth of focally thickened oral epithelium into the underlying mesenchyme to form the dental lamina. As this is occurring, the local ectomesenchyme of neural crest origin participates in further tissue organization, leading to orderly tooth development. The dental lamina provides positional information, facilitating the formulation of discrete dental units by ectomesenchymal components. Induction of cell adhesion molecules and substrate adhesion molecules within the adjacent ectomesenchymal components is important in this process (5).

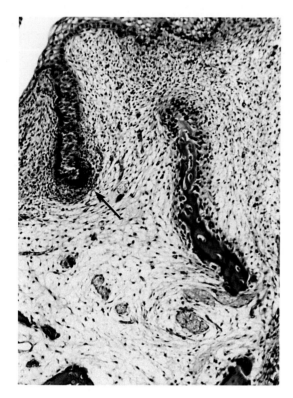

Figure 1-1
DENTAL LAMINA IN BUD STAGE

Downgrowth of the narrow strand of dental lamina (arrow) extends from surface oral ectoderm into the mesenchyme. Induced proliferation of mesenchymal cells around the deep segment of the dental lamina is characteristic of the early bud stage (X80). (Fig. 2 from Fascicle 24, 2nd Series.)

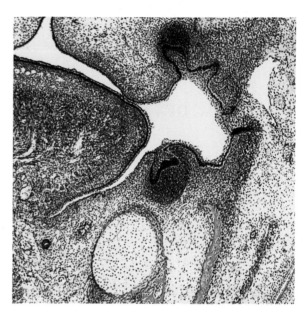

Figure 1-2
CAP STAGE OF ODONTOGENESIS

At the superior portion of the forming alveolus is a dense mesenchymal cell aggregation covered with a cap of odontogenic epithelium in this coronal section of an embryo at approximately 9 weeks of gestation.

As early as 28 days, small elevations of oral epithelium are present within the maxillary and mandibular arches as well as in the frontonasal processes. By 6 weeks, localized proliferations of dental lamina within the elevations of these arches (fig. 1-1) produce the soon to be recognized tooth bud. The dental papilla and dental sac components of the tooth bud subsequently are formed by proliferation and concentration of adjacent ectomesenchymal cells.

Differentiation of the Enamel Organ

The earliest stage of enamel organ development is the bud stage, followed by the formation of a cap-shaped enamel organ which is superimposed over the dental papilla (fig. 1-2). The second morphologic phase of enamel organ formation, the so-called bell stage, involves the formation of a concavity along the inner surface of the enamel organ which houses the dental papilla (fig. 1-3). In the bell stage, an inner enamel epithelium, a stratum intermedium, a stellate reticulum, and an outer enamel epithelium can be recognized. Surrounding the entire enamel organ is the dental sac, which is separated from the outer enamel epithelium by a discrete basement membrane. Between the inner and outer enamel epithelia are clusters of star-shaped cells that comprise the stellate reticulum. These cells are characterized by long, slender cytoplasmic extensions, wide intercellular spaces, and numerous gap junctions and desmosomes. Approaching the inner enamel epithelium is a narrow zone of cuboidal cells, the stratum intermedium, which separates the stellate reticulum from the inner enamel epithelium. This stratum intermedium is most evident prior to ameloblastic differentiation.

The cells of the inner enamel epithelium are columnar, and are bordered at one end by the stratum intermedium and at the other end by ectomesenchymal cells, the latter destined to become odontoblasts (fig. 1-4). Thin aperiodic fibrils

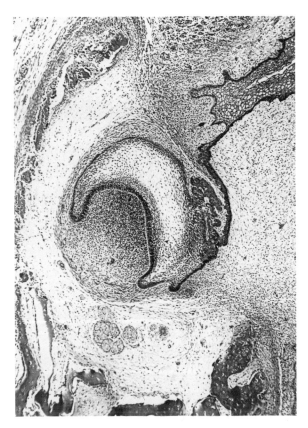

Figure 1-3
BELL STAGE OF ODONTOGENESIS
The early bell stage shows the relationship between the cell-rich dental papilla being encircled by the odontoblastic layer which in turn is surrounded by the dental sac. The dental lamina may be seen connecting the overlying oral cavity to the forming tooth.

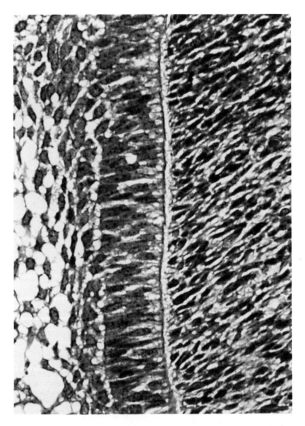

Figure 1-4
INNER ENAMEL EPITHELIUM
AND STRATUM INTERMEDIUM
The early inner enamel epithelium is columnar and situated between the dental papilla along its basal aspect and the stratum intermedium on the opposite end of the cell. The stratum intermedium in turn contacts the stellate reticulum where wide intercellular spaces are clearly evident.

and a basement membrane zone or lamina densa separate the forming odontoblasts from the inner enamel epithelial cells. A specific directional orientation is noted in the cytodifferentiation of odontoblasts and ameloblasts, with the process beginning at the tip of future cusps. This differentiation is under the influence of stimuli from within the inner enamel epithelium allowing the preodontoblasts to differentiate. These, in turn, stimulate cells of the inner enamel epithelium to form a single layer of taller cells (ameloblasts), which secrete enamel matrix. The secretory stage of the odontoblast begins prior to ameloblastic secretion of enamel matrix material. A complex interaction of cell membrane receptors, growth factors, and matrix molecules within the inner enamel epithelial basement membrane zone helps control the differentiation of both amelo-

blasts and odontoblasts from the inner enamel epithelium and outer cells of the dental papilla. In this early phase of development, cells in both the preameloblast and preodontoblast compartments cease division and differentiate into matrix-forming elements. A thin layer of predentin, secreted by odontoblasts, is formed prior to the formation of the enamel matrix (fig. 1-5). The most numerous and rapid cell division occurs at the cervical loop; cells then extend along the length of the enamel organ until they reach their mature state during the bell phase of enamel organ development (fig. 1-6).

Recent experimental data have provided insight into the informational exchange that occurs between the ectomesenchymal and epithelial components of odontogenesis. Within the

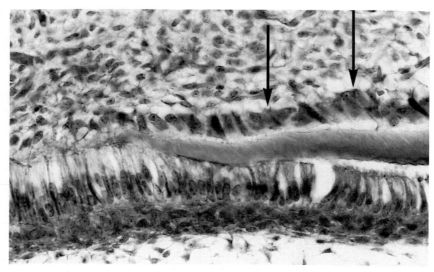

Figure 1-5
MATURE AMELOBLASTS
The nuclei of mature ameloblasts polarize toward the stratum intermedium. Note odontoblasts producing dentin (arrows)
(X425). (Fig. 7 from Fascicle 24,
2nd Series.)

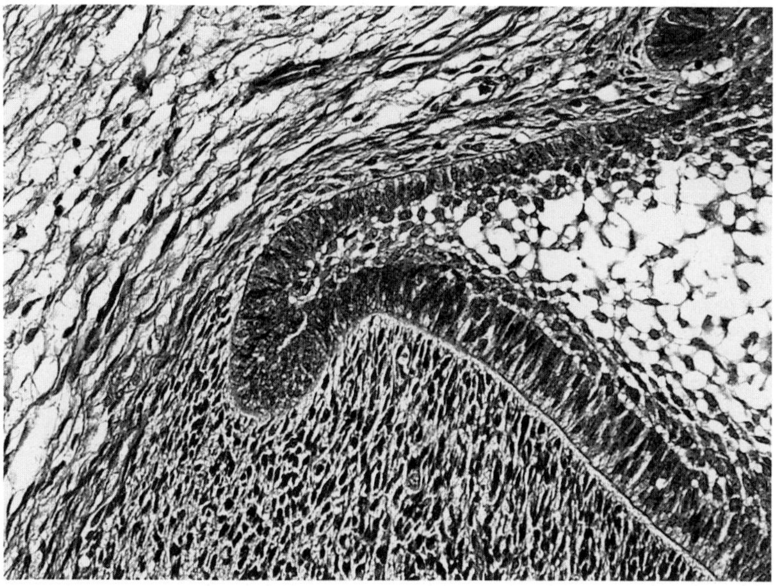

Figure 1-6
CERVICAL LOOP OF
ENAMEL ORGAN
The cervical loop region of the enamel
organ proliferates apically to ultimately
form Hertwig's root sheath and represents the junction of the inner and outer
enamel epithelium.

basement membrane, several constituents of matrix-mediated signaling occur. Cell membrane receptors read the information, while receptor-ligand interactions influence cytoskeleton and cytoplasmic enzymes, thus controlling transcriptional and post-transcriptional events. Soluble substances that participate in the signaling function during odontogenesis include fibronectin and their receptors, tenascin and syndecan (11). A simple demonstration of the instructive influence of mesenchyme over epithelium is best seen in organ culture, where dental epithelium recombined with skin mesenchyme leads to the development of skin epidermis, while skin epithelium cultured in contact with dental mesenchyme results in tooth formation. Slavkin and coinvestigators (9) have shown that developing tooth explants can undergo complete cell differentiation, with subsequent matrix mineralization, within a chemically defined medium. They concluded that autocrine and paracrine factors help coordinate the sequence of discrete cellular differentiation events during tooth development.

Many soluble factors, including transforming growth factor beta 2, contribute to normal growth and differentiation of this structure (3). Vitamin A analogs, including the parent vitamin, retinol, and retinoic acid, play a critical role in the regulation of epithelial proliferation and differentiation in concert with their role in influencing critical factors in craniofacial development (1–3,6). The effect of retinoic acid and derivatives is dependent initially upon their binding to nuclear transcription factors which are specifically controlled on various target genes. The cellular retinol and retinoic acid binding proteins control the level of free retinoic acid available to interact with nuclear retinoic acid receptors. The binding of retinoic acid to nuclear retinoic acid receptors controls the coding of epidermal growth factors. Epidermal growth factor plays a major role in the control of cell proliferation within the dental lamina and early stages of tooth development in a paracrine or autocrine manner. Subsequent to achieving the cap stage of development, the level of epidermal growth factor decreases within the epithelial component, but persists within the ectomesenchymal elements of the dental papilla.

An additional important genetic expression during tooth development occurs when the midkine (MK) protein becomes preferentially located at sites of epithelial mesenchymal interaction in embryonal tissues. This protein stimulates cell proliferation and is found in greatest concentration in the inner enamel epithelium, the basal lamina, and the dental papilla during periods of odontoblastic differentiation. This protein seems to be of particular importance in epithelial mesenchymal interactions (7). Early signaling events are initiated by matrix molecules which behave as growth factors. Research related to these matrix molecules will lead to a greater understanding of tooth development and associated pathologic events (9).

OVERVIEW

The clinical correlation of the cellular and molecular events in odontogenesis concerns itself with the development of human dentition (4). The initial evidence of tooth formation occurs at approximately 4 weeks' gestation by way of a thickening of the oral epithelium within the maxillary, mandibular, and median nasal processes,

when the human embryo is 8 to 9 mm in body length. At 11 to 14 mm, the overlying epithelium (a stomodeal ectodermal derivative) invaginates into the underlying cell-rich mesenchyme to form the dental lamina. The dental lamina represents a linear aggregation of epithelial knots or clusters which form as a result of differential cell proliferation, beginning in the most distal or molar region and progressing anteriorly toward the midline. Individual tooth bud formation is preceded by dental lamina enlargement and condensation of the ectomesenchyme of neural crest origin. These condensations ultimately produce 20 deciduous tooth elements consisting of 8 incisors, 4 canines, and 8 molars. The three remaining dental lamina structures in each quadrant, which ultimately form the permanent molars, form from a distal extension of the dental lamina known as the accessional lamina. Permanent tooth buds which derive from the deciduous dental lamina are positioned lingual to the primary precursors in the premolar, canine, and incisor areas.

As the early or cap stage of odontogenesis evolves, the bell stage forms, creating the basic outline of the tooth and initiating the morphodifferentiation stage. As the bell stage continues, the dental lamina begins to fragment, resulting in small clusters or rests of residual odontogenic epithelium. These persist both in the alveolar mucosa between the periosteum of the jaws and in alveolar bone. The soft tissue remnants of the dental lamina are known as rests of Serres.

An additional source of epithelial rest tissue is the Hertwig epithelial root sheath which forms from the cervical loop subsequent to the completion of root formation. In this structure, inner and outer enamel epithelia are juxtaposed, with the absence of an intervening stellate reticulum and stratum intermedium component. The residual small rests reside within the periodontal ligament as the so-called rests of Malassez (fig. 1-7). These epithelial rests are located in the interface between the bone and cemental surface of the root throughout a person's lifetime, or until the tooth is extracted and periodontal ligament structures resorb along with the epithelial rests. Both the rests of Malassez and the dental lamina rests (Serres) as well as any residua of the enamel organ may give rise to odontogenic cysts and/or tumors, beginning in the postnatal period and continuing throughout life.

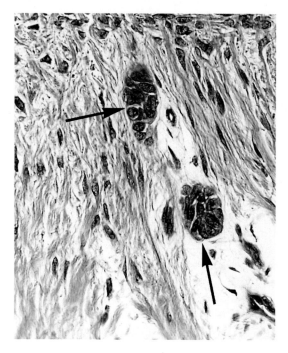

Figure 1-7
PERIODONTAL LIGAMENT AND
ODONTOGENIC EPITHELIAL RESTS

This high-power view illustrates the attachment of the periodontal ligament to the cementum of the root of an erupted tooth. Odontogenic rests (arrows), the so-called rests of Malassez (remnants of Hertwig's root sheath) are seen. (Fig. 9 from Fascicle 24, 2nd Series.)

JAW DEVELOPMENT AND ORIGIN OF NONODONTOGENIC EPITHELIAL RESTS

Epithelial rests of ectodermal origin which do not possess odontogenic potential are also found enclaved within jaw structures, usually at developmental fusion sites. They possess the ability to form intraosseous lesions which are not developmentally related to dental structures. A brief review of the development of the face and oral cavity provides a basis for understanding the origin of these nonodontogenic ectodermal rests.

At about the third week of embryogenesis, the future face consists of a rounded prominence containing the forebrain (prosencephalon). Caudal to this rounded prominence is a deep groove, the primary oral fossa (oral plate or stomodeal pit), which is bounded below by the first branchial arch (mandibular arch) and laterally by the maxillary processes (fig. 1-8). The stomodeal pit, or oral fossa, invaginates to meet the anterior blind end of the foregut, a double-lined ectodermal layer, referred to as the buccopharyngeal membrane. An ectodermal ingrowth (Rathke's pouch) is formed in the roof of the primitive oral cavity, derived from the stomodeal ectoderm, which subsequently gives rise to the anterior

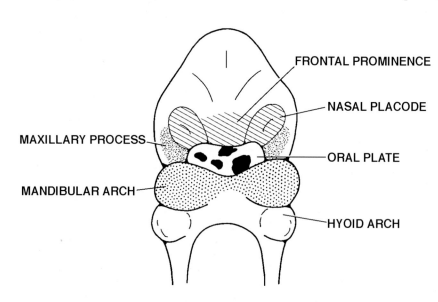

Figure 1-8
PRIMARY ORAL FOSSA

This is a schematic representation of the early fetal face and the primary oral fossa or plate. Note that it is bound caudally by the mandibular arch (first branchial arch) and laterally by the maxillary processes. (Fig. 10 from Fascicle 24, 2nd Series.)

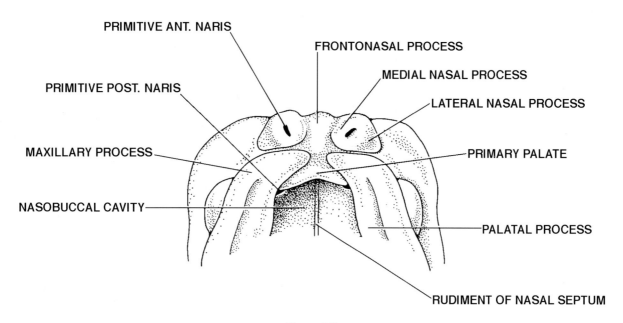

PRIMITIVE ANT. NARIS

FRONTONASAL PROCESS

MEDIAL NASAL PROCESS

PRIMITIVE POST. NARIS

LATERAL NASAL PROCESS

MAXILLARY PROCESS

PRIMARY PALATE

NASOBUCCAL CAVITY

PALATAL PROCESS

RUDIMENT OF NASAL SEPTUM

Figure 1-9
PRIMARY PALATE FORMATION
This schematic representation illustrates the formation of the primary palate. It is formed by the fusion of portions of the medial and lateral nasal processes with the maxillary processes. Thus, the upper lip and the anterior portion of the maxillary alveolar process are formed. (Fig. 11 from Fascicle 24, 2nd Series.)

lobe of the pituitary gland. Since the stomodeum is lined by ectoderm, all other paraoral structures that eventually develop will be of ectodermal origin, such as the lining of the nasal and oral cavities, the enamel of the teeth, and the salivary glands.

The face is derived from seven primordial tissues: two maxillary process, two mandibular processes, two lateral nasal processes, and the medial nasal process. The maxillary and mandibular processes originate from the first branchial arch, while the medial and two lateral nasal processes arise from the frontonasal process. The frontonasal process gives rise to most of the structures of the upper and middle portions of the face. The rounded anterolateral corners of the medial nasal process are known as the globular processes and form the upper portion of the oral orifice. They unite with the maxillary processes on both sides of the midline. The lateral nasal processes do not contribute to the upper boundary of the oral orifice.

The primary palate forms during the fifth and sixth weeks of intrauterine development. It gives rise to the upper lip and the anterior portion of the maxillary alveolar process. It is formed by a union of the inferomedial portion of the medial nasal process with the lateral nasal process and the maxillary process. Thus, the nasal cavity and anterior portion of the oral cavity are separated by this primary palate.

When the primary palate is completed, the primary nasal cavity exists as a short duct leading from the nostril into the primitive oral cavity. Its outer and inner openings (primary choanae) are separated from the face and oral cavity by the primary palate. As the primitive oral cavity increases in height, the tissue that separates the right and left primitive nostrils grows backward and downward to form the future nasal septum. The oral cavity now has an incomplete, horseshoe-shaped roof formed anteriorly by the primary palate and laterally by the oral surface of the maxillary processes (fig. 1-9). On either side of the septum, the oral cavity communicates with the nasal cavities (fig. 1-10, left).

Folds develop from the medial edges of the maxillary processes at the lateral portions of the oral roof. They grow downward, almost vertically, on either side of the tongue as the palatine processes, extending posteriorly to the lateral walls of the pharynx. At this stage of development,

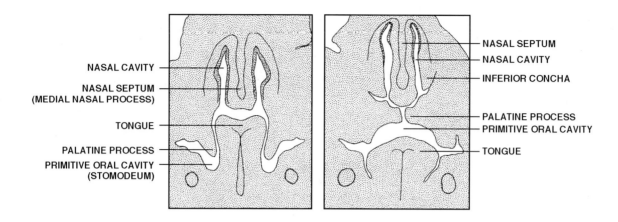

Figure 1-10
SECONDARY PALATE FORMATION
This illustration depicts the descent of the tongue from the primitive nasal cavity (left) into the widened mandibular arch space of the oral cavity (right). Thus, the oral and nasal cavities are separated by the formation of the secondary palate. (Fig. 12 from Fascicle 24, 2nd Series.)

the tongue is narrow and high and reaches the nasal septum. The secondary palate, which is destined to separate the oral and nasal cavities posterior to the primary palate, is formed by a union of the two palatine processes after the tongue assumes a more inferior position and the palate processes rotate approximately 90° to assume a horizontal position. Soon after, the new horizontal processes merge and ultimately join in the midline. This transposition and subsequent union of the palatine processes can occur only when the tongue has moved downward, evacuating the space between the palatine processes (fig. 1-10, right). This occurs simultaneously with a marked growth spurt of the mandible, in both length and width. When the palatine processes assume their horizontal position, they touch the lower border of the nasal septum, but are still separate from each other by a median cleft that is wider posteriorly than it is toward the anterior aspect. Closure occurs in an anterior to posterior direction as the proliferating mesoderm from each of the palatine processes crosses over and enters the other, affecting fusion. During this process the ectoderm lining their medial aspects breaks down, thereby facilitating the crossover. Although most of these lining barriers are destroyed in this process, residual nests persist along the fused junctional sites (figs. 1-11, 1-12). The palatine processes

give rise to the soft palate and the central portions of the hard palate.

In the anterior portion of the primitive stomodeum, where the anterior borders of the palatine processes unite with and overgrow the oral aspect of the primary palate, two strands of ectoderm form. They extend from the nasal cavity to the oral cavity on each side of the midline. These are the primordia of the nasopalatine ducts. In lower animals, these ducts serve as necessary organs of smell (Jacobsen's vomeronasal organ). In humans, they are vestigial and as such break down, leaving ectodermal rests of the aborted nasopalatine ducts.

It is evident that the nonodontogenic epithelial rests in the jaws are derived from the breakdown of ectodermal lining cells during the union or fusion of the various embryonic processes in direct relation to mesodermal proliferation at each fusion locus. These entrapped rests may serve as sites for the future development of nonodontogenic central and parosteal lesions of the jaws. In addition, an extraosseous epithelial remnant, the organ of Chievitz, lies in close proximity to the posterior mandible and maxilla, usually along the ascending ramus of the mandible. There is usually intimate association with peripheral nerve tissue (fig. 1-13) which may be mistaken for metastatic or infiltrative carcinoma (8,10).

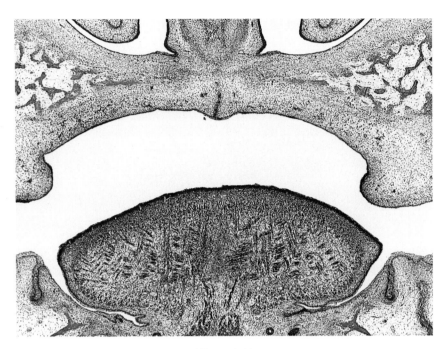

Figure 1-11
DEVELOPMENT OF THE SECONDARY PALATE
Mandibular growth has enlarged the arch space, allowing the tongue to descend, thereby evacuating the space it formerly occupied between the palatal processes. These processes now have grown together and are fused at the midline, closing off the nasal cavity from the oral cavity. Fusion has also occurred with the nasal septum. The secondary palate is now complete (X30). (Fig. 13 from Fascicle 24, 2nd Series.) (Figures 1-11 and 1-12 are from the same patient.)

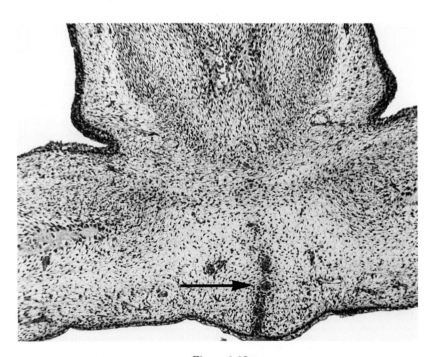

Figure 1-12
DEVELOPMENT OF PALATAL PROCESSES
This is a higher power view of the fusion site between the right and left palatal processes and nasal septum. Note the residual nonodontogenic ectodermal remnants at the midline (arrow) (X80). (Fig. 14 from Fascicle 24, 2nd Series.)

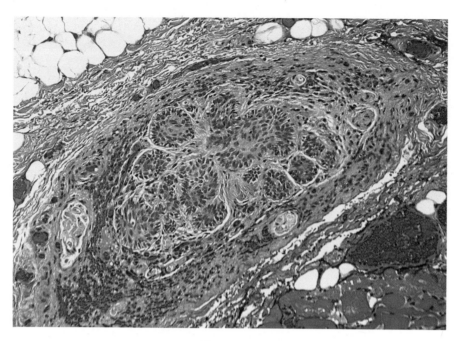

Figure 1-13
ORGAN OF CHIEVITZ

Clustered islands of epithelial cells are in close association with peripheral nerve elements. The specimen was obtained from the medial aspect of the mandibular ramus adjacent to the lingula.

REFERENCES

1. Block-Zupan A, Decimo D, Loriot M, Mark MP, Ruch JV. Expression of nuclear retinoic acid receptors during mouse odontogenesis. Differentiation 1994;57:195–203.
2. Block-Zupan A, Mark MP, Weber B, Ruch JV. In vitro effect of retinoic acid on mouse incisor development. Arch Oral Biol 1994;38:891–900.
3. Chai Y, Mah A, Crohin C. Specific transforming growth factor-B subtypes regulate embryonic mouse Meckel's cartilage and tooth development. Dev Biol 1994;162:85–103.
4. Garant PR. Introduction to cell and tissue biology of the oral cavity (in press).
5. Lunsden AG. Spatial organization of the epithelium and the role of neural crest cells in the initiation of the mammalian tooth germ. Development 1988;103:155–69.
6. Mark MP, Block-Zupan A, Ruch JV. Effects of retinoids on tooth morphogenesis and cytodifferentiation in vitro. In J Dev Bio 1992;36:517–26.
7. Mitsiadis TA, Muramatsu T, Muramatsu H, Thesleff I. Midkine (MK), a heparin-binding growth/differentiation factor, is regulated by retinoic acid and epithelial-mesenchymal interactions in the developing mouse tooth and affects cell proliferation and morphogenesis. J Cell Biol 1995;129:267–81.
8. Sciubba JJ, Sachs SA. Schwannoma of the inferior alveolar nerve in association with the organ of Chievitz. J Oral Pathol 1980;9:16–28.
9. Slavkin HC. Molecular determinants during dental morphogenesis and cytodifferentiation: a review. J Craniofac Genet Dev Biol 1991;11:338–49.
10. Tschen JA, Fechner RE. The juxtaoral organ of Chievitz. Am J Surg Pathol 1979;3:147–50.
11. Vainio S, Thesleff I. Sequential induction of syndecan, tenascin and cell proliferation associated with mesenchymal cell condensation during early tooth differentiation. Differentiation 1992;50:97–105.

2
CLASSIFICATION OF CYSTS AND TUMORS OF THE JAWS

Many classification schemes for odontogenic tumors have been proposed that have been based upon an understanding of dental precursors, including their origin, interactions, and developmental sequencing. The basis for most modern odontogenic tumor classification schemes was published by Thoma and Goldman in 1946 (6). They divided odontogenic tumors into ectodermal, mesenchymal, and mixed types, reflective of their putative origin. Other, more developmentally based schemes, were simply reflective of the obvious or dominant tumor cell type(s) or the presumed interactions of the tumor cells and more passive elements, which result in some form of embryonal induction (3). Using the induction formulation as a basis, Gorlin et al. (1) suggested a modified scheme in which absent or minimal to marked inductive changes in connective tissue were used to characterize epithelial odontogenic tumors. The first World Health Organization (WHO) classification scheme published in 1971 (4) categorized odontogenic tumors into benign and malignant forms, with no attempt to reflect cell of origin, induction, or developmental relationships, or the predominant structure formed or mimicked. Rather, all cementum-forming lesions were included, including dysplastic conditions, as well as a lesion of neural crest origin, the melanotic neuroectodermal tumor of infancy.

The most recent WHO classification of odontogenic tumors (2) is based on earlier recognized schemes and emphasizes the complex interaction at the inductive level between epithelium (when present) and associated ectomesenchyme. Included from the earlier WHO classification as major categories, however, are the benign and malignant categories (Table 2-1). Emphasis has been placed on tumor behavior, with subdivisions predicated upon the odontogenic tissue types involved including ectomesenchymal and odontogenic epithelium in all permutations. Extremely rare entities such as ameloblastic fibrodentinosarcoma and odontogenic carcinosarcoma are not included in this classification.

As with odontogenic tumors, odontogenic cysts (Table 2-2) have been variously classified,

with the current WHO classification (2) defining and listing "true" or epithelial-lined cysts under two categories: inflammatory and developmental. Nonodontogenic cysts are considered as developmental cysts, and include the nasopalatine duct cyst, the nasoalveolar cyst, the epithelial-lined palatal cyst of infancy, and the surgical cyst of the maxillary sinus. Nonepithelial cystic defects have been grouped under pseudocysts, the solitary bone cyst, or as miscellaneous entities which include the lingual mandibular salivary

Table 2-1

WHO CLASSIFICATION OF ODONTOGENIC TUMORS

Benign Odontogenic Tumors
Odontogenic epithelium without odontogenic mesenchyme
  ameloblastoma
  squamous odontogenic tumor
  calcifying epithelial odontogenic tumor
Odontogenic epithelium with odontogenic mesenchyme, with or without dental hard tissue formation
  ameloblastic fibroma
  ameloblastic fibro-odontoma
  odontoameloblastoma
  adenomatoid odontogenic tumor
  calcifying odontogenic cyst/odontogenic ghost cell tumor
  odontoma
Odontogenic mesenchyme with or without odontogenic epithelium
  odontogenic fibroma
  odontogenic myxoma/fibromyxoma
  benign cementoblastoma

Malignant Odontogenic Tumors
Odontogenic carcinomas
  malignant ameloblastoma
  primary intraosseous carcinoma
  clear cell odontogenic carcinoma
  malignant counterparts of other epithelial tumors
  malignant transformation of odontogenic cysts
Odontogenic sarcomas
  ameloblastic fibrosarcoma

Table 2-2

CYSTS OF THE JAWS

Odontogenic Cysts
    Inflammatory
        radicular cyst
            residual cyst
        paradental cyst
            inflammatory buccal cyst
    Developmental
        dentigerous cyst
            eruption cyst
        lateral periodontal cyst
        botryoid odontogenic cyst
        odontogenic keratocyst
            primordial cyst
        glandular odontogenic cyst
        calcifying odontogenic cyst
        gingival cyst of adults
        gingival cyst of infants

Nonodontogenic Cysts, Pseudocysts, and
  Miscellaneous Entities
    Developmental
        nasopalatine duct cyst
        nasoalveolar (nasolabial) cyst
        palatal cysts of infants
        lingual mandibular salivary gland depression
    Other
        surgical ciliated cyst
        solitary bone cyst
        focal osteoporotic marrow defect

Table 2-3

NEOPLASMS AND OTHER LESIONS RELATED TO BONE

Fibro-osseous Lesions
    Fibrous dysplasia
    Ossifying (cemento-ossifying) fibroma
    Juvenile ossifying fibroma
    Periapical cemental dysplasia
    Florid osseous (cemento-osseous) dysplasia
        familial gigantiform cementoma
Nonodontogenic Lesions of the Jaws
    Giant cell lesions
        giant cell granuloma
        cherubism
        aneurysmal bone cyst
    Osseous lesions
        osteoma
        osteoblastoma/osteoid osteoma
        osteosarcoma
    Cartilaginous lesions
        osteochondroma
        chondroblastoma
        chondromyxoid fibroma
        chondrosarcoma
    Fibrous lesions
        desmoplastic fibroma
        fibrosarcoma
        myofibromatosis
    Hematopoietic, lymphoid, histiocytic lesions
        Langerhans' cell histiocytosis
        myeloma
        leukemia
        lymphoma
    Vascular lesions
        angioma
        angiosarcoma
    Synovial lesions
        synovial chondromatosis
        pigmented villonodular synovitis
    Neuroectodermal
        neuroectodermal tumor of infancy

gland depression and the focal osteoporotic marrow defect.

Special consideration has been applied to the calcifying odontogenic cyst. While often cystic and nonaggressive, its solid presentation, at times with attendant aggressive behavior, has led to its placement into the tumor category by the WHO. This is supported by the studies of Praetorius and colleagues (5) who showed that infiltrative growth may be present. Further emphasizing the neoplastic quality of this entity is its malignant counterpart, the odontogenic ghost cell carcinoma, which currently is not considered within the WHO odontogenic tumor classification. We have chosen to include the solid form of the calcifying odontogenic cyst under the benign tumor classification, however, its placement remains controversial.

Lesions of bone include neoplasms and dysplastic conditions reported in the jaws, with a wide spectrum of entities represented (Table 2-3). Expansion of the fibro-osseous category includes not only fibrous dysplasia and ossifying (cemento-ossifying) fibroma but also dysplastic cementum-forming lesions. The melanotic neuroectodermal tumor of infancy represents a tumor of primitive neural crest origin, rather than one of odontogenic origin. Earlier classifications considered this to represent a form of pigmented ameloblastoma prior to an improved understanding that neuroblastic cells cluster in an alveolar pattern, mimicking follicular ameloblastoma.

REFERENCES

1. Gorlin RJ, Chaudhry AP, Pindborg JJ. Odontogenic tumors. Classification, histopathology and clinical behavior in man and domesticated animals. Cancer 1961;14:73–101.
2. Kramer IR, Pindborg JJ, Shear M. Histologic typing of odontogenic tumors, 2nd edition. Geneva: World Health Organization, 1992.
3. Pindborg JJ, Clausen F. Classification of odontogenic tumors: suggestion. Acta Odont Scand 1958;16:293–301.
4. Pindborg JJ, Kramer IR. Histological typing of odontogenic tumours, jaw cysts, and allied lesions. Geneva: World Health Organization, 1971.
5. Praetorius F, Hjorting-Hansen E, Gorlin RJ, Vickers RA. Calcifying odontogenic cyst. Range, variations and neoplastic potential. Acta Odont Scand 1981;39:227–40.
6. Thoma KH, Goldman HM. Odontogenic tumors: classification based on observation of epithelial, mesenchymal and mixed varieties. Am J Path 1946;22:433–71.

3
ODONTOGENIC CYSTS

INFLAMMATORY ODONTOGENIC CYSTS

Radicular Cyst

Definition. The radicular cyst arises from epithelial odontogenic rests (rests of Malassez) in the periodontal ligament, secondary to inflammation, following necrosis of the dental pulp. The terms *periapical* and *lateral radicular cyst* indicate the location of the cyst.

Clinical and Radiologic Features. The radicular cyst is invariably associated with a nonvital tooth. Consequently, this cyst is associated with teeth that have extensive caries or a history of physical or chemical trauma that results in pulpal necrosis. The radicular cyst is the most common cyst of the jaws, comprising 52.3 percent of jaw cysts in the series of Shear (7), 56.9 percent in that of Kreidler et al. (3), and 65.15 percent in that of Daley et al. (1). Approximately 60 percent of cases occur in the maxilla, mostly involving the anterior maxilla (7). Peak incidence occurs in patients in the third through the sixth decades (7); there is a slight male predilection.

The radicular cyst is rarely seen in the primary dentition. The cyst is often noted as an incidental finding on routine dental radiographic examination. Pain and swelling are common symptoms. As these cysts expand, resorption of bone occurs and the cyst may even perforate into soft tissues. This is frequently the case with radicular cysts of the anterior maxilla because of the thin cortical bone in this anatomic site. There may be a significant periosteal reaction. Rarely, a fistula develops in the overlying mucosa. A mobile tooth results if the cyst is of sufficient size.

These cysts are usually associated with the apical foramen of the nonvital tooth, hence the periapical designation. However, they can occur on the lateral root surface, presumably associated with a lateral root canal. Thus the term radicular, indicating association with any portion of the tooth root, is preferable.

The radiographic pattern is similar to that of a periapical granuloma: a radiolucency at the root apex (fig. 3-1, left) or less commonly along the lateral root surface. There is loss of lamina dura adjacent to the tooth root. Root resorption is a possible sequela. If the tooth has been treated endodontically, extruded filling material might be identified radiographically within or adjacent to the cyst. Radiographically, a radicular cyst cannot be distinguished from a periapical granuloma.

Pathologic Findings. Grossly, the radicular cyst frequently demonstrates the presence of cholesterol in the cyst lumen and wall (fig. 3-1, right). These cysts often are submitted in fragments, as they are surgically curetted from bone. The cyst wall is usually quite thick. Posterior maxillary cysts may have attached antral tissue at the periphery. Pigment and fragments of endodontic filling material, most commonly gutta percha and silver points, sometimes are noted on gross examination.

The radicular cyst is lined by proliferative epithelium of the nonkeratinizing stratified type. There is an intense inflammatory infiltrate composed of plasma cells, lymphocytes, and macrophages. The macrophages frequently cluster and exhibit a foamy appearance. In many of these cysts cholesterol crystal clefts are identified (fig. 3-2). Foreign body type giant cells and foamy macrophages accompany the cholesterol crystal clefts. Radicular cysts can have mucous cells admixed with the lining squamous cells; ciliated cells are less commonly noted. Dystrophic calcification of individual epithelial cells may also occur. Intraepithelial hyaline (Rushton) bodies are occasionally identified within the epithelial lining (fig. 3-3) (4,6). These bodies are not specific to radicular cysts but have also been noted in dentigerous and odontogenic keratocysts. Theories as to their origin include a cell product of odontogenic epithelial cells, basement membrane material, dental matrix protein, hyalinized capillaries, or degenerate erythrocytes (5).

Radicular cyst development is likely preceded by a periapical granuloma, an inflammatory focus at the root surface without evidence of cystic epithelium (fig. 3-4). This inflammatory focus results in a proliferation of the epithelial

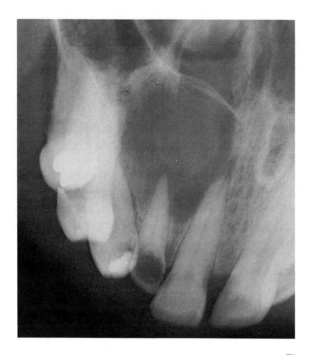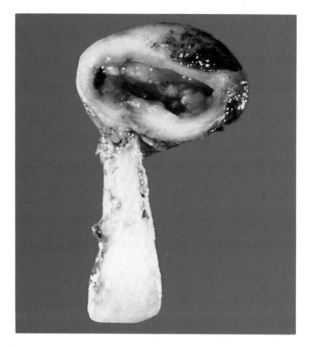

Figure 3-1
RADICULAR CYST
Left: A radiolucent lesion is present at the apex of a carious anterior maxillary tooth.
Right: Gross specimen of radicular cyst attached to root apex of tooth. (Courtesy of Dr. D.R. Weathers, Atlanta, GA.)

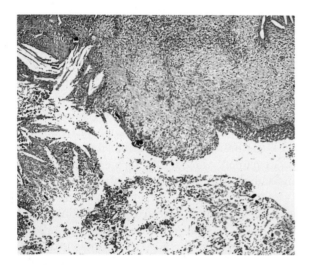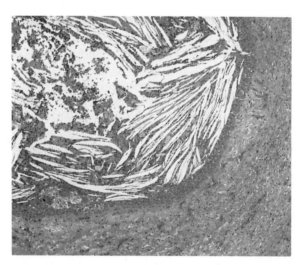

Figure 3-2
RADICULAR CYST
Left: An inflamed radicular cyst with cholesterol in the cyst lumen and a connective tissue wall.
Right: A radicular cyst with cholesterol crystal clefts in the cyst lumen. The wall of the cyst exhibits minimal inflammation.

odontogenic rests that reside in the periodontal ligament. These epithelial residues proliferate in this inflammatory milieu (fig. 3-5) and eventually form the cyst. Maxillary cysts can encroach upon antral or nasal mucosa and inflamed cyst lining may be seen in association with respiratory mucosa (fig. 3-6). The walls of some cysts may exhibit an exuberant epithelial

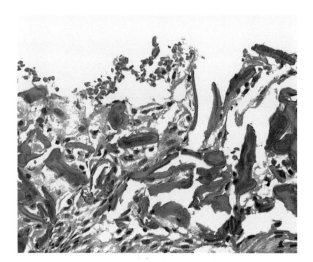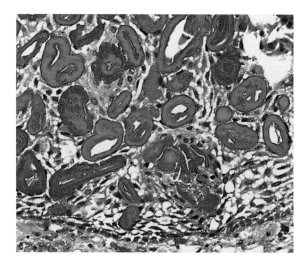

Figure 3-3
RADICULAR CYST
Radicular cyst with intraepithelial hyaline bodies, which are linear and curved (left) and ring shaped (right).

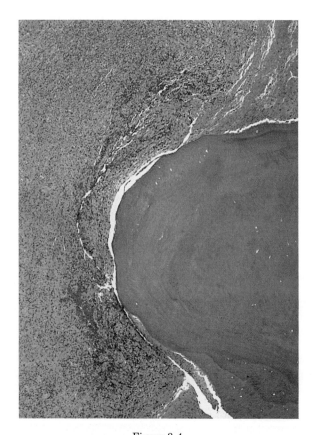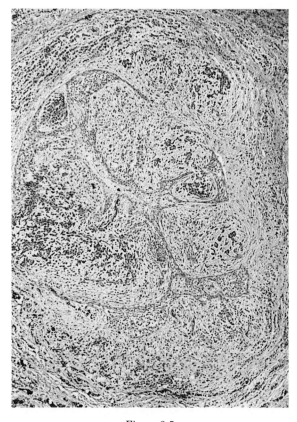

Figure 3-4
PERIAPICAL GRANULOMA
Root apex with associated periapical inflammation (peri-apical granuloma).

Figure 3-5
RADICULAR CYST
Proliferative epithelium and early radicular cyst formation.

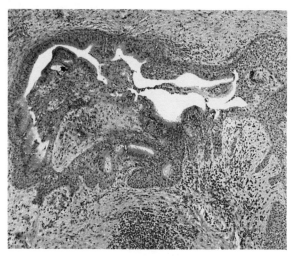

Figure 3-6
RADICULAR CYST
Radicular cyst in continuity with antral mucosa.

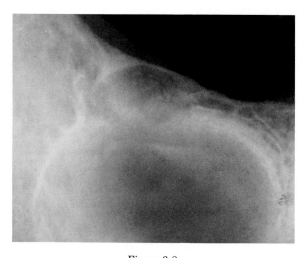

Figure 3-8
RESIDUAL CYST
Well-defined radiolucency in the posterior edentulous mandible.

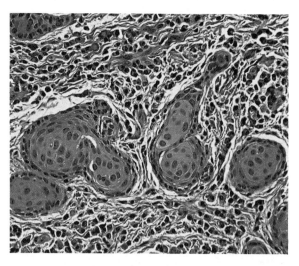

Figure 3-7
RADICULAR CYST
Squamous odontogenic tumor-like islands in the wall of a radicular cyst.

proliferation that can simulate a squamous odontogenic tumor (fig. 3-7) (8). Rare cases of carcinoma arising in radicular cysts have been reported (7).

The cause for the proliferation of odontogenic epithelium is poorly understood. Gao and colleagues (2) demonstrated an induction of keratinocyte growth factor by the stromal cells of periapical lesions. This may play a role in stimulating epithelial proliferation.

Treatment and Prognosis. Since there is no reliable way to distinguish, clinically or radiographically, periapical granuloma from radicular cyst, conservative nonsurgical endodontic therapy is the usual approach for most lesions. Should the area in question not exhibit radiographic resolution after nonsurgical treatment, biopsy is recommended.

Residual Cyst

Definition. The residual cyst is a radicular cyst that is retained in the jaws after removal of the associated tooth.

Clinical and Radiologic Features. The residual cyst usually does not cause symptoms and is identified on routine radiographic examination of an edentulous area. The radiographic presentation is that of a well-defined radiolucency with sclerotic borders (fig. 3-8). Although these lesions can attain considerable size, expansion of the jaws is unusual (fig. 3-9).

Pathologic Findings. The histopathology of the residual cyst is similar to that of the radicular cyst. There is typically less inflammation (fig. 3-10A) and the epithelial proliferation may not be as prominent as in the radicular cyst. Epithelial dysplasia and carcinoma arising in residual cysts have been reported (12).

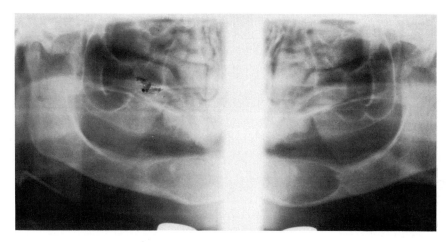

Figure 3-9
RESIDUAL CYST
The large radiolucency involving the anterior mandible was diagnosed as a residual cyst.

Residual cysts, as well as other odontogenic cysts, may exhibit connective tissue hyaline bodies in the cyst wall (fig. 3-10B,C). Since the lesions associated with these bodies resemble a vegetable granuloma (pulse granuloma), it is thought that vegetable material is introduced via an extraction socket and the bodies are thus derived from the implanted vegetable material (10,11). Alternatively, these structures may result from the pooling of extravasated serum followed by fibrosis (9). The literature on the nature of these connective tissue hyaline bodies has been reviewed by Matthews (10).

Paradental Cyst

Definition. The paradental cyst is an inflammatory odontogenic cyst occurring on the lateral or other aspect of a tooth root, often secondary to an inflammatory process in a periodontal pocket.

Clinical and Radiologic Features. Craig (14) coined the term "paradental cyst" in 1976, for a cyst located distal, buccal, or rarely, mesial to a partially erupted third molar tooth with an associated pericoronitis. Main (19) first described this type of cyst in 1970 and used the terms "inflammatory collateral cyst" and "inflammatory lateral periodontal cyst." This lesion was then described in teeth other than the third molar (13), in particular the buccal aspect of the mandibular first or second molar in children (21). Stoneman and Worth (22) designated this lesion "mandibular infected buccal cyst." The "buccal bifurcation cyst" (18) is another term that has been suggested for a cyst associated with a multi-rooted molar tooth that exhibits cervical enamel extension toward the furcation area.

The teeth associated with paradental cysts are vital. Most cysts occur in males, are 1 to 2 cm in size, and are usually attached to the coronal third of the tooth root and the cementoenamel junction. This type of cyst is probably more common than the literature indicates. The pathogenesis appears to be related to inflammation of the odontogenic epithelium of the superficial aspect of the periodontal ligament (13,15,17) or epithelial rests of Malassez, or unilateral expansion of the dental follicle secondary to inflammatory destruction of bone (16). Developmental enamel anomalies may influence the development of the paradental cyst.

There appear to be two distinct clinical circumstances associated with paradental cysts: in one, a radiolucent lesion most often involves the buccal or distal aspect of a partially erupted third molar in an adult (fig. 3-11) (13,16,17,25) and in the other, a buccally located radiolucency involves the first or second permanent molar in a child (fig. 3-12) (15,21,24,26). Martinez-Conde et al. (20) reported bilateral paradental cysts involving the second molars. The term "paradental" encompasses both clinical circumstances and is the preferred term for this cyst. Those cysts that are associated with the distal portion of a partially erupted third molar tooth may be difficult to separate clinically, radiographically, and histologically from pericoronitis. Swelling and pain of the involved area is the most common clinical finding. A radiolucency with distinct

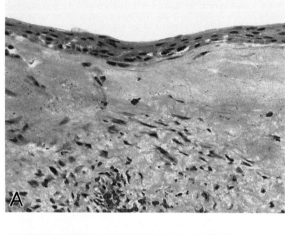

Figure 3-10
RESIDUAL CYST AND
CONNECTIVE TISSUE HYALINE BODIES

Thin cyst lining with hyalinization of the cyst wall and minimal inflammation (A). An additional case of residual cyst with multiple spherical hyaline bodies and an inflammatory background (B). Higher power demonstrates a centrally located, multinucleated giant cell surrounded by a hypocellular hyaline zone and granulation tissue (C). Hyaline bodies (B,C) were identified in the wall of an inflamed residual cyst.

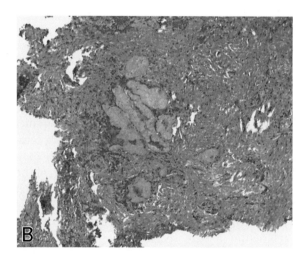

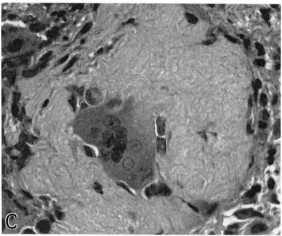

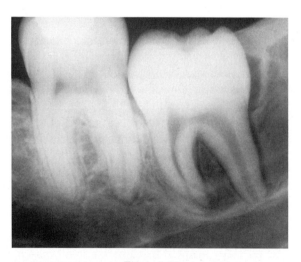

Figure 3-11
PARADENTAL CYST

The radiolucency is associated with the crown of a mandibular third molar tooth. The paradental cyst was located on the buccal and distal aspect of the tooth.

borders is typical of a paradental cyst associated with the distal portion of the third molar tooth, whereas a cyst that occurs buccal to a mandibular first or second molar tooth is less distinct in routine dental and panoramic films (26). The periodontal ligament space is not widened when the lesion is superimposed on the buccal aspect of the root and the lamina dura can be traced around the root of the tooth. An occlusal radiograph and computed tomogram or magnetic resonance imaging study may better define the presence of a cystic process (23).

Pathologic Findings. Histologically, paradental cysts are lined by proliferative nonkeratinized epithelium (fig. 3-13A,B) through which inflammatory cells migrate. The connective tissue adjacent to the cyst exhibits a marked inflammatory cell infiltrate consisting of plasma cells, lymphocytes, macrophages, and neutrophils.

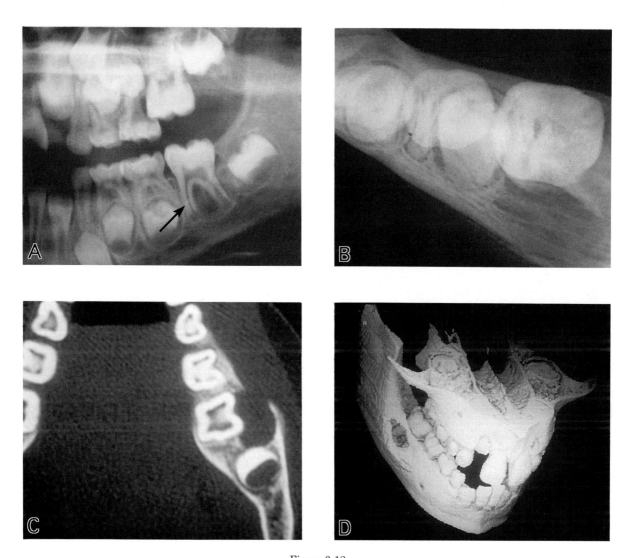

Figure 3-12
PARADENTAL CYST
A: Panoramic radiograph shows a radiolucency associated with the permanent mandibular first molar.
B: Occlusal view shows buccal expansion.
C: Computed tomography shows buccal expansion.
D: Three-dimensional image of the paradental cyst.

This histologic picture is similar to that noted in radicular cysts and inflamed dentigerous cysts. The clinical presentation, coupled with the radiographic features, is necessary to arrive at the appropriate designation. Those lesions that occur on the buccal aspect of first and second molars in children are usually associated with a proliferative periostitis characterized by parallel spicules of reactive bone. This reactive bone should not be confused with neoplastic bone or fibrous dysplasia (fig. 3-13C).

Treatment and Prognosis. Enucleation of the cyst is the treatment of choice; third molar teeth should be extracted with the cyst. In children, cyst removal without extraction of the first or second molar tooth is recommended. Clinical circumstances particular to each case will dictate appropriate treatment. Recurrences are not expected.

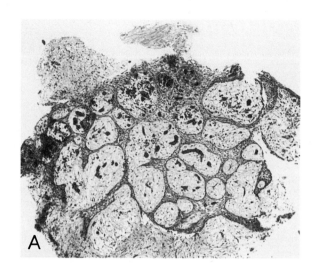

Figure 3-13
PARADENTAL CYST
Low- (A) and intermediate- (B) power views of lesion seen in figure 3-12 shows epithelial proliferation with inflamed fibrous connective tissue. Reactive bone is peripheral to the cystic process (C).

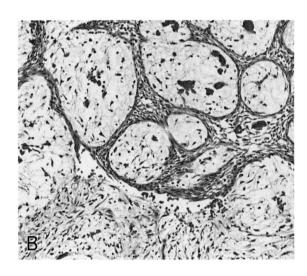

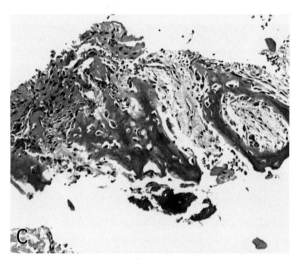

DEVELOPMENTAL ODONTOGENIC CYSTS

Dentigerous Cyst

Definition. The dentigerous cyst surrounds the crown of an impacted tooth, and is attached to the tooth at the crown root junction. Formation of the cyst is due to expansion of the follicle that surrounds the impacted tooth. *Follicular cyst* is a synonymous term.

Clinical and Radiologic Features. This cyst occurs in association with the more commonly impacted teeth, namely, the mandibular third molar, maxillary canine and third molar, and the mandibular premolars (32). However, any tooth, supernumerary tooth, mesiodens, and odontoma can exhibit an associated dentigerous cyst. The cyst occurs over a wide age range but is typically diagnosed during the second to fourth decades (33). The lesion is somewhat more common in males. It is the most common noninflammatory odontogenic cyst of the jaws, accounting for 21.3 (31) to 24 percent (28) of such cysts.

This cyst probably develops as a result of fluid accumulation between the reduced enamel epithelium and the tooth crown (27,33). An origin from odontogenic rests in the follicle and cystification of the enamel organ is unlikely.

The dentigerous cyst is usually asymptomatic and discovered during radiographic examination, however, large destructive cysts can cause symptoms due to cyst expansion. The pathologic sequelae of impacted third molars have been addressed by Stanley et al. (34). A review of their large population of 11,598 patients revealed

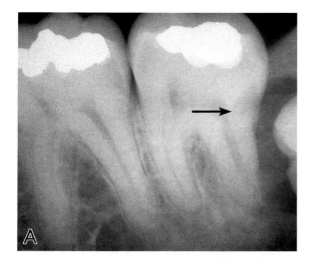

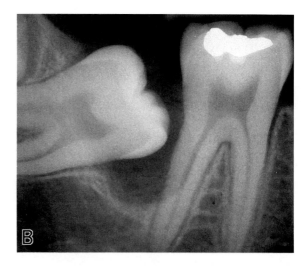

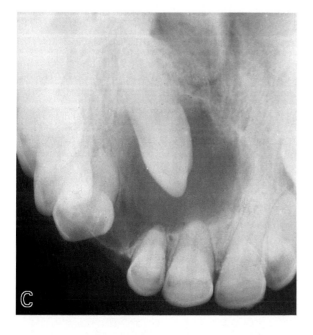

Figure 3-14
DENTIGEROUS CYST
Dentigerous cysts are characterized by radiolucencies surrounding the crowns of: a horizontally impacted third molar (A); mesioangular impacted third molar (B); and impacted maxillary canine tooth (C).

1,756 to have 3,702 impacted third molars; dentigerous cysts occurred in association with 30 of the 3,702 impacted teeth (0.81 percent).

It is important to recognize that other odontogenic cysts and tumors as well as nonodontogenic processes can exhibit a similar relationship to the involved tooth. These include odontogenic keratocyst, paradental cyst, ameloblastoma, and adenomatoid odontogenic tumor.

Radiographically, the dentigerous cyst is a well-defined unilocular lesion associated with the crown of an impacted tooth (fig. 3-14). Rarely, it may appear multiloculated but is always uni-

locular on gross and histologic examination. The borders are usually sclerotic unless infected, in which case margins become less defined. The cyst symmetrically surrounds the associated tooth, however, asymmetric cysts are more common in partially erupted teeth (33). It may cause significant tooth displacement and root resorption of adjacent teeth (34).

A follicular space surrounds unerupted teeth. According to Shear (33) this does not signify the presence of a cyst unless the pericoronal width is at least 3 to 4 mm. Daley and Wysocki (27) addressed the diagnostic dilemma of distinguishing a small dentigerous cyst from a large follicle radiologically and histologically. They concluded that the presence of a cystic cavity at the time of surgery might be the only reliable distinguishing feature.

Pathologic Findings. Surgical removal of the impacted tooth typically results in separation of the tooth from the surrounding cyst, so that this relationship is rarely appreciated at the time of extraction (fig. 3-15). The noninflamed dentigerous cyst has a thin epithelial lining composed of two to three layers of cuboidal or ovoid epithelial cells (fig. 3-16, left). This epithelium may resemble reduced enamel epithelium (fig. 3-16, right). Mucous cells are frequently encountered within the epithelial lining (fig. 3-17) and ciliated cells less frequently. The cyst lining may be focally keratinized. Dystrophic calcification of epithelial cells is sometimes noted (fig. 3-18). The subjacent connective tissue may be fibrous or fibromyxomatous (fig. 3-19). Epithelial odontogenic rests, which appear inactive, are often present within this connective tissue (fig. 3-20). In areas where the lining epithelium is attcnuated or absent, the lesion may resemble an odontogenic fibroma or myxoma. Dental follicular tissue may be misinterpreted as an odontogenic tumor (30).

Many dentigerous cysts are inflamed. This results in a proliferation of the epithelium and a migration of the inflammatory component through the epithelium and into the cyst lumen (fig. 3-21). The inflamed dentigerous cyst resembles a radicular cyst with the accumulation of cholesterol and epithelial (Rushton) or connective tissue hyaline bodies. However, the dentigerous cyst and radicular cyst can be distinguished clinically and radiographically.

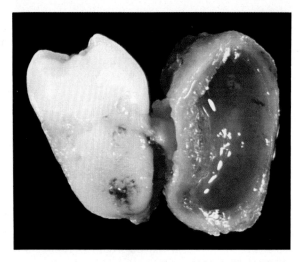

Figure 3-15
DENTIGEROUS CYST
Gross photograph of a dentigerous cyst that surrounded the crown of this impacted molar tooth. The cyst was partially dislodged from the crown root junction upon removal.

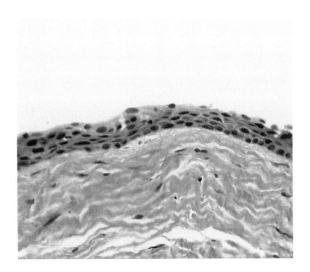 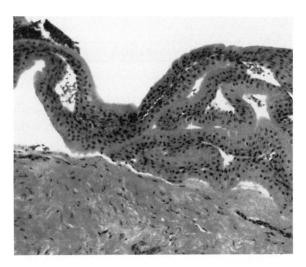

Figure 3-16
DENTIGEROUS CYST
Thin epithelial lining of a dentigerous cyst (left) contrasts with reduced enamel epithelium of a dental follicle (right).

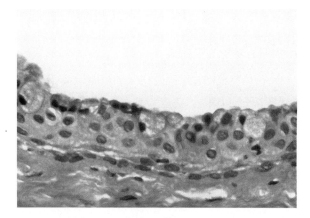

Figure 3-17
DENTIGEROUS CYST
Mucous cells within the lining of dentigerous cyst.

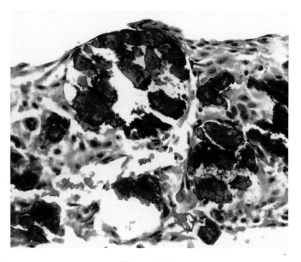

Figure 3-18
DENTIGEROUS CYST
Numerous dystrophic calcifications in the lining of a
dentigerous cyst.

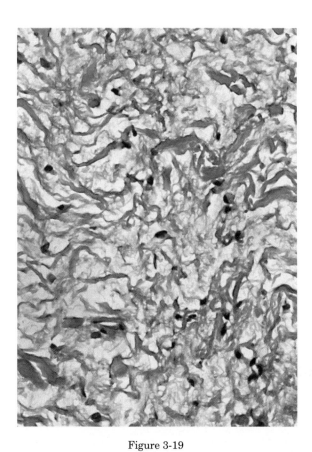

Figure 3-19
DENTIGEROUS CYST
A fibromyxomatous wall of a dentigerous cyst can be
misinterpreted as an odontogenic myxoma.

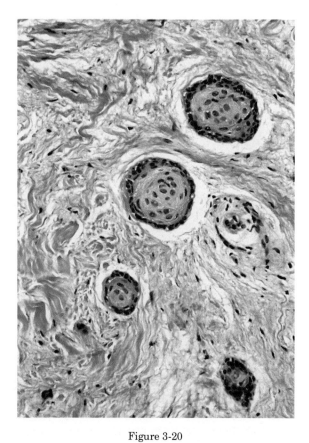

Figure 3-20
DENTIGEROUS CYST
Epithelial odontogenic rests in the connective tissue wall
of a dentigerous cyst.

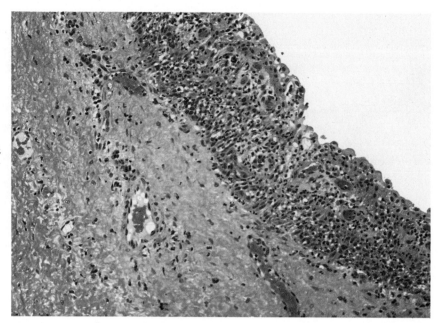

Figure 3-21
DENTIGEROUS CYST
An inflamed dentigerous cyst is histologically similar to a radicular cyst.

Neoplastic transformation rarely complicates a dentigerous cyst. Reported neoplasms include ameloblastoma (29), squamous cell carcinoma, and central mucoepidermoid carcinoma (35) (vide infra, benign and malignant odontogenic tumors).

Treatment and Prognosis. The recommended treatment is enucleation of the cyst and removal of the associated tooth (33). However, in some circumstances, such as with an impacted maxillary canine in a young patient, enucleation of the cyst with preservation of the tooth is preferred. Marsupialization of large cysts is also an effective treatment, provided biopsy has established a diagnosis of dentigerous cyst and excluded other aggressive cystic or neoplastic lesions.

Eruption Cyst

Definition. The eruption cyst is a variant of the dentigerous cyst that surrounds the crown of an erupting tooth. This cyst can impede eruption of the associated tooth.

Clinical and Radiologic Features. The eruption cyst is identified in children and can involve either primary or permanent dentition (36). It causes a fluctuant swelling of the overlying gingiva and is either of normal color or bluish (fig. 3-22, left). The term *eruption hematoma* is a clinical term that refers to extravasated blood within an eruption cyst. Most of these cysts spontaneously rupture so that their frequency is difficult to assess. Radiographically, the associated tooth lies immediately below a soft tissue shadow and there is no evidence of overlying bone (fig. 3-22, right).

Pathologic Findings. These cysts demonstrate a close relationship of cystic epithelium to surface epithelium (fig. 3-23). An inflammatory infiltrate is often present within the cyst lining.

Treatment and Prognosis. The eruption cyst may be marsupialized. This exposes the crown of the tooth and allows for its rapid eruption.

Lateral Periodontal Cyst

Definition. The lateral periodontal cyst is developmental and occurs on the lateral aspect or between the roots of vital teeth. It arises from odontogenic epithelial remnants.

Clinical and Radiologic Features. The lateral periodontal cyst is a developmental odontogenic cyst (37). It is derived from dental lamina (49,52), reduced enamel epithelium (39), or rests of Malassez. It forms along the lateral periodontium or within bone between the roots of erupted vital teeth. These lesions most frequently occur in the mandibular premolar region but other sites, including the maxilla, have been reported. The incidence of this cyst in a series of jaw cysts was reported as less than 1 percent (45). The lateral periodontal cyst is more prevalent in adults (fifth to seventh decades) and appears to have no racial

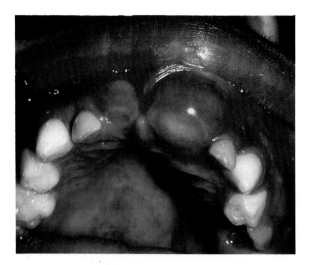 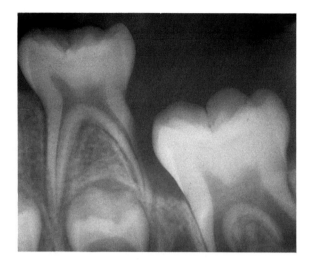

Figure 3-22
ERUPTION CYST
Left: Gingival swelling characterizes an eruption cyst overlying an erupting maxillary central incisor.
Right: Radiograph of an unerupted mandibular first molar tooth that had an associated soft tissue swelling. The lesion was marsupialized and diagnosed as an eruption cyst.

or gender predilection (37,38,41,42,47,49). The majority of the patients are asymptomatic and lesions are identified radiographically (47).

Infrequently, expansion of mandibular bone is observed. Perforation of cortical bone with involvement of the overlying gingiva can lead to difficulty in distinguishing a lateral periodontal cyst from a gingival cyst. Laterally positioned inflammatory cysts secondary to pulpal or periodontal disease, odontogenic keratocysts (43), and calcifying odontogenic cysts (44) arising in the lateral periodontium can all have a similar clinical presentation. A lateral periodontal cyst and a gingival cyst have been reported in the same patient (50).

The *botryoid odontogenic cyst* is considered by several investigators to represent a polycystic variant of the lateral periodontal cyst (42,51,52). This cyst, however, appears to have a potential for recurrence and more rapid growth (49).

Radiographically, the lateral periodontal cyst presents as a well-delineated radiolucency on the lateral surface of a tooth root between the alveolar crest and the root apex (47). The lesions are unilocular and often exhibit a thin opaque border of sclerotic bone (fig. 3-24). Occasionally, the lesion creates a pear-shaped radiolucency that causes root divergence of the associated teeth. Root resorption of adjacent teeth is rarely encountered. The cyst is usually less than 1 cm in diameter (fig. 3-25).

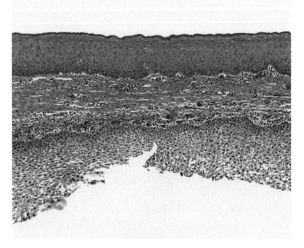

Figure 3-23
ERUPTION CYST
Photomicrograph of an eruption cyst showing surface mucosa and an underlying inflamed cyst lining.

Pathologic Findings. The histology of these cysts is unique, although similar to that of the gingival cyst of the adult (52). It is lined by an attenuated, nonkeratinized epithelium that often consists of a single or double layer of cells (fig. 3-26, left) (48). Focal, plaque-like epithelial thickenings are often noted (fig. 3-26, right). Clear cells, which presumably are glycogen rich, can be observed in the cyst lining. Sometimes the plaque-like areas

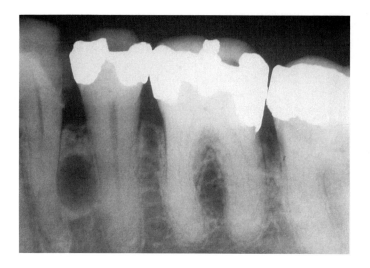

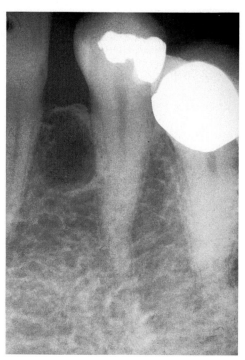

Figure 3-24
LATERAL PERIODONTAL CYST
Above: The radiolucency involves alveolar bone between the mandibular premolar teeth. Note the sclerotic border surrounding this lateral periodontal cyst.
Right: Radiolucency of a typical lateral periodontal cyst at the crest of the alveolar bone.

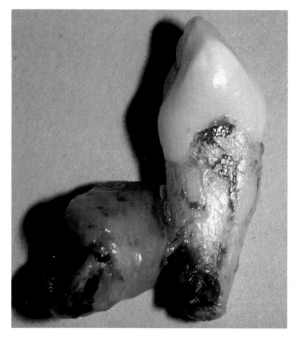

Figure 3-25
LATERAL PERIODONTAL CYST
This lateral periodontal cyst is attached to a vital canine tooth. The histologic features were typical for a developmental lateral periodontal cyst. The reason for tooth extraction was not given when the specimen was submitted for histologic examination.

have a whorled appearance. The epithelial lining is surrounded by fibrous connective tissue devoid of any significant inflammatory component. Infrequently, an acellular, hyalinized connective tissue band is observed immediately beneath the cyst lining. Separation of the epithelial lining from the underlying connective tissue is sometimes evident. Microscopic examination is necessary to distinguish the lateral periodontal cyst from cysts of either pulpal or periodontal origin, the odontogenic keratocyst (43), and other pathologic processes that can occur in the same anatomic region. Melanin pigment has been reported in the epithelial cyst lining (40). A rare case of squamous cell carcinoma arising in a lateral periodontal cyst has been reported (39).

Treatment and Prognosis. The lateral periodontal cyst is treated by local excision (enucleation) without extraction of adjacent teeth. Enucleation of cysts that are more apically located can lead to devitalization of pulpal tissue, thereby necessitating endodontic treatment. There is no reported tendency for recurrence. Complete bone remodeling at the surgical site is expected. Freeze dried bone graft has been used for a lateral periodontal cyst that perforated buccal

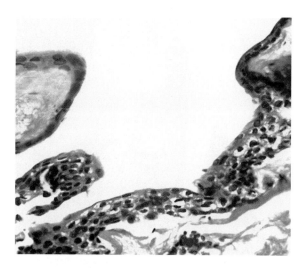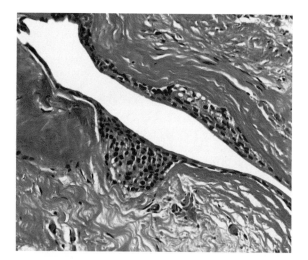

Figure 3-26
LATERAL PERIODONTAL CYST
Cyst showing thin odontogenic epithelium (left) with focal plaque-like thickenings (right).

and lingual cortex (46). The polycystic variant of the lateral periodontal cyst appears to behave more aggressively and tends to recur (37,41,49).

Botryoid Odontogenic Cyst

Definition. Botryoid odontogenic cyst is a polycystic lesion that is histologically similar to the lateral periodontal cyst. It may be locally aggressive and can recur.

Clinical and Radiologic Features. Since the initial report of two botryoid odontogenic cysts by Weathers and Waldron (71) and a possible similar lesion reported by Shafer and Standish (69) in their series of lateral periodontal cysts, there have been limited numbers of case reports (53,55,58,60–62,66,67) and fewer reports of series (56,57) of this uncommon odontogenic cyst. The cysts are most commonly seen in the mandible and in patients over 50 years of age with no sex predilection. Patients tend to be asymptomatic but the cyst may expand bone. The clinical presentation is similar to that of the lateral periodontal cyst, with the exception that botryoid odontogenic cyst is seen in a somewhat older age group (54,57).

The radiographic features are variable (fig. 3-27): some lesions present as unilocular radiolucencies with a thin sclerotic bony margin and others as multilocular lesions larger than 2 cm. Root resorption is not a characteristic find-

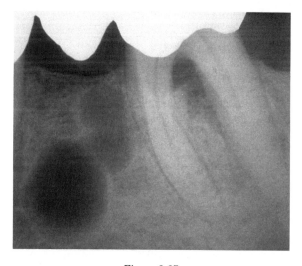

Figure 3-27
BOTRYOID ODONTOGENIC CYST
Radiograph showing a multiloculated radiolucency adjacent to the mesial root of the first molar tooth and in the vicinity of the missing second premolar tooth.

ing. One of the lesions reported by Greer and Johnson (56) presented as a unilocular radiolucency measuring 4.5 cm.

Lynch and Madden (62) described a botryoid variant of a gingival cyst that perforated cortical bone. They proposed that the term botryoid odontogenic cyst be reserved for those lateral periodontal and gingival cysts that are multilocular and have a lobulated appearance clinically

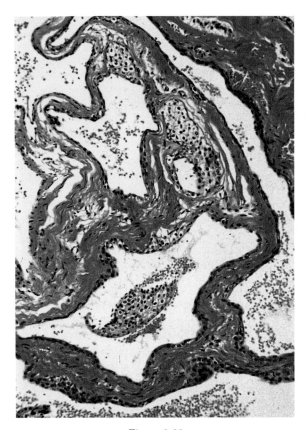

Figure 3-28
BOTRYOID ODONTOGENIC CYST
Low-power photomicrograph demonstrates the poly-cystic nature of the lesion.

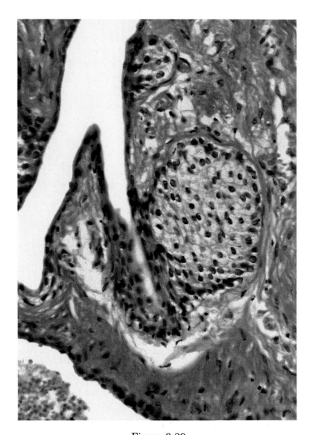

Figure 3-29
BOTRYOID ODONTOGENIC CYST
Focal plaque-like thickening of clear odontogenic epithe-lial cells is seen.

and grossly (62). Kaugars (60) proposed the following criteria for the diagnosis of botryoid odontogenic cyst: 1) histologic features similar to lateral periodontal cyst and demonstration of multiple cystic areas; 2) a multilocular radiographic pattern; and 3) no evidence of an inflammatory origin from pulpal or periodontal elements.

Pathologic Findings. The multicystic lesion is lined by compressed epithelium that is only one to three cell layers thick (fig. 3-28). Several foci of epithelial plaque-like thickenings may be present (fig. 3-29). In addition, glycogen-containing clear cells can be identified. In the series of Gurol et al. (57), 31 of 33 cases contained glycogen-rich clear cells. The histologic picture is quite similar to that of lateral periodontal cyst except for the polycystic character (54,57,70,72). Clusters of epithelial odontogenic rests are sometimes present in the connective tissue adjacent to the cyst wall. There are also similarities

to gingival cyst (64) and the glandular odontogenic cyst because of the polycystic quality and the epithelial plaque-like thickenings of the cyst lining (59,63,65,68).

Treatment and Prognosis. Surgical removal by curettage is the recommended treatment. The initial report of this entity suggested a potential for recurrence because of "buds" and islands of glycogen-rich epithelial clusters that extended into the connective tissue. Weathers and Waldron (71) concluded, however, that these lesions are unlikely to be aggressive and that simple enucleation is adequate therapy. Subsequently, Kaugars (60) reported three cases of botryoid odontogenic cyst, one of which recurred 9 years after the initial surgical removal. Phelan and colleagues (66) similarly reported a case of recurrent botryoid odontogenic cyst. Greer and Johnson (56) reported 10 cases, three of which recurred 8, 10, and 10 years after surgery; some of these exhibited significant destructive behavior. A likely explanation for this potential to recur is inadequate removal of a lesion with multiple compartments. Alternatively, etiologic factors that promote cyst formation in odontogenic epithelium may continue after removal of the initial lesion. Redman et al. (67) reported a case with histologic evidence of a multicentric origin. Additional studies have documented the recurrent potential of the botryoid odontogenic cyst (57,58,70). Thus, long-term follow-up is recommended.

Glandular Odontogenic Cyst

Definition. The glandular odontogenic cyst arises in tooth-bearing areas of the jaws, is lined by cuboidal to columnar epithelial cells, and exhibits crypt-like and microcystic spaces often lined by mucous cells.

Clinical and Radiologic Features. The intraosseous glandular odontogenic cyst was first reported by Padyachee and van Wyk in 1992 (89). The lesion shares some histologic features with botryoid odontogenic cyst and mucoepidermoid tumor or carcinoma (88,89,92,99). Padyachee and van Wyk suggested the term "sialo-odontogenic cyst" on the basis of their analysis of two mandibular lesions. The terms *sialo-odontogenic cyst* and *mucus-producing cyst* had been previously discussed by Gardner (79). Gardner et al. (80) published eight cases which they referred to as glandular odontogenic cyst. Additional terms used to describe this cyst are *mucoepidermoid odontogenic cyst* (92) and *polymorphous odontogenic cyst* (83). This latter term introduced by High et al. (83) encompasses the varied histologic appearance of these cysts. Since these initial reports, a number of cases have been documented (73–76,78,82–88,90–100).

A case report and review of the literature by Ramer et al. (91) revealed the following: 34 of 39 (87.2 percent) glandular odontogenic cysts occurred in the mandible (74 percent in the anterior mandible), and 5 of 39 (12.8 percent) in the maxilla (all 5 in the anterior segment). The average age at time of diagnosis was 49.5 years. There was a slight male predilection (55.3 percent). Symptoms included painless swelling (48 percent), painful swelling (32 percent), pain alone (12 percent), and no symptoms (8 percent). The lesions range in size from 1 cm to some that involve the entire

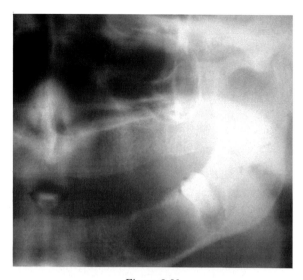

Figure 3-30
GLANDULAR ODONTOGENIC CYST
A radiolucent lesion in the body of the mandible is adjacent to impacted molar.

mandible. Lesions of the anterior mandible frequently cross the midline (77,81,83,91). They have presented in a lateral periodontal location (95) and as dentigerous cysts (85).

Radiologically, these lesions are usually multilocular and radiolucent (81,83,87,91). The review of Ramer et al. (91) indicated the presence of a unilocular radiolucency in 13 of 34 (38.2 percent) cases and a multilocular radiolucency in 21 of 34 (61.8 percent) cases. Occasionally, the lesion border is sclerotic although some cases have ill-defined peripheral margins. Radiographic features of three separate glandular odontogenic cysts are presented in figures 3-30–3-32.

Pathologic Findings. The histologic features include: 1) a multicystic lesion partially lined by nonkeratinized epithelium with focal plaque-like thickenings which may have a swirled appearance similar to that seen in lateral periodontal and botryoid odontogenic cysts (80,89); 2) a surface epithelial layer that may include eosinophilic cuboidal cells and cilia (74); and 3) mucous cells and mucin pools in microcystic areas resulting in a glandular appearance (fig. 3-33) (75). The histopathologic findings are similar to those seen in lateral periodontal and botryoid odontogenic cysts and in low-grade central mucoepidermoid carcinoma (77,88,89,92,99). Waldron and Koh (99) noted

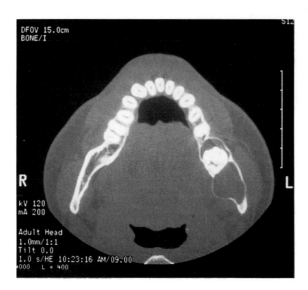
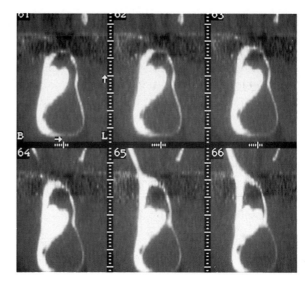

Figure 3-31
GLANDULAR ODONTOGENIC CYST
Left: Computed tomographic axial view of glandular odontogenic cyst associated with an impacted molar.
Right: Dental scan of same lesion showing the relationship to molar tooth.

that in selected fields, the latter may be histologically identical to glandular odontogenic cyst; they considered that the distinction between these two lesions was largely dependent on the degree of epithelial proliferation. Cytokeratin 7, 13, 14, and 19 expression within the glandular odontogenic cyst has been reported (75,94). Hyaline bodies have also been noted (85). Ramer et al. (91) reported the presence of ghost cells in a cyst wall that otherwise exhibited the classic features of glandular odontogenic cyst.

As mentioned previously, these cysts have microscopic features similar to those of lateral periodontal and botryoid odontogenic cysts, supporting an odontogenic origin. The presence of mucous cells does not detract from an odontogenic origin as this feature has been reported in a variety of odontogenic cysts, most notably in dentigerous and radicular cysts. The glandular odontogenic cyst may represent a developmental odontogenic cyst that either initially or over time exhibits glandular differentiation. The histologic similarity to low-grade cystic central mucoepidermoid carcinoma may result in a significant misdiagnosis. The histogenesis of the latter in the jaw is unknown; however, origin from the epithelial lining of odontogenic cysts that exhibit mucous metaplasia or entrapment of salivary gland tissue within the jaws has been proposed. Waldron and Koh (99) have

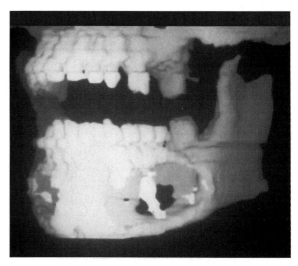

Figure 3-32
GLANDULAR ODONTOGENIC CYST
Computed tomographic, three-dimensional reconstruction of glandular odontogenic cyst, which crossed the midline and involved the entire anterior mandible.

emphasized that the degree of epithelial proliferation may be the only distinguishing feature that allows separation of glandular odontogenic cyst from central mucoepidermoid carcinoma. Whether glandular odontogenic cyst represents a distinct lesion or part of a spectrum of central

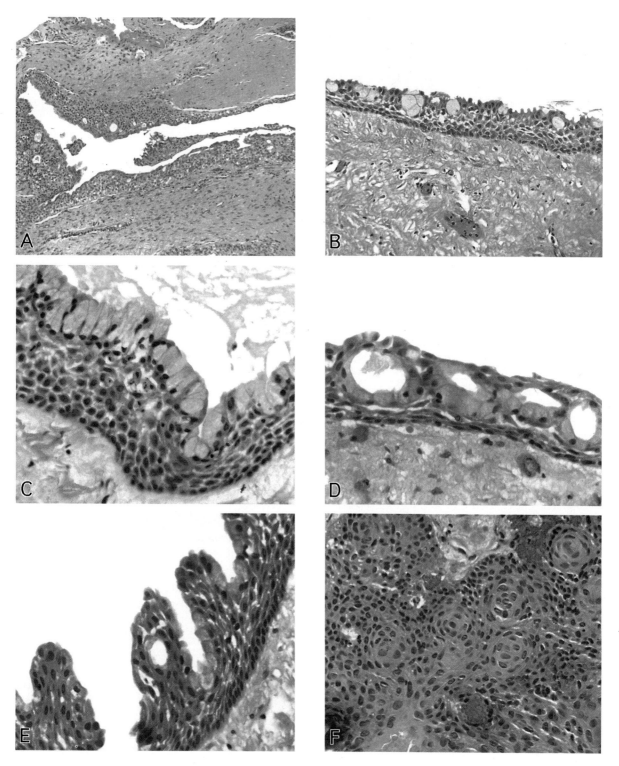

Figure 3-33
GLANDULAR ODONTOGENIC CYST

Cystic lesion showing variable thickness of the lining epithelium (A); mucous cells and apocrine-like changes of luminal epithelial cells (B); ciliated epithelium, mucous cells, and apocrine-like change (C); microcystic area rimmed by mucous cells (D); papillary epithelial projections into cyst lumen lined by mucous cells (E); and thickened epithelial lining resulting in a whorled appearance (F).

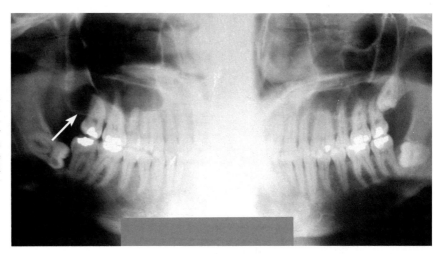

Figure 3-34
PRIMORDIAL CYST
Panoramic radiograph of an adult patient with three impacted third molar teeth. There is a discrete radiolucency in the maxillary right third molar area; no tooth is present. The histopathology of the lesion was that of a noninflamed odontogenic cyst without any evidence of keratinization.

mucoepidermoid lesions of the jaws remains to be determined. However, the designation "glandular odontogenic cyst" should be applied when the classic features of mucoepidermoid carcinoma are absent. Caution should be exercised when rendering a diagnosis of glandular odontogenic cyst based on a limited biopsy from a large radiolucent lesion. Controversial entities such as median mandibular cyst and globulomaxillary cyst may be examples of glandular odontogenic cyst.

Treatment and Prognosis. This lesion should be considered locally aggressive, as Gardner and Morency (81) have documented recurrences. They suggested that a marginal resection was the recommended treatment but did not exclude curettage or enucleation, and emphasized the need for careful follow-up.

Primordial Cyst

The primordial cyst is extremely rare and is considered to originate from cystic degeneration of the enamel organ prior to the formation of any dental hard tissue. It is lined by nonkeratinized squamous epithelium.

The designation "primordial cyst" remains controversial (101,105,107). It is frequently used synonymously with odontogenic keratocyst (102,105) and this has caused considerable confusion since the diagnosis of odontogenic keratocyst is based on specific histologic criteria (102,105,107). The term primordial cyst was introduced by Robinson in 1945 (104), for "those closed epithelial lined sacs formed through degeneration of the stellate reticulum in the enamel organs before any calcified

structures have been laid down." Robinson, Koch, and Kolas (106) later stated that the primordial cyst is differentiated from a residual cyst only after careful review of the dentition history.

Philipsen (103), who first described the odontogenic keratocyst, considered it to be primordial in origin so that the terms primordial cyst and odontogenic keratocyst came to be used synonymously. Odontogenic keratocysts may occur in a dentigerous relationship to teeth, at the apex, in the lateral periodontium, or in a primordial location where a tooth might otherwise be present. The World Health Organization (WHO) Histological Typing of Odontogenic Tumors, 1992 (102), lists odontogenic keratocyst as the preferred term for cysts with a keratinized lining but still lists primordial cyst as synonymous. We believe that the designation primordial cyst should be applied to those cysts that do not have the histologic features of an odontogenic keratocyst but occur in an area where a missing tooth would otherwise be expected.

The nonkeratinized primordial cyst is an extremely rare entity, seldom referred to in the literature. Figures 3-34 and 3-35 show a radiograph and photomicrograph of a case in which the cystic process is lined by a double row of nonkeratinizing epithelial cells.

Odontogenic Keratocyst

Definition. The odontogenic keratocyst is a distinctive developmental odontogenic jaw cyst characterized by a parakeratinized, stratified, squamous epithelial lining.

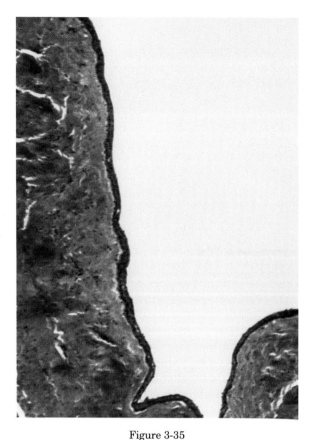

Figure 3-35
PRIMORDIAL CYST
An odontogenic cyst is lined by a double row of epithelial cells. Note the absence of keratin.

Clinical and Radiologic Features. The term odontogenic keratocyst was first introduced by Philipsen in 1956 (142). This cyst may be associated with an erupted or unerupted tooth or occur in a nontooth-bearing area of the jaw; peripheral odontogenic keratocysts involving gingival tissue have also been reported (116,120). The cyst may be aggressive (109,121) and has a high recurrence rate compared to other odontogenic cysts (112,118, 127,158). Thus, a diagnosis of keratocyst necessitates long-term clinical and radiographic follow-up. Those cysts that exhibit a parakeratinized surface behave more aggressively and have a higher recurrence rate (5 to 62 percent) than orthokeratinized variants (113,118,158,163). The orthokeratinized variant has also been referred to as an *orthokeratinized odontogenic cyst* and histologically resembles an epidermal inclusion cyst (163). Both cyst types have usually been dealt with together in the literature. The orthokera-

tinized odontogenic cyst is discussed in a separate section.

The odontogenic keratocyst is a component of the nevoid basal cell carcinoma syndrome (Gorlin-Goltz syndrome), and a diagnosis of an odontogenic keratocyst, especially multiple cysts, should raise the suspicion of this syndrome (110,115). Approximately 5 percent of odontogenic keratocysts are associated with the nevoid basal cell carcinoma syndrome. However, multiple cysts have been reported in patients without the syndrome as well.

The odontogenic keratocyst probably originates from the dental lamina or its residues; however, origin from reduced enamel epithelium cannot be entirely excluded. The term primordial cyst has been used synonymously with odontogenic keratocyst, but this adds confusion to the jaw cyst classification scheme (146), since diagnosis of the keratocyst is based purely on histology.

The odontogenic keratocyst represents approximately 4 to 10 percent of all odontogenic cysts (112,118,119). Analysis of data from large series indicates a peak incidence in the second to fourth decades, and an age range from infancy (126) to 93 years. The cyst is slightly more common in males than females. Caucasians are more commonly affected than blacks, Orientals, and Indians. Odontogenic keratocysts occur twice as frequently in the mandible as in the maxilla. Posterior regions of the jaws, specifically the third molar area of either jaw and the ramus area of the mandible, are the most common locations. These cysts can cross the midline and maxillary cysts can involve the antra (132) and floor of the nose.

The odontogenic keratocyst can present in a dentigerous (associated with the crown of an impacted tooth), a primordial (in an area related to an undeveloped tooth), a residual (in an area where a tooth was previously present), a lateral periodontal, a globulomaxillary, or a nasopalatine location (112,118,140,161).

Most keratocysts do not cause symptoms. However, swelling, pain, discomfort, and intraoral drainage have been noted. The presence of neurologic symptoms is dependent on the location of the keratocyst. Buccal and lingual expansion with possible bony perforation can be expected in the more aggressive cysts (137). Keratinaceous material is often identified at time of surgery (see fig. 3-3).

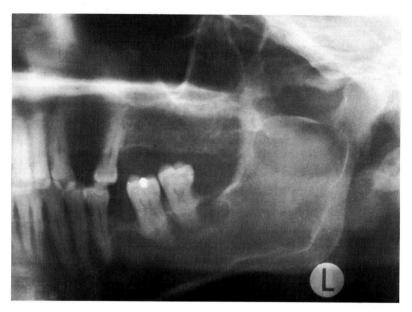

Figure 3-36
ODONTOGENIC KERATOCYST
Panoramic radiograph of a large cyst involving the body and ramus of the mandible.

Most keratocysts are radiographically unilocular. However, multiloculation (125) is more common with larger lesions (fig. 3-36). The borders are smooth or scalloped and corticated. Larger lesions can cause bony expansion with or without perforation of the cortical plates. Displacement of adjacent teeth is more common than resorption. The radiographic features are not pathognomonic and the presentation can be similar to that of other odontogenic cysts or jaw tumors (fig. 3-37). Keratin in the cyst lumen may result in a cloudy radiographic appearance. Computed tomography and three-dimensional reconstruction may aid in surgical planning (164).

Pathologic Findings. Grossly, the keratocyst is filled with keratin (fig. 3-38). The histologic features were first described by Philipsen (142). The basal cells of the lining epithelium are palisaded and columnar or cuboidal, above which are several layers of polyhedral squamous cells that mature to a parakeratotic surface (fig. 3-39A,B). The nuclei of these parakeratinized cells demonstrate a wavy pattern. Keratin in the cyst lumen may not contain nuclei. Thus, the distinction between parakeratinized and orthokeratinized variants requires analysis of the superficial layer of the cyst lining and not the luminal contents. Rarely, a cyst may exhibit both orthokeratin and parakeratin (113,118,163). Reversed polarity of the nuclei of the basal cells may be noted. Cyst epithelium and the basal lamina complex fre-

quently separate from the underlying connective tissue (fig. 3-39C); this has been documented with ultrastructural studies (160).

The epithelial lining of an odontogenic keratocyst lacks rete pegs; however, if the cyst is inflamed, rete pegs may form and focal areas of the cyst then resemble a common inflammatory odontogenic cyst (fig. 3-40) (147). Satellite cysts (fig. 3-41, left), solid epithelial proliferations, odontogenic rests, and basal budding (fig. 3-41, above) have been described in association with odontogenic keratocysts. Ameloblastomatous proliferation within the lining of these cysts has also been reported as has a combined ameloblastoma and odontogenic keratocyst (152). These features, including ameloblastic transformation, are more common in keratocysts associated with the nevoid basal cell carcinoma syndrome (145). Mineralization in the fibrous connective tissue cyst wall occurs and probably represents calcification of odontogenic rests. This is not a feature peculiar to the odontogenic keratocyst and is found also in dentigerous cysts and apical periodontal cysts. Cholesterol accumulation and epithelial hyaline bodies (Rushton bodies) may be present. Melanocytes and melanin pigment have been noted within keratocysts (133,157). Respiratory type epithelium has also been noted in direct continuity with a mandibular keratocyst (143). When respiratory type epithelium is present, the glandular odontogenic cyst should be excluded

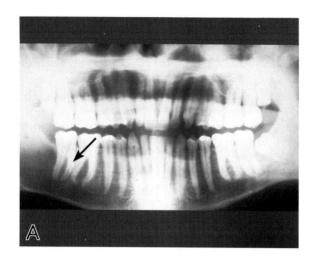

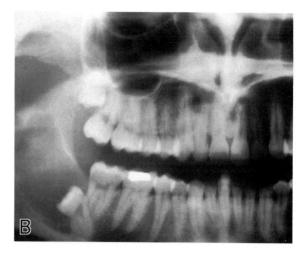

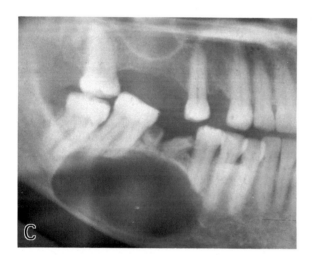

Figure 3-37
ODONTOGENIC KERATOCYST
Radiographs of odontogenic keratocysts located in a primordial (A); dentigerous (B); periapical (C); lateral periodontal (D); and globulomaxillary position (E).

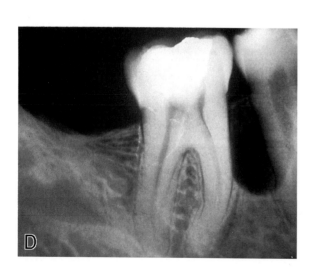

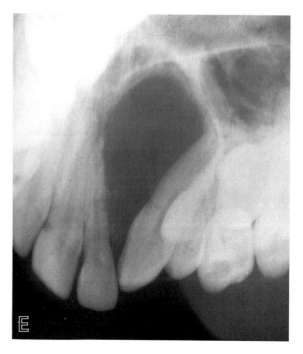

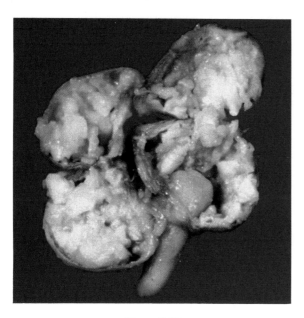

Figure 3-38
ODONTOGENIC KERATOCYST
Keratin fills the lumen of an odontogenic keratocyst surrounding the crown of a premolar tooth. (Courtesy of D. R. Weathers, Atlanta, GA.)

Figure 3-39
ODONTOGENIC KERATOCYST
A: Low-power photomicrograph of an odontogenic keratocyst. Note lack of rete pegs.
B: Higher power showing palisading of the basal cells and the epithelium maturing to a parakeratotic surface.
C: The epithelial lining separates from the connective tissue, a common feature of the keratocyst.

as a diagnostic possibility. Cases of odontogenic keratocyst containing cartilage in the cyst wall (128,139) and a keratocyst associated with an intramandibular chondroma (111) have been reported. Mast cells have been documented (155). An odontogenic keratocyst occurred simultaneously with a traumatic (simple) bone cyst, resulting in a pathologic fracture (135).

Epithelial dysplasia and squamous cell carcinoma have occurred in odontogenic keratocysts (110,123,124,134,153). There is also a case of synchronous verrucous carcinoma and squamous cell carcinoma arising in an odontogenic keratocyst (110). The veterinary literature cites the occurrence of an odontogenic keratocyst in a dog (144).

Using autoradiography and DNA cytomorphometry, Scharffetter et al. (149) demonstrated

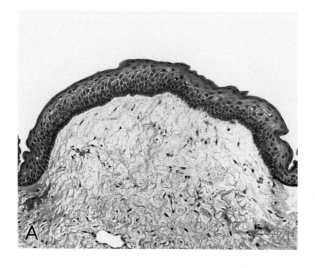

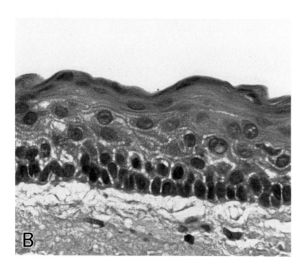

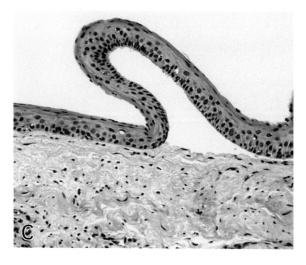

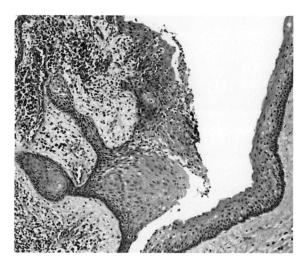 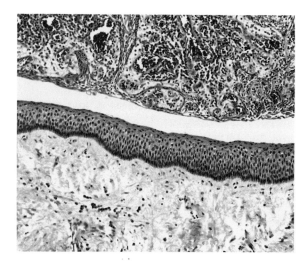

Figure 3-40
ODONTOGENIC KERATOCYST

Odontogenic keratocyst is adjacent to an area of inflammation. The cyst lining has the appearance of an inflammatory odontogenic cyst.

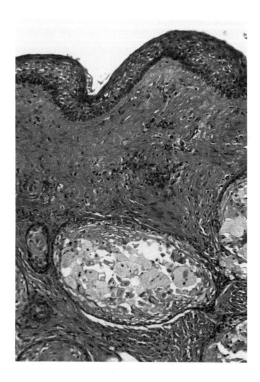 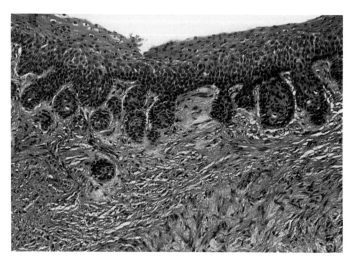

Figure 3-41
ODONTOGENIC KERATOCYST

Left: Satellite cysts within the connective tissue wall of an odontogenic keratocyst.

Above: Budding of keratocyst epithelium along the basal cell layer in a patient with nevoid basal cell carcinoma syndrome.

that the proliferation of both epithelium and connective tissue is higher in a keratocyst than in a reference radicular cyst. Studies using lectin histochemistry suggest that the positive binding of *Ulex europaeus* agglutinin I and *Bandeirea simplicifolia* agglutinin I to jaw cysts, including the odontogenic keratocyst, may be a useful histologic aid

for differentiating between cystic ameloblastoma and non-neoplastic jaw cysts (108,148). No positive reactions were obtained with the two lectins to the epithelial components of ameloblastoma. High levels of lactoferrin have been demonstrated in the fluid of odontogenic keratocysts, but these levels were not statistically significant.

Intermediate filament keratin proteins have been identified in parakeratinized odontogcnic keratocysts, specifically the high molecular weight cytokeratins, K10/11 and cytokeratin K19 (136, 150). However, to date, keratin profiles have not aided in the histologic diagnosis of keratocysts. The p53 protein has been demonstrated in odontogenic keratocysts although a specific genetic mutation has not been identified (131,141,154). Growth factor receptors have been identified in odontogenic cysts including the odontogenic keratocyst (129,151). Immunohistochemical expression of transforming growth factor-alpha, epidermal growth factor in the epithelial lining of odontogenic cysts, and transforming growth factor-beta in the extracellular matrix of the fibrous connective tissue wall of these cysts have been documented by Li et al. (130). Human papillomavirus type 16 DNA has been noted in one case (117). Lo Muzio et al. (131a) have studied the cellular proliferation rate (proliferating cell nuclear antigen), the p53 tumor suppressor gene, and expression of oncoproteins bcl-1 and bcl-2 (cyclin D1) in sporadic odontogenic keratocysts and keratocysts associated with nevoid basal cell carcinoma syndrome.

Treatment and Prognosis. The keratocyst is treated surgically; however, some controversy exists as to the optimal method employed to treat such cysts. This is likely related to the high recurrence rate compared to most odontogenic cysts. Important features that dictate a conservative or aggressive approach include location, size of lesion, relationship to tooth roots, and perforation of cortical bone with or without soft tissue extension (114,159). Enucleation, aggressive or nonaggressive curettage, decompression (114), marsupialization, and a modified Brosch procedure (122) are the more conservative surgical procedures (138) while resection, with or without a continuity defect and disarticulation are the more aggressive. Some may require a supraperiosteal dissection in continuity with adjacent soft tissues. Recurrent lesions have been reported in the soft tissues (156,162).

Nevoid Basal Cell Carcinoma Syndrome

Definition. The nevoid basal cell carcinoma syndrome (NBCCS) is an autosomal dominant disorder characterized by numerous basal cell carcinomas of the skin, odontogenic keratocysts of the jaws, and skeletal abnormalities, specifically an enlarged calvarium and bifid ribs, and less frequently, neoplasms such as ovarian fibroma and medulloblastoma (167–170).

General Features. The syndrome was first delineated in the 1950s (170) and 1960s (168). The condition has been variously known as *basal cell nevus syndrome, Gorlin-Goltz syndrome, Gorlin syndrome,* and *NBCCS* (167). The prevalence has been estimated at 1 per 56,000 (166).

Malformations such as calcification of the falx cerebri (fig. 3-42A), palmar and plantar pits (fig. 3-42B), cleft palate, and generalized overgrowth are components of the syndrome (165,167,168). Also, neoplasms such as fibrosarcoma, meningioma, rhabdomyosarcoma, and cardiac fibroma probably occur in excess in this syndrome (166,174).

Kimonis et al. (171) carried out a detailed analysis of 105 patients with the syndrome who were examined at the National Institutes of Health since 1985. There were 57 females and 48 males. Eighty percent of affected whites and 38 percent of blacks had at least one basal cell carcinoma, the initial neoplasm occurring at a mean age of 23 and 21 years, respectively. The number of basal cell carcinomas ranged from 1 to greater than 1,100 with a median of 8 in whites, and 1 to 3 with a median of 2 in blacks. Jaw cysts occurred in 74 percent; the median number of jaw cysts was three. Eighty percent had their first lesion by 20 years of age. Palmar and plantar pits were seen in 87 percent of patients. Ovarian fibromas were identified by ultrasound in 17 percent of the females. Medulloblastoma was diagnosed in four patients at a mean age of 2.3 years. Three patients had cleft lip or palate. Radiographic findings included calcification of the falx cerebri in 65 percent, calcification of the tentorium cerebelli in 20 percent, a bridged sella in 68 percent, bifid ribs in 26 percent, hemivertibrae in 15 percent, fusion of vertebral bodies in 10 percent, and flame-shaped lucencies of the phalanges, metacarpals, and carpal bones of the hand in 30 percent. Previously considered components of the syndrome which were not found to be significantly increased included short fourth metacarpal, scoliosis, cervical ribs and spina bifida occulta.

The gene for this syndrome is located on chromosome 9q22 and probably functions as a tumor suppressor gene, since deletion of this region is

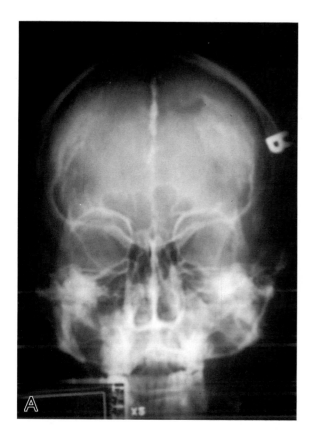

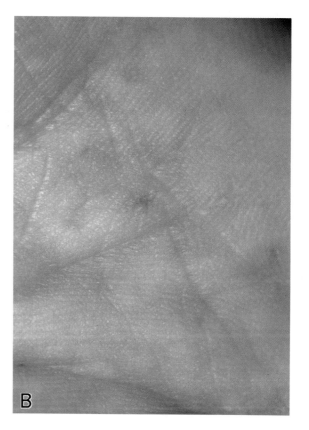

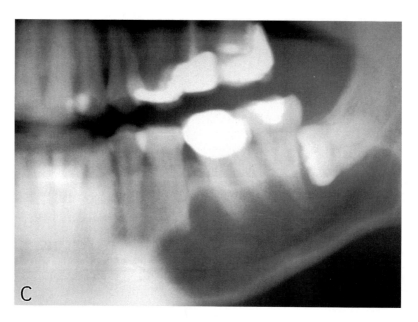

Figure 3-42
NEVOID BASAL CELL CARCINOMA SYNDROME
Radiograph demonstrating calcification of the falx cerebri (A) and palmar pits (B) in a patient with NBCCS. Panoramic radiograph
of an adult patient with stigmata of NBCCS and a biopsy of proven odontogenic keratocyst of the mandible (C).

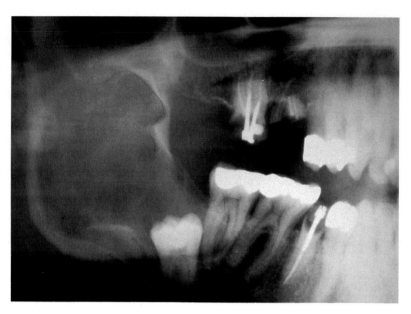

Figure 3-43
ORTHOKERATINIZED
ODONTOGENIC CYST
Large radiolucency is enveloping the crown of an impacted mandibular molar and extends into the ramus and sub-condylar region.

found in many neoplasms related to the syndrome (174). Patched (PTCH) is the tumor suppressor gene located on chromosome 9q22.3 and functions as a cell cycle regulator. A detailed discussion of the molecular biology of the PTCH gene and the hedgehog signaling network in NBCCS has been presented by Cohen (165a).

The odontogenic keratocyst in the syndrome is of the parakeratinized type. These cysts are considered to develop during the first decade of life and are usually identified radiographically during the second and third decades (fig. 3-42C). The jaw cysts, like neoplasms in other cancer predisposition syndromes, are often multiple and appear in a random pattern. However, similar isolated defects are seen in the general population. Levant et al. (173) presented molecular evidence of a two-hit mechanism, similar to the Knudson model for neoplasia (172), for the pathogenesis of keratocysts, with allelic loss of chromosome 9q22. This data indicates that loss of heterozygosity is significantly less common in sporadic than in hereditary cysts (173).

Orthokeratinized Odontogenic Cyst

Definition. The orthokeratinized odontogenic cyst is a cyst that microscopically has a uniform, orthokeratinized epithelial lining. These cysts are different histologically and are less likely to recur than the parakeratinized odontogenic keratocyst.

Clinical and Radiologic Features. The orthokeratinized odontogenic cyst can have a variable clinical presentation (184). Most patients are asymptomatic, however presenting signs and symptoms include pain, swelling, infection, and expansion of the involved jaw (175–179,181–184). Most are associated with the crown of an impacted mandibular molar tooth (fig. 3-43) and may present clinically and radiographically as a radicular or residual cyst. Vuhahula et al. (183) reported 12 orthokeratinized cysts, 8 in the mandible and 4 in the maxilla, with a mean patient age of 25 years; 9 were associated with an impacted tooth. Two-thirds of orthokeratinized cysts occur in the molar region (179); the following jaw locations are affected less commonly and in descending order of frequency: anterior, ramus, premolar, and tuberosity regions. The average size of these cysts was 5.9 cm in one study (179).

Wright in 1981 (184) proposed the term *odontogenic keratocyst (orthokeratinized variant)* and suggested that this cyst be separated from its parakeratinized counterpart to emphasize their histologic and clinical differences. The orthokeratinized odontogenic cyst is not associated with the nevoid basal cell carcinoma syndrome (177,181,184).

Pathologic Findings. The orthokeratinized odontogenic cyst is characterized by stratified squamous epithelium, with a cuboidal or flattened basal cell layer that matures to an orthokeratinized

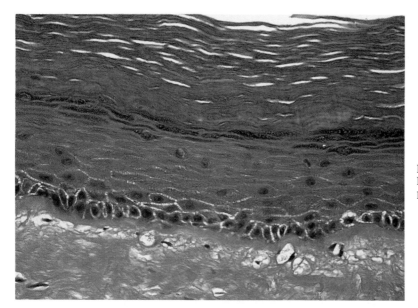

Figure 3-44
ORTHOKERATINIZED
ODONTOGENIC CYST
Orthokeratin is overlying a granular
layer. The basal layer is well defined but
lacks the characteristic palisading of the
parakeratinized odontogenic keratocyst.

surface (fig. 3-44). The basal layer does not demonstrate the classic palisading that characterizes
the parakeratinized variety. A granular layer is
noted immediately below the orthokeratinized surface. Occasionally, cysts demonstrate both a parakeratinized and orthokeratinized surface (177,
179,184). In an analysis of both jaw cysts, Brannon
(177) found 83.2 percent were parakeratinized,
9.7 percent were orthokeratinized, and 7.1 percent had features of both. Those with combined
orthokeratin and parakeratin features should be
treated as parakeratinized odontogenic keratocysts since they have a higher tendency to recur
than the orthokeratinized odontogenic cyst but
a lower recurrence rate than uniformly parakeratinized odontogenic keratocysts (176).

Keratin metaplasia in other odontogenic cysts
must be distinguished from the orthokeratinized
odontogenic cyst. This type of metaplasia is usually focal compared to the more extensive keratinization in the orthokeratinized odontogenic
cyst. Areas of nonkeratinized cyst lining may be
observed in areas where there is subepithelial
inflammation. Epidermal appendages such as
sebaceous glands (183, case 11), hair, and sweat
glands (183, case 12) have been noted in orthokeratinized jaw cysts, and are probably best
subclassified as dermoid cysts of the jaw. Use of
various cytokeratin markers has not proved reliable in differentiating various odontogenic and
nonodontogenic cysts (180).

Treatment and Prognosis. Enucleation of
the cyst with curettage is the recommended treatment. Extraction of teeth may be required to allow
for surgical access to the lesion. Wright (184) reported a recurrence rate of 4.2 percent (1 of 24
cases) and Crowley et al. (179) 2.2 percent (1 of 45
cases). Anand et al. (175) documented the highest
recurrence rate of 36 percent (5 of 14 cases).

Calcifying Odontogenic Cyst

Definition. The calcifying odontogenic cyst is
an odontogenic lesion with variable histologic features that include columnar basal cells, epithelial
cells that resemble stellate reticulum, and ghost
cells in the cyst lining or connective tissue capsule. Calcification of these ghost cells, along with
dentin or enamel matrix similar to that noted in
odontoma, is frequently seen. Cystic and solid
variants are recognized and malignant counterparts have been reported.

General Features. In 1962, Gorlin et al. (195)
coined the term calcifying odontogenic cyst and
noted the similarity of this lesion to the calcifying
epithelioma of Malherbe. In 1963 Gold (194) referred to this same lesion as keratinizing and
calcifying odontogenic cyst. As more cases were
reported, a variety of clinical and histologic features were appreciated (185,187,192,198,201,204).
Both intraosseous (187,193) and extraosseous
(188,193) lesions were recognized. Most lesions
are cystic but solid neoplastic-appearing forms

Table 3-1

CLASSIFICATION SCHEMES OF THE CALCIFYING ODONTOGENIC CYST (COC)*

Praetorius, 1981 (201)
Type 1. Cystic type
           simple unicystic type
           odontoma-producing type
           ameloblastomatous proliferating
              type
Type 2. Neoplastic type: dentinogenic ghost
              cell tumor

Buchner, 1991 (187)
Peripheral (extraosseous) COC
   cystic variant
   neoplastic solid variant
Central (intraosseous) COC
   cystic variant
      simple (unicystic or multicystic)
      associated with an odontoma
      associated with odontogenic tumors
         (other than odontoma)
      other variants (such as clear cell variant,
         pigmented variant)
   neoplastic (solid) variant: dentinogenic ghost
      cell tumor or epithelial odontogenic
      ghost cell tumor
   malignant COC

Hong et al., 1991 (198)
Type 1. Cystic
           nonproliferative
           proliferative
           ameloblastomatous
           associated with odontoma
Type 2. Neoplastic
           ameloblastomatous ex COC
           peripheral epithelial odontogenic
             ghost cell tumor
           central epithelial odontogenic
             ghost cell tumor

Toida, 1998 (204)
Cyst: calcifying ghost cell odontogenic cyst
   (CGCOC)
Neoplasm:
   benign: calcifying ghost cell odontogenic
      tumor (CGCOT)
      cystic variant: cystic CGCOT
      solid variant: solid CGCOT
   malignant CGCOT
Combined lesion: each of the categories described
   above (CGCOC, CGCOT and malignant
   CGCOT) associated with the following lesions
      odontoma
      ameloblastoma
      other odontogenic lesions

*Adapted from reference 204.

have been reported (185,190,191,196,198,201, 204). This resulted in additional modifications in terminology: calcifying ghost cell odontogenic tumor by Fejerskov and Krogh in 1972 (192), and cystic calcifying odontogenic tumor by Freedman et al. in 1975 (193). In 1981 Praetorius (201) classified these lesions as being either cystic (type 1) or solid (type 2). This and subsequent classification schemes by Buchner (187), Hong et al. (198), and Toida (204) address the diversity of histologic subtypes, including cystic, solid, and malignant variants (Table 3-1). In 1992 the WHO (199) classified calcifying odontogenic cyst as an odontogenic tumor. The solid neoplastic variants are discussed in the benign and malignant odontogenic tumor section of this Fascicle.

Clinical and Radiologic Features. These lesions are seen in both the maxilla and mandible in approximately equal distribution (187). Maxillary lesions occur more commonly in the anterior region and are rare in the posterior maxilla. Mandibular lesions likewise favor an anterior location but premolar and molar regions of the mandible are not uncommon sites (185,187,193,194,195 204). There is no gender predilection. A wide age range is noted, with the peak incidence in the second and third decades. This cyst has been reported in all races. The lesion may present as an asymptomatic radiolucency of the affected jaw, with or without expansion (fig. 3-45A,B).

The radiographic features of the calcifying odontogenic cyst are those of a unilocular or multilocular radiolucency, without (fig. 3-45C) or with (fig. 3-46) radiopacities (185). Those with an odontoma component have radiopaque foci (197). The lesions are often associated with an unerupted tooth (205), but may be located in a periapical or lateral periodontal relationship to adjacent teeth (187).

Pathologic Findings. The epithelial lining of the cyst is of variable thickness and composed of flattened or columnar basal cells that resemble ameloblasts (fig. 3-47A). The suprabasal epithelial cells exhibit features of stellate reticulum or "ghost cell" formation (fig. 3-47B). Ghost cells are characterized by sharply outlined eosinophilic cytoplasm with an absence of nuclei (fig. 3-47C). Calcification of the ghost cells is a frequent finding (fig. 3-47D). In addition, dentin-like material and enamel matrix may be present in juxtaposition to the epithelial components. Chen and

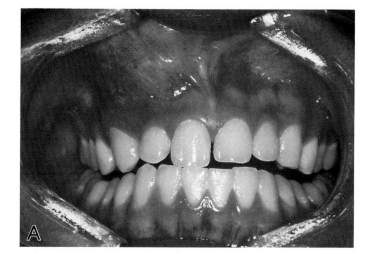

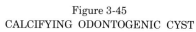

Figure 3-45
CALCIFYING ODONTOGENIC CYST
A: Calcifying odontogenic cyst expands the right anterior maxilla and involves the maxillary vestibule.
B: Occlusal view of calcifying odontogenic cyst depicted in A showing palatal expansion.
C: Radiolucency of the anterior maxilla with root divergence of the lateral incisor and canine teeth. (Courtesy of Dr. G. Wysocki, London, Ontario, Canada.)

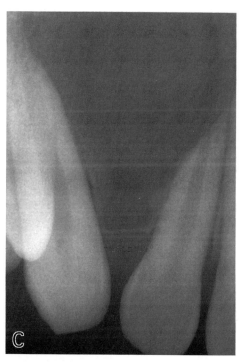

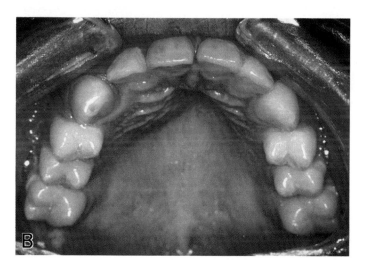

Figure 3-46
CALCIFYING
ODONTOGENIC CYST
Calcifying odontogenic cyst involving the anterior mandible. Note the calcification within the radiolucency. (Courtesy of Dr. Y. Tajima, Saitama, Japan.)

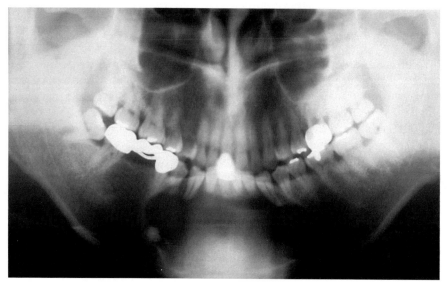

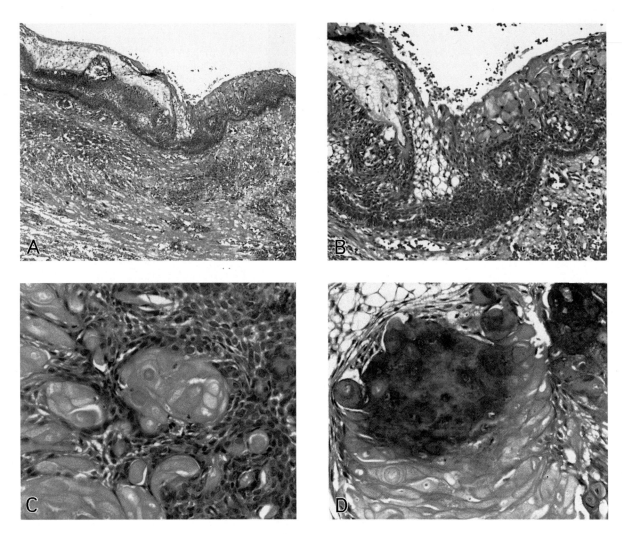

Figure 3-47
CALCIFYING ODONTOGENIC CYST
Low-power photomicrograph of calcifying odontogenic cyst exhibiting proliferative epithelium resembling ameloblastoma (A); higher power demonstrates evidence of ghost cells (B). Ghost cell clusters are associated with basaloid odontogenic epithelium (C) and mineralization (D).

Miller (189) identified four ultrastructural cell types: a basal cell and stellate reticulum type cell, both of which contained tonofilament bundles; the ghost cell, with coarse bundles of tonofilaments; and the hornified cell with densely packed tonofilaments. Calcification of the ghost cell and hornified cell with concomitant calcification of adjacent collagen was also identified. The ghost cells express little or no immunoreactivity to cytokeratins, a feature that prompted Hong et al. (198) to suggest that ghost cells result from coagulative necrosis of odontogenic epithelium. Subsequently, Lukinmaa et al. (200) reported immunohistochemical staining with monoclonal antibody to high and low molecular weight cytokeratins, and immunoreactive patterns with the matrix glycoprotein tenascin C, suggesting that the calcifying odontogenic cyst represents the pathologic counterpart of normal odontogenesis.

This may explain the histologic diversity and reported association of calcifying odontogenic cyst with other odontogenic tumors, including odontogenic adenomatoid tumor (206), odontoameloblastoma, ameloblastic fibroma, ameloblastic fibro-odontoma (202), odontoma (197,201), and ameloblastoma (203). Also of note is the similarity of the solid (neoplastic) variant of the calcifying odontogenic cyst to craniopharyngioma (186).

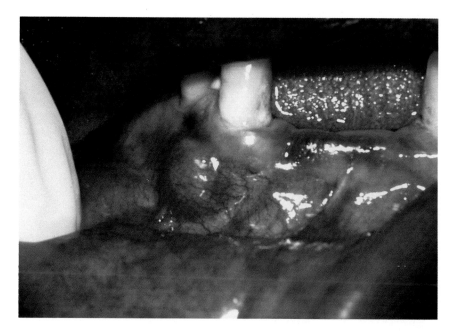

Figure 3-48
GINGIVAL CYST
A well-defined swelling of the mandibular gingiva is located between the mandibular cuspid and first premolar tooth.

Treatment and Prognosis. Surgical enucleation is the treatment of choice for the cystic variant of this entity unless it is associated with a more aggressive odontogenic tumor such as an ameloblastoma, in which case a more aggressive approach is warranted. Recurrence after surgical intervention, although rare, has been reported (205).

Gingival Cyst of Adults

Definition. The gingival cyst arises from epithelial remnants and lies within the connective tissues of gingival mucosa.

Clinical and Radiologic Features. These cysts are well circumscribed and typically occur on the attached gingiva. They are most frequently located in the mandibular buccal gingiva (fig. 3-48), in the area of canine and premolar teeth (217). Some may involve alveolar mucosa. Gingival cysts rarely exceed 1 cm in diameter, and most are smaller. Multiple (221) and bilateral (211,218) gingival cysts have been documented. The larger, longstanding cysts may cause pressure resorption of underlying cortical bone, with slight shadowing noted radiographically. Some may have the normal color of the overlying gingiva, and others may have a bluish hue. These lesions are uncommon and most are identified in adults during the fifth and sixth decades. No significant sex predilection has been established; however, seven of eight patients reported by Bell et al. (207) were female.

Pathologic Findings. Histologically, these are unicystic and lined by thin epithelium of one to three cell layers. Some resemble reduced enamel epithelium (217). They are located immediately below the surface epithelium (fig. 3-49). The layer of flattened epithelium may be overlooked in a fragmented specimen (fig. 3-50A); in addition, separation of the epithelium from the surrounding connective tissue wall is common (fig. 3-50B). Multiple sections may be required to identify the cyst lining in small, collapsed, or fragmented specimens. Focal epithelial plaques or thickenings with a whorled pattern are a frequent finding (fig. 3-50C). The cytoplasm of some epithelial cells has a clear cell morphology. Some gingival cysts are histologically similar to lateral periodontal cysts, and there is a report of a lateral periodontal cyst and a gingival cyst occurring in the same patient (220). The surrounding fibrous connective tissue does not generally exhibit inflammation. Cysts in close proximity to the gingival crevicular epithelium may exhibit a localized inflammatory cell infiltrate (209). Polycystic lesions (213,217) are rare, but if encountered, have been designated *gingival botryoid odontogenic cyst* (213). Cysts that are histologically similar to the odontogenic keratocyst (210) should be designated as such and not as a gingival cyst. Moskow and Baden

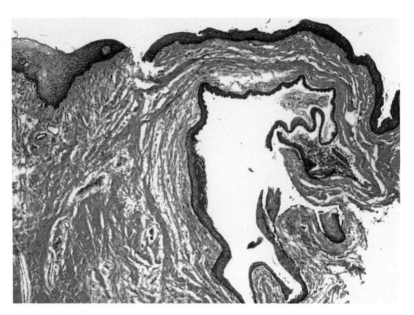

Figure 3-49
GINGIVAL CYST
Photomicrograph shows the relationship of gingival cyst to surface epithelium.

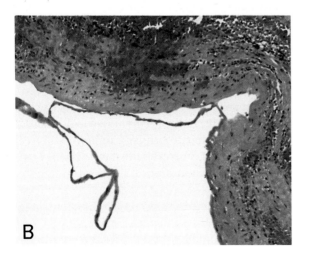

Figure 3-50
GINGIVAL CYST
A: Thin epithelial lining of a gingival cyst.
B: Thin epithelial lining detached from the underlying connective tissue.
C: Focal thickenings of the epithelial lining of a gingival cyst.

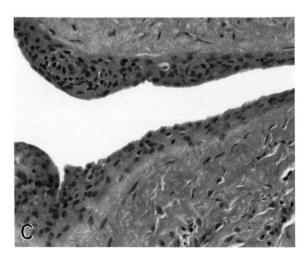

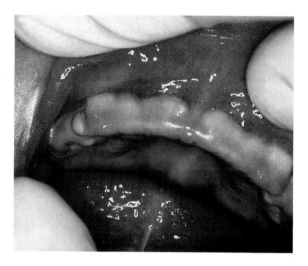
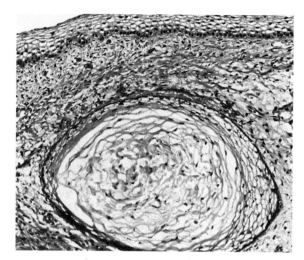

Figure 3-51
GINGIVAL CYST OF INFANCY
Left: Newborn with small white nodule in the crest of the maxillary alveolar ridge; this regressed at 1 month. (Courtesy of Dr. Paul Crespi, New Hyde Park, NY.)
Right: Keratin-filled cyst below the gingival mucosa.

(214) described a gingival salivary gland choristoma in association with a gingival cyst, and Young et al. (223) documented a gingival cyst lined by respiratory epithelium. Rare lesions may be histologically similar to the keratin-filled gingival cyst of infants (212).

This cyst most probably originates from odontogenic rests of the dental lamina (215,216,222). Traumatic implantation of surface epithelium or cystification of elongated projections of surface epithelium are alternative etiologies. Shear (219) states that the close proximity of some gingival cysts to junctional epithelium supports an origin from this reduced enamel epithelial-derived tissue. A gingival "surgical cyst" developing secondarily to a subepithelial connective tissue graft has been documented (208).

Treatment and Prognosis. Simple excision with minimal margins is recommended. Recurrence is not expected.

Gingival Cyst of Infants

Definition. The gingival cyst of infancy is a superficial microcyst that arises from embryonic rests located in alveolar mucosa.

Clinical Features. This developmental odontogenic cyst of newborn infants occurs on the alveolar ridge of the maxilla (fig. 3-51) or less

commonly, the mandible and originates from dental lamina rests (224,225,229). Similar type cysts occur along the midline of the palate and are also known as *Epstein pearls* (227). Moreillon and Schroeder (228) demonstrated microcysts associated with the dental lamina in a detailed study of human fetuses. Gingival cysts may be single or multiple, 1 to 3 mm, white to yellow nodules. They usually undergo involution or spontaneous rupture, are rarely identified after 3 months of age, and are rarely viewed microscopically. The exact incidence is unknown. Clinically, they can simulate natal or neonatal teeth. Conversely, such teeth may be misconstrued as gingival cysts. Lymphangiomas have been reported on the alveolar ridges of neonates and should not be clinically confused with the gingival cyst of infants (226). Like gingival cysts, these lymphangiomas can regress spontaneously.

Pathologic Findings. These cysts are located immediately below the epithelium of the mucosa and are lined by a thin layer of stratified squamous epithelium with flattened basal cells and a parakeratinized surface (fig. 3-51, right). Keratin fills the lumen and this is responsible for the white to yellow appearance.

Treatment and Prognosis. There is no reason to treat these cysts as involution or rupture occurs shortly after their discovery.

REFERENCES

Radicular Cyst

1. Daley TD, Wysocki GP, Pringle GA. Relative incidence of odontogenic tumors and oral and jaw cysts in a Canadian population. Oral Surg Oral Med Oral Pathol 1994;77:276–80.
2. Gao Z, Flaitz CM, Mackenzie IC. Expression of keratinocyte growth factor in periapical lesions. J Dent Res 1996;75:1658–63.
3. Kreidler JF, Raubenheimer EJ, van Heerden WF. A retrospective analysis of 367 cystic lesions of the jaws—the Ulm experience. J Cranio Maxillofac Surg 1993;21:339–41.
4. Matthews JB. Hyaline bodies in the wall of odontogenic cysts. In: Browne RM. Investigative pathology of the odontogenic cysts. Boca Raton: CRC Press, 1991:191–209.
5. Morgan PR, Johnson NW. Histological, histochemical and ultrastructural studies on the nature of hyaline bodies in odontogenic cysts. J Oral Pathol 1974;3:127–47.
6. Rushton MA. Hyaline bodies in the epithelium of dental cysts. Proc Royal Soc Med 1955;48:407–9.
7. Shear M. Cysts of the oral regions. 3rd ed. Oxford: Wright, 1992;136–62.
8. Wright JM. Squamous odontogenic tumorlike proliferations in odontogenic cysts. Oral Surg Oral Med Oral Pathol 1979;47:354–8.

Residual Cyst

9. Chen SY, Fantasia JE, Miller AS. Hyaline bodies in the connective tissue wall of odontogenic cysts. J Oral Pathol 1981;10:147–57.
10. Matthews JB. Hyaline bodies in the wall of odontogenic cysts, In: Browne RM. Investigative pathology of the odontogenic cysts. Boca Raton: CRC Press, 1991:191–209.
11. Talacko AA, Radden BG. Oral pulse granuloma: clinical and histologic features. Int J Maxillofac Surg 1988;17:343–6.
12. van der Waal I, Rauhamaa R, van der Kwast WA, Snow GB. Squamous cell carcinoma arising in the lining of odontogenic cysts. Report of five cases. Int J Oral Surg 1985;14:146–52.

Paradental Cyst

13. Ackermann G, Cohen MA, Altini M. The paradental cyst: a clinicopathologic study of 50 cases. Oral Surg Oral Med Oral Pathol 1987;64:308–12.
14. Craig GT. The paradental cyst. A specific inflammatory odontogenic cyst. Br Dent J 1976;141:9–14.
15. el Magboul K, Duggal MS, Pedlar J. Mandibular infected buccal cyst or a paradental cyst?: report of a case. Br Dent J 1993;175:330–2.
16. Fowler CB, Brannon RB. The paradental cyst: a clinicopathologic study of six new cases and review of the literature. J Oral Maxillofac Surg 1989;47:243–8.
17. Magnusson B, Borrman H. The paradental cyst: a clinicopathologic study of 26 cases. Swed Dent J 1995;19:1–7.
18. Main DM. Epithelial jaw cysts: 10 years of the WHO classification. J Oral Pathol 1985;14:1–7.
19. Main DM. Epithelial jaw cysts: a clinicopathologic reappraisal. Br J Oral Surg 1970;8:114–25.
20. Martinez-Conde R, Aquirre JM, Pindborg JJ. Paradental cyst of the second molar: report of a bilateral case. J Oral Maxillofac Surg 1995;53:1212–4.
21. Packota GV, Hall JM, Lanigan DT, Cohen MA. Paradental cysts on mandibular first molars in children: report of five cases. Dentomaxillofac Radiol 1990;19:126–32.
22. Stoneman DW, Worth HM. The mandibular infected buccal cyst—molar area. Dent Radiog Photog 1983;56:1–14.
23. Thompson IO, de Waal J, Nortje CJ. Mandibular infected buccal cyst and paradental cyst: the same or separate entities? J Dent Assoc S Afr 1997;52:503–6.
24. Thurnwald GA, Acton CH, Savage NW. The mandibular infected buccal cyst, a reappraisal. Ann R Australas Coll Dent Surg 1994;12:255–63.
25. Vedtofte P, Praetorius F. The inflammatory paradental cyst. Oral Surg Oral Med Oral Pathol 1989;68:182–8.
26. Wolf J. Hietanen J. The mandibular infected buccal cyst (paradental cyst). A radiographic and histologic study. Br J Oral Maxillofac Surg 1990;28:322–5.

Dentigerous Cyst

27. Daley TD, Wysocki GP. The small dentigerous cyst. Oral Surg Oral Med Oral Pathol Oral Radiol Endod 1995;79:77–81.
28. Daley TD, Wysocki GP, Pringle GA. Relative incidence of odontogenic tumors: oral and jaw cysts in a Canadian population. Oral Surg Oral Med Oral Pathol 1994;77:276–80.
29. Holmlund A, Anneroth G, Lundquist G, Nordenram A. Ameloblastoma originating from odontogenic cysts. J Oral Pathol Med 1991;20:318–21.
30. Kim J, Ellis GL. Dental follicular tissue: misinterpretation as odontogenic tumors. J Oral Maxillofac Surg 1993;51:762–7.
31. Kreidler JF, Raubenheimer EJ, van Heerden WF. A retrospective analysis of 367 cystic lesions of the jaw—the Ulm experience. J Cranio Maxillofac Surg 1993;21:339–41.
32. Regezi JA, Sciubba JJ. Oral pathology: clinical pathologic correlations, 3rd ed. Philadelphia: Saunders, 1999;291–6.
33. Shear M. Cysts of the oral regions, 3rd ed. Oxford: Wright, 1992:75–98.

34. Stanley HR, Alattar M, Collet WK, Stringfellow HR Jr, Spiegel EH. Pathological sequelae of "neglected" impacted third molars. J Oral Path Med 1988;17:113–7.
35. Waldron CA, Koh ML. Central mucoepidermoid carcinoma of the jaws: report of four cases with analysis of the literature and discussion of the relationship to mucoepidermoid, sialodontogenic, and glandular odontogenic cysts. J Oral Maxillofac Surg 1990;48:871–7.

Eruption Cyst

36. Shear M. Cysts of the oral regions, 3rd ed. Oxford: Wright, 1992:99–101.

Lateral Periodontal Cyst

37. Altini M, Shear M. The lateral periodontal cyst: an update. J Oral Pathol Med 1992;21:245–50.
38. Angelopoulou E, Angelopoulos AP. Lateral periodontal cyst. Review of the literature and report of a case. J Periodontol 1990;61:126–31.
39. Baker RD, D'Onofriio ED, Corio RL, Crawford BE, Terry BC. Squamous cell carcinoma arising in a lateral periodontal cyst. Oral Surg Oral Med Oral Pathol 1979;47:495–9.
40. Buchner A, David R, Carpenter W, Leider A. Pigmented lateral periodontal cyst and other pigmented odontogenic lesions. Oral Dis 1996;2:299–302.
41. Carter LC, Carney Yl, Perez-Pudlewski D. Lateral periodontal cyst. Multifactorial analysis of a previously unreported series. Oral Surg Oral Med Oral Pathol Oral Radiol Endod 1996;81:210–6.
42. Cohen DA, Neville BW, Damm DD, White DK. The lateral periodontal cyst. A report of 37 cases. J Periodontal 1984;55:230–4.
43. Fantasia JE. Lateral periodontal cyst. An analysis of forty-six cases. Oral Surg Oral Med Oral Pathol 1979;48:237–43.
44. Huang YL, Lin LM, Lin CC, Yan YH. Calcifying odontogenic cyst presenting as a lateral periodontal cyst, a case report. Chung hua Ya I Hseuh Hui Tsa Chih 1990;9:42–5.
45. Kreidler JF, Raubenheimer EJ, van Heerden WF. A retrospective analysis of 367 cystic lesions of the jaw—the Ulm experience. J Craniomaxillofac Surg 1993;21:339–41.
46. Lehrhaupt NB, Browstein CN, Deasy MJ. Osseous repair of a lateral periodontal cyst. J Periodontol 1997;68:608–11.
47. Rasmusson LG, Magnusson BC, Borrman H. The lateral, periodontal cyst. A histopathologic and radiographic study of 32 cases. Br J Oral Maxillofac Surg 1991;21:54–7.
48. Shear M, Pindborg JJ. Microscopic features of the lateral periodontal cyst. Scand J Dent Res 1975;83:103–10.
49. Suljak JP, Bohay RN, Wysocki GP. Lateral periodontal cyst: a case report and review of the literature. J Can Dent Assoc 1998;64:48–51.
50. Tolson GE, Czuszak Ca, Billman MA, Lewis DM. Report of lateral periodontal cyst and gingival cyst occurring in the same patient. J Periodontol 1996;67:541–4.
51. Weathers DR, Waldron CA. Unusual multilocular cysts of the jaws (botryoid odontogenic cysts). Oral Surg Oral Med Oral Pathol 1973;36:235–41.
52. Wysocki GP, Brannon RB, Gardner DG, Sapp P. Histogenesis of the lateral periodontal cyst and the gingival cyst of the adult. Oral Surg Oral Med Oral Pathol 1980;50:327–34.

Botryoid Odontogenic Cyst

53. Barone R, Ficarra G, Cudia G. Odontogenic botryoid cyst. Minerva Stomatol 1990;39:69–72.
54. Cohen DA, Neville BW, Damm DD, White DK. The lateral periodontal cyst. A report of 37 cases. J Periodontol 1984;55:230–4.
55. de Sousa SO, Campos AC, Santiago JL, Jaeger RG, de Araujo VC. Botryoid odontogenic cyst: report of a case with clinical and histogenetic considerations. Brit J Oral Maxillofac Surg 1990;28:275–6.
56. Greer RO Jr, Johnson M. Botryoid odontogenic cyst: clinicopathologic analysis of ten cases with three recurrences. J Oral Maxillofac Surg 1988;46:574–9.
57. Gurol M, Burkes EJ, Jacoway J. Botryoid odontogenic cyst: analysis of 33 cases. J Periodontol 1995;66:1069–73.
58. Heikinheimo K, Happonen RP, Forssell K, Kussilehto A, Virtanen I. A botryoid odontogenic cyst with multiple recurrences. Int J Oral Maxillofac Surg 1989;18:10–3.
59. High AS, Main DM, Khoo SP, Pedlar J, Hume WJ. The polymorphous odontogenic cyst. J Oral Pathol Med 1996;25:25–31.
60. Kaugars GE. Botryoid odontogenic cyst. Oral Surg Oral Med Oral Pathol 1986;62:555–9.
61. Lindh C, Larsson A. Unusual jaw-bone cysts. J Oral Maxillofac Surg 1990;48:258–63.
62. Lynch DP, Madden CR. The botryoid odontogenic cyst. Report of a case and review of the literature. J Periodontol 1985;56:163–7.
63. Manojlovic S, Grgurevic J, Knezevic G, Kruslin B. Glandular odontogenic cyst: a case report and clinicopathologic analysis of the relationship to central mucoepidermoid carcinoma. Head Neck 1997;19:227–31.
64. Nxumalo TN, Shear M. Gingival cyst in adults. J Oral Pathol Med 1992;21:309–13.
65. Padayachee A, Van Wyk CW. Two cystic lesions with features of both botryoid odontogenic cyst and the central mucoepidermoid tumour: sialo-odontogenic cyst? J Oral Pathol 1987;16:499–504.
66. Phelan JA, Kritchman D, Fusco-Ramer M, Freedman PD, Lumerman H. Recurrent botryoid odontogenic cyst (lateral periodontal cyst). Oral Surg Oral Med Oral Pathol 1988;66:345–8.
67. Redman RS, Whitestone BW, Winne CE, Hudec MW, Patterson RH. Botryoid odontogenic cyst. Report of case with evidence of multicentric origin. Int J Oral Maxillofac Surg 1990;19:144–6.

68. Sadeghi EM, Weldon LL, Kwon PH, Sampson E. Mucoepidermoid odontogenic cyst. Int J Oral Maxillofac Surg 1991;20:142–3.
69. Standish SM, Shafer WG. The lateral periodontal cyst. J Periodontal 1958;29:27–33.
70. van der Waal I. Lateral periodontal cystlike lesion; a discussion on the so-called botryoid odontogenic cyst. J Dent Assoc S Afr 1992;47:231–3.

71. Weathers DR, Waldron CA. Unusual multilocular cysts of the jaws (botryoid odontogenic cysts). Oral Surg Oral Med Oral Pathol 1973;36:235–41.
72. Wysocki GP, Brannon RB, Gardner DG, Sapp P. Histogenesis of the lateral periodontal cyst of the adult. Oral Surg Oral Med Oral Pathol 1980;50:327–34.

Glandular Odontogenic Cyst

73. Baliga M, Aby J, Vidya M. Glandular odontogenic cyst. A case report. Indian J Dent Res 1997;8:82–4.
74. de Carvalho YR, Kimaid A, Cabral LA, Nogueira T. The glandular odontogenic cyst: a case report. Quintessence Int 1994;25:351–4.
75. de Sousa SO, Cabezas NT, de Oliveira PT, de Araujo VC. Glandular odontogenic cyst: report of a case with cytokeratin expression. Oral Surg Oral Med Oral Pathol Oral Radiol Endod 1997;83:478–83.
76. Economopoulou P, Patrikiou A. Glandular odontogenic cyst of the maxilla: report of a case. J Oral Maxillofac Surg 1995;53:834–7.
77. Fantasia JE. Lateral periodontal cyst, botryoid odontogenic cyst, and glandular odontogenic cyst. In: Assael LA, ed. Benign lesions of the jaws. Oral Maxillofac Surg Clin N Am 1991;3:127–36.
78. Ficarra G, Chou L, Panzoni E. Glandular odontogenic cyst (sialo-odontogenic cyst): a case report. Int J Oral Maxillofac Surg 1990;19:331–3.
79. Gardner DG. Unusual odontogenic cyst (mucus-producing odontogenic cyst). Presented at the International Association of Oral Pathology. Noordwijkerhout, The Netherlands, 1984.
80. Gardner DG, Kessler HP, Morency R, Schaffner DL. The glandular odontogenic cyst: an apparent entity. J Oral Pathol 1988;17:359–66.
81. Gardner DG, Morency R. The glandular odontogenic cyst: a rare lesion that tends to recur. J Can Dent Assoc 1993;59:929–30.
82. Gunzl HJ, Horn H, Vesper M. Hellner D. Diagnosis and differential diagnosis of sialo-odontogenic (glandular odontogenic) cyst. Pathologe 1993;14:346–50.
83. High AS, Main DM, Khoo SP, Pedlar J, Hume WJ. The polymorphous odontogenic cyst. J Oral Pathol Med 1996;25:25–31.
84. Hussain K, Edmonson HD, Browne RM. Glandular odontogenic cysts: diagnosis and treatment. Oral Surg Oral Med Oral Pathol Oral Radiol Endod 1995;79:593–602.
85. Ide F, Shimoyama T, Horie N. Glandular odontogenic cyst with hyaline bodies: an unusual dentigerous presentation. J Oral Pathol Med 1996;25:401–4.
86. Lindh C, Larsson A. Unusual jawbone cysts. J Oral Maxillofac Surg 1990;48:258–63.
87. Magnusson B, Goransson L, Odesjo B, Grondahl K, Hirsch JM. Glandular odontogenic cyst. Report of seven cases. Dentomaxillofac Radiol 1997;26:26–31.

88. Manojlovic S, Grgurevic J, Knezevic G, Kruslin B. Glandular odontogenic cyst: a case report and clinicopathologic analysis of the relationship to central mucoepidermoid carcinoma. Head Neck 1997;19:227–31.
89. Padayachee A, Van Wyk CW. Two cystic lesions with features of both the botryoid cyst and the central mucoepidermoid tumor: sialo-odontogenic cyst. J Oral Pathol 1987;16:499–504.
90. Patron M, Colmenero C, Larrauri J. Glandular odontogenic cyst: clinicopathologic features and analysis of three cases. Oral Surg Oral Med Oral Pathol 1991;72:71–4.
91. Ramer M, Montazem A, Lane SL, Lumerman H. Glandular odontogenic cyst. Report of a case and review of the literature. Oral Surg Oral Med Oral Pathol Oral Radiol Endod 1997;84:54–7.
92. Sadeghi EM, Weldon LL, Kwon PH, Sampson E. Mucoepidermoid odontogenic cyst. Int J Oral Maxillofac Surg 1991;20:142–3.
93. Savage NW, Joseph BK, Monsour PA, Young WG. The glandular odontogenic jaw cyst: report of a case. Pathology 1996;28:370–2.
94. Semba I, Kitano M, Mimura T, Sonoda S, Miyawaki A. Glandular odontogenic cyst: analysis of cytokeratin expression and clinicopathologic features. J Oral Pathol Med 1994;23:377–82.
95. Takeda Y. Glandular odontogenic cyst mimicking a lateral periodontal cyst: a case report. Int J Oral Maxillofac Surg 1994;23:96–7.
96. Toida H, Nakashima E, Okumura Y, Tatematsu N. Glandular odontogenic cyst: a case report and review of the literature. J Oral Maxillofac Surg 1994;52:1312–6.
97. Van Heerden WF, Raubenheimer EJ, Turner ML. Glandular odontogenic cyst. Head Neck 1992;14:316–20.
98. Vesper M, Gunzl J, Hellner D, Schmelzle R. Die sialoodontogene (glandular odontogene) Zyste. Dtsch Z Mund Kiefer Gesichtschir 1994;18:254.
99. Waldron CA, Koh ML. Central mucoepidermoid carcinoma of the jaws: report of four cases with analysis of the literature and discussion of the relationship to mucoepidermoid, sialodontogenic and glandular odontogenic cysts. J Oral Maxillofac Surg 1990;48:871–7.
100. Wang SZ, Chen XM, Li Y. Clinicopathologic analysis of glandular odontogenic cyst. Chung Hua Kou Chiang Hsueh Tsa Chih 1994;29:329–31.

Primordial Cyst

101. Daley TD, Wysocki GP. New developments in selected cysts of the jaws. J Can Dent Assoc 1997;63:526–32.

102. Kramer IR, Pindborg JJ, Shear M. Histological typing of odontogenic tumors. World Health Organization, 2nd ed. Berlin: Springer-Verlag, 1992:35.

103. Philpsen HP. Om keratocystes (kolesteatomer). I Kaeberne, Tandlaegebladet 1956;60:963–80.

104. Robinson HB. Classification of cysts of the jaws. Am J Orthod Oral Surg 1945;31:370–5.

105. Robinson HB. Primordial cyst versus keratocyst. Oral Surg Oral Med Oral Pathol 1975;40:362–4.

106. Robinson HB, Koch WE, Kolas S. Radiographic interpretation of oral cysts. Dent Radiogr Photogr 1956; 29:61–68.

107. Waldron CA. Odontogenic cysts and tumors, In: Neville BW, Damm DD, Allen CA, Bouquot JE, eds. Oral & maxillofacial pathology. Philadelphia: WB Saunders, 1995:496–7.

Odontogenic Keratocyst

108. Aguirre A, Takai Y, Meenaghan M, Neiders M, Natiella JR. Lectin histochemistry of ameloblastoma and odontogenic keratocysts. J Oral Pathol Med 1989;18:68–73.

109. Ahlors E, Larsson A, Sjogren S. The odontogenic keratocyst: a benign cystic tumor? J Oral Maxillofac Surg 1984;42:10–9.

110. Anand VK, Arrowood JP Jr, Krolls SO. Malignant potential of the odontogenic keratocyst. Otolaryngol Head Neck Surg 1994;111:124–9.

111. Arwill T, Kahnberg KE. Odontogenic keratocyst associated with an intramandibular chondroma. J Oral Surg 1977;35:64–7.

112. Brannon RB. The odontogenic keratocyst. A clinicopathologic study of 312 cases. Part I. Clinical features. Oral Surg Oral Med Oral Pathol 1976;42:54–72.

113. Brannon RB. The odontogenic keratocyst. A clinicopathologic study of 312 cases. Part II. Histologic features. Oral Surg Oral Med Oral Pathol 1977;43:233–55.

114. Brondum N, Jensen VJ. Recurrence of keratocysts and decompression treatment. A long-term follow-up of forty-four cases. Oral Surg Oral Med Oral Pathol 1991;72:265–9.

115. Browne RM. The pathogenesis of odontogenic cysts: a review. J Oral Pathol 1975;4:31–46.

116. Chehade A, Daley TD, Wysocki GP, Miller AS. Peripheral odontogenic keratocyst. Oral Surg Oral Med Oral Pathol 1994;77:494–7.

117. Cox M, Eveson J, Scully C. Human papilloma virus type 16 DNA in an odontogenic keratocyst. J Oral Pathol Med 1991;20:143–5.

118. Crowley TE, Kaugars GE, Gunsolley JC. Odontogenic keratocysts: a clinical and histologic comparison of the parakeratin and orthokeratin variants. J Oral Maxillofac Surg 1992;50:22–6.

119. Daley TD, Wysocki GP, Pringle GA. Relative incidence of odontogenic tumors and jaw cysts in a Canadian population. Oral Surg Oral Med Oral Pathol 1994:77:276–80.

120. Dayan D, Buchner A, Gorsky M, Harel-Raviv M. The peripheral odontogenic keratocyst. Int J Oral Maxillofac Surg 1988;17:81–3.

121. DeGould MD, Goldberg JS. Recurrence of an odontogenic keratocyst in a bone graft. Report of a case. Int J Oral Maxillofac Surg 1991;20:9–11.

122. Ephros H, Lee HY. Treatment of a large odontogenic keratocyst using the Brosch procedure. J Oral Maxillofac Surg 1991;49:871–4.

123. Foley WL, Terry BC, Jacoway JR. Malignant transformation of an odontogenic keratocyst: report of a case. J Oral Maxillofac Surg 1991;49:768–71.

124. Hennis HL, Stewart WC, Neville B, O'Connor KF. Carcinoma arising in an odontogenic keratocyst with orbital invasion. Doc Ophthalmol 1991;77:73–9.

125. Katz JO, Underhill TE. Multilocular radiolucencies. Dent Clin North Am 1994;38:63–81.

126. Khalique N, Rippin JW. Odontogenic keratocyst in an infant. Br Dent J 1992;172:282–3.

127. Kondell PA, Wiberg J. Odontogenic keratocysts. A follow-up study of 29 cases. Swed Dent J 1988;12:57–62.

128. Kratochvil FJ, Brannon RB. Cartilage in the walls of odontogenic keratocyst. J Oral Pathol Med 1993;22:282–5.

129. Li TJ, Browne RM, Matthews JB. Expression of epidermal growth factor receptors by odontogenic jaw cysts. Virchows Arch [A] 1993;423:137–44.

130. Li TJ, Browne RM, Matthews JB. Immunocytochemical expression of growth factors by odontogenic jaw cysts. Mol Pathol 1997;50:21–7.

131. Li TJ, Browne RM, Prime SS, Paterson IC, Matthews JB. p53 expression in odontogenic keratocyst epithelium. J Oral Pathol Med 1996;25:245–55.

131a. Lo Muzio L, Staibiano S, Pannone G, et al. Expression of cell cycle and apoptosis related proteins in sporadic odontogenic keratocysts and odontogenic keratocysts associated with the nevoid basal cell carcinoma syndrome. J Dent Res 1999;78:1345–53.

132. MacDonald–Jankowski DS. The involvement of the maxillary antrum by odontogenic keratocyst. Clin Radiol 1992;45:31–3.

133. Macleod RI, Fanibunda KB, Soames JV. A pigmented odontogenic keratocyst. Br J Oral Maxillofac Surg 1985;23:216–9.

134. MacLeod RI, Soames JV. Squamous cell carcinoma arising in an odontogenic keratocyst. Br J Oral Maxillofac Surg 1988;26:52–7.

135. Matise JL, Beto LM, Fantasia JE, Fielding AF. Pathologic fracture of the mandible associated with simultaneous occurrence of an odontogenic keratocyst and traumatic bone cyst. J Oral Maxillofac Surg 1987;45:69–71.

136. Matthews JB, Mason GI, Browne RM. Epithelial cell markers and proliferating cells in odontogenic jaw cysts. J Pathol 1988;156:283–90.

137. Meara JG, Shah S, Li KK, Cunningham MJ. The odontogenic keratocyst: a 20-year clinicopathologic review. Laryngoscope 1998;108:280–3.

138. Meiselman F. Surgical management of the odontogenic keratocyst: conservative approach. J Oral Maxillofac Surg 1994;52:960–3.

139. Mosqueda-Taylor A, de la Piedra-Garza JM, Troncozo-Vazquez F. Odontogenic keratocyst with chondroid fibrous wall. A case report. Int J Oral Maxillofac Surg 1998;27:58–60.

140. Neville BW, Damm DD, Brock T. Odontogenic keratocysts of the midline maxillary region. J Oral Maxillofac Surg 1997;55:340–4.

141. Ogden GR, Chilsom DM, Kiddie RA, Lane DP. p53 protein in odontogenic cysts. Increased expression in some odontogenic keratocysts. J Clin Pathol 1992;45:1007–10.

142. Philipsen HP. Om keratocysts (Kolesteatomer) I Kaeberne, Tandlaegebladet 1956;60:963–80.

143. Piecuch JF, Eisenberg E, Segal D, Carlson R. Respiratory epithelium as an integral part of an odontogenic keratocyst: report of a case. J Oral Surg 1980;38:445–7.

144. Poulet FM, Valentine BA, Summers BA. A survey of epithelial odontogenic tumors and cysts in dogs and cats. Vet Pathol 1992;29:369–80.

145. Rippin JW, Woolgar JA. Odontogenic keratocyst in basal cell nevus syndrome and non-syndrome patients. In: Browne RM, ed. Investigative pathology of the odontogenic cysts. Boca Raton: CRC Press, 1991;211–32.

146. Robinson HB. Primordial cyst versus keratocyst. Oral Surg Oral Med Oral Pathol 1975;40:362–4.

147. Rodu B, Tate AL, Martinez MG Jr. The implications of inflammation in odontogenic keratocysts. J Oral Pathol 1987;16:518–21.

148. Saku T, Shibata Y, Koyama Z, Cheng J, Okabe H, Yeh Y. Lectin histochemistry of cystic jaw lesions: an aid for differential diagnosis between cystic ameloblastoma and odontogenic cysts. J Oral Pathol Med 1991;20:108–13.

149. Scharffetter K, Balz-Herrmann C, Lagrange W, Koberg W, Mittermayer C. Proliferation kinetics study of the growth of keratocysts. Morpho-functional explanation of recurrences. J Craniomaxillofac Surg 1989;17:226–33.

150. Schuler CF, Shriver BJ. Identification of intermediate filament keratin proteins in parakeratinized odontogenic keratocysts. A preliminary study. Oral Surg Oral Med Oral Pathol 1987;64:439–44.

151. Shrestha P, Yamada K, Higashiyama H, et al. Epidermal growth factor receptor in odontogenic cysts and tumors. J Oral Pathol Med 1992;21:314–7.

152. Siar CH, Ng KH. Combined ameloblastoma and odontogenic keratocyst or keratinizing ameloblastoma. Br J Oral Maxillofac Surg 1993;31:183–6.

153. Siar CH, Ng KH. Squamous cell carcinoma in an orthokeratinised odontogenic keratocyst. Int J Oral Maxillofac Surg 1987;16:95–8.

154. Slootweg PJ. p53 and Ki-67 reactivity in epithelial odontogenic lesions. An immunohistochemical study. J Oral Pathol Med 1995;24:393–7.

155. Smith G, Smith AJ, Basu MK. Mast cells in human odontogenic cysts. J Oral Pathol Med 1989;18:274–8.

156. Stoelinga PJ. Recurrent odontogenic keratocyst within the temporalis muscle [Letter]. Br J Oral Maxillofac Surg 1992;30:277–8.

157. Takeda Y, Kuroda M, Kuroda M, Suzuki A, Fujioka Y. Melanocytes in odontogenic keratocyst. Acta Pathol Jpn 1985;35:899–903.

158. Vedtofte P, Praetorius F. Recurrence of the odontogenic keratocyst in relation to clinical and histological features. A 20-year follow-up study of 72 patients. Int J Oral Surg 1979;8:412–20.

159. Williams TP, Connor FA Jr. Surgical management of the odontogenic keratocyst: aggressive approach. J Oral Maxillofac Surg 1994;52:964–6.

160. Wilson DF, Ross AS. Ultrastructure of odontogenic keratocysts. Oral Surg Oral Med Oral Pathol 1978;45:887–93.

161. Woo SB, Eisenbud L, Kleiman M, Assael N. Odontogenic keratocysts in the anterior maxilla: report of two cases, one simulating a nasopalatine cyst. Oral Surg Oral Med Oral Pathol 1987;64:463–5.

162. Worrall SF. Recurrent odontogenic keratocyst within the temporalis muscle. Br J Oral Maxillofac Surg 1992;30:59–62.

163. Wright JM. The odontogenic keratocyst: orthokeratinized variant. Oral Surg Oral Med Oral Pathol 1981;51:609–18.

164. Yoshiura K, Higuchi Y, Araki K, et al. Morphologic analysis of odontogenic cysts with computed tomography. Oral Surg Oral Med Oral Pathol Radiol Endod 1997;83:712–8.

Nevoid Basal Cell Carcinoma Syndrome

165. Bale SJ, Amos CI, Parry DM, Bale AE. The relationship between head circumference and height in normal adults and in the nevoid basal cell carcinoma syndrome and neurofibromatosis type 1. Am J Med Genet 1991;40:206–10.

165a. Cohen MM Jr. Nevoid basal cell carcinoma syndrome: molecular biology and new hypotheses. Int J Oral Maxillofac Surg 1999;28:216–23.

166. Evans DG, Fardon PA, Burnell LD, Gattamaneni HR, Birch JM. The incidence of Gorlin syndrome in 173 consecutive cases of medulloblastoma. Br J Cancer 1991;64:959–61.

167. Gorlin RJ. Nevoid basal cell carcinoma syndrome. Dermatol Clin 1995;13:113–25.

168. Gorlin RJ. Nevoid basal-cell carcinoma syndrome. Medicine 1987;66:98–113.

169. Gorlin RJ, Goltz RW. Multiple nevoid basal-cell epithelioma, jaw cysts and bifid rib: a syndrome. N Engl J Med 1962;262:908–12.

170. Howell B, Caro MR. The basal cell nevus: its relationship to multiple cutaneous cancers and associated anomalies of development. Arch Dermatol 1959:15:67–80.

171. Kimonis VE, Goldstein AM, Pastakia B, et al. Am J Med Genet 1997;69:299–308.

172. Knudson AG. Mutation and cancer: statistical study of retinoblastoma. Proc Natl Acad Sci USA 1971;68:820–3.

173. Levanat S, Gorlin RJ, Fallet S, Johnson DR, Fantasia JE, Bale AE. A two-hit model for developmental defects in Gorlin syndrome. Nature Genet 1996;12:85–7.

174. Wicking C, Bale AE. Molecular basis of the nevoid basal cell carcinoma syndrome. Curr Opin Pediatr 1997;9:630–5.

Orthokeratinized Odontogenic Cyst

175. Anand VK, Arrowood JP Jr, Krolls SO. Odontogenic keratocysts: a study of 50 patients. Laryngoscope 1995;105:14–6.

176. Brannon RB. The odontogenic keratocyst: a clinicopathological study of 312 cases. Part 1: Clinical features. Oral Surg Oral Med Oral Pathol 1976;42:54–72.

177. Brannon RB. The odontogenic keratocyst: a clinicopathological study of 312 cases. Part 2: Histologic features. Oral Surg Oral Med Oral Pathol 1977;43:233–55.

178. Cohen MA, Shear M. Comparison of parakeratinized and orthokeratinized primordial cysts (keratocysts). J Dent Assoc S Afr 1980;35:161–8.

179. Crowley TE, Kaugars GE, Gunsolley JC. Odontogenic keratocysts: a clinical and histologic comparison of the parakeratin and orthokeratin variants. J Oral Maxillofac Surg 1992;50:22–6.
180. Matthews JB, Browne RM. Diagnostic importance of cytokeratin expression in linings of odontogenic cysts. J Clin Pathol 1990;43:84–5.
181. Payne TF. An analysis of the clinical and histologic parameters of the odontogenic keratocyst. Oral Surg Oral Med Oral Pathol 1972;33:538–46.
182. Siar CH, Ng KH. Orthokeratinized odontogenic keratocysts in Malaysians. Br J Oral Maxillofac Surg 1988;26:215–20.
183. Vuhahula E, Nikai H, Ijuhin N, et al. Jaw cysts with orthokeratinization: analysis of 12 cases. J Oral Pathol Med 1993;22:35–40.
184. Wright JM. The odontogenic keratocyst: orthokeratinized variant. Oral Surg Oral Med Oral Pathol 1981;51:609–18.

Calcifying Odontogenic Cyst

185. Altini M, Farman AG. The calcifying odontogenic cyst. Eight new cases and a review of the literature. Oral Surg Oral Med Oral Pathol 1975;40:751–9.
186. Badger KV, Gardner DG. The relationship of adamantinomatous craniopharyngioma to ghost cell ameloblastoma of the jaws: a histopathologic and immunohistochemical study. J Oral Pathol Med 1997;26:349–55.
187. Buchner A. The central (intraosseous) calcifying odontogenic cyst: an analysis of 215 cases. J Oral Maxillofac Surg 1991;49:330–9
188. Buchner A, Merrell PW, Hansen LS, Leider AS. Peripheral (extraosseous) calcifying odontogenic cyst. Oral Surg Oral Med Oral Pathol 1991;72:265–70.
189. Chen SY, Miller AS. Ultrastructure of the keratinizing and calcifying odontogenic cyst. Oral Surg Oral Med Oral Pathol 1975;39:769–80.
190. Colmenero C, Patron I, Colmenero B. Odontogenic ghost cell tumors. The neoplastic form of calcifying odontogenic cyst. J Craniomaxillofac Surg 1990;18:215–8.
191. Ellis GL, Shmookler BH. Aggressive (malignant?) epithelial odontogenic ghost cell tumor. Oral Surg Oral Med Oral Pathol 1986;61:471–8.
192. Fejerskov O, Krogh J. The calcifying ghost cell odontogenic tumor—or the calcifying odontogenic cyst. J Oral Pathol 1972;1:273–87.
193. Freedman PD, Lummerman H, Gee JK. Calcifying odontogenic cyst: a review and analysis of seventy cases. Oral Surg Oral Med Oral Pathol 1975;40:93–105.
194. Gold L. The keratinizing and calcifying odontogenic cyst. Oral Surg Oral Med Oral Pathol 1963;16:1414–24.
195. Gorlin RJ, Pindborg JJ, Clausen FP, Vickers RA. The calcifying odontogenic cyst—a possible analogue of the cutaneous calcifying epithelioma of Malherbe. An analysis of fifteen cases. Oral Surg Oral Med Oral Pathol 1962;15:1235–43.
196. Grodjsek JE, Dolinsky HB, Schneider LC, Dolinsky EH, Doyle JL. Odontogenic ghost cell carcinoma. Oral Surg Oral Med Oral Pathol 1987;63:576–81.
197. Hirschberg A, Kaplan I, Buchner A. Calcifying odontogenic cyst associated with odontoma: a possible separate entity (odontocalcifying odontogenic cyst). J Oral Maxillofac Surg 1994;52:555–8.
198. Hong SP, Ellis GL, Hartman KS. Calcifying odontogenic cyst. A review of ninety-two cases with reevaluation of their nature as cysts or neoplasms, the nature of ghost cells, and subclassification. Oral Surg Oral Med Oral Pathol 1991;72:56–64.
199. Kramer IR, Pindborg JJ, Shear M. Histological typing of odontogenic tumours, 2nd ed. WHO International Histologic Classification of Tumours. Berlin: Springer-Verlag, 1992:20–1.
200. Lukinmaa PL, Leppaniemi A, Hietanen J, Allemanni G, Zardi L. Features of odontogenesis and expression of cytokeratins and tenascin-C in three cases of extraosseous and intraosseous calcifying odontogenic cyst. J Oral Pathol Med 1997;26:265–72.
201. Praetorius F, Hjorting Hansen E, Gorlin RJ, Vickers RA. Calcifying odontogenic cyst. Range, variations and neoplastic potential. Acta Odontol Scand 1981;39:227–40.
202. Shear M. Developmental odontogenic cysts. An update. J Oral Pathol Med 1994;23:1–11.
203. Tajima Y, Sakamoto E, Yamamoto T. Ameloblastoma arising in calcifying odontogenic cyst. Oral Surg Oral Med Oral Pathol 1992;74:776–9.
204. Toida M. So-called calcifying odontogenic cyst: review and discussion on the terminology and classification. J Oral Pathol Med 1998;27:49–52.
205. Wright BA, Bhardwaj AK, Murphy D. Recurrent calcifying odontogenic cyst. Oral Surg Oral Med Oral Pathol 1984;58:579–83.
206. Zeitoun IM, Dhanrajani PJ, Mosadomi HA. Adenomatoid odontogenic tumor arising in a calcifying odontogenic cyst. J Oral Maxillofac Surg 1996;54:634–7.

Gingival Cyst of Adults

207. Bell RC, Chauvin PJ, Tyler MT. Gingival cyst of the adult: a review and a report of eight cases. J Can Dent Assoc 1997;63:533–5.
208. Breault LG, Billman MA, Lewis DM. Report of the gingival "surgical cyst" developing secondarily to a subepithelial connective tissue graft. J Periodontol 1997;68:392–5.
209. Buchner A, Hansen LS. The histomorphologic spectrum of the gingival cyst of the adult. Oral Surg Oral Med Oral Pathol 1979;48:532–9.
210. Chehade A, Daley TD, Wysocki GP, Miller AS. Peripheral odontogenic keratocyst. Oral Surg Oral Med Oral Pathol 1994;77:494–7.

211. Dent CD, Rubis EJ, MacFarland PJ. Bilateral gingival swellings in the mandibular canine-premolar areas. J Am Dent Assoc 1990;120:71–2.

212. Garlick JA, Calderon S, Metzker A, Rotem A, Abramovici A. Simultaneous occurrence of a congenital lateral upper lip sinus and gingival cyst: a case report and discussion of pathogenesis. Oral Surg Oral Med Oral Pathol 1989;68:317–23.

213. Lynch DP, Madden CR. The botryoid odontogenic cyst. Report of a case and review of the literature. J Periodontol 1985;56:163–7.

214. Moskow BS, Baden E. Gingival salivary gland choristoma. Report of a case. J Clin Periodontol 1986; 13:720–4.

215. Moskow BS, Bloom A. Embryogenesis of the gingival cyst. J Clin Periodontol 1983;10:119–30.

216. Moskow BS, Weinstein MM. Further observations on the gingival cyst. Three case reports. J Periodontol 1975;46:178–82.

217. Nxumalo TN, Shear M. Gingival cysts in adults. J Oral Pathol Med 1992;21:309–13.

218. Shade NL, Carpenter WM, Delzer DD. Gingival cyst of the adult. Case report of a bilateral presentation. J Periodontol 1987;58:796–9.

219. Shear M. Developmental odontogenic cysts. An update. J Oral Pathol Med 1994;23:1–11.

220. Tolson GE, Czusazak CA, Billman MA, Lewis DM. Report of a lateral periodontal cyst and gingival cyst occurring in the same patient. J Periodontol 1996;67:541–4.

221. Westcott WB, Correll RW, Craig RM. Two fluid-filled gingival lesions of the mandibular canine–first premolar area. J Am Dent Assoc 1984;108:653–4.

222. Wysocki GP, Brannon RB, Gardner DG, Sapp P. Histogenesis of the lateral periodontal cyst and the gingival cyst of the adult. Oral Surg Oral Med Oral Path 1980; 50:327–34.

223. Young LL, Reeve CM, Frantzis TG. Gingival cyst lined by respiratory epithelium: report of a case. J Periodontol 1972;43:490–1.

Gingival Cyst of Infants

224. Cataldo E, Berkman MD. Cysts of the oral mucosa in newborns. Am J Dis Child 1968;116:44–8.

225. Ikemura K, Kakinoki Y, Nishio K, Suenaga Y. Cysts of the oral mucosa in newborns: a clinical observation. Sangyo Ika Daigaku Zasshi 1983:5:163–8.

226. Levin LS, Jorgenson RJ, Jarvey BA. Lymphangiomas of the alveolar ridge in neonates. Pediatrics 1976;58:881–4.

227. Monteleone L, McLellan, MS. Epstein's pearls (Bohn's nodules) of the palate. J Oral Surg 1964;22:301–4.

228. Moreillon MC, Schroeder HE. Numerical frequency of epithelial abnormalities, particularly microkeratocysts, in the developing human oral mucosa. Oral Surg Oral Med Oral Pathol 1982;53:44–55.

229. Rivers JK, Frederiksen PC, Dibdin C. A prevalence survey of dermatoses in the Australian neonate. J Am Acad Dermatol 1990;23:77–81.

❖❖❖

4

NONODONTOGENIC CYSTS, PSEUDOCYSTS, AND MISCELLANEOUS ENTITIES

NONODONTOGENIC CYSTS

Nasopalatine Duct Cyst

Definition. The nasopalatine duct cyst is a developmental cyst arising from epithelial remnants within the nasopalatine canal, which is located in the midline of the anterior maxilla between and posterior to the central incisor teeth. *Incisive canal cyst* is a synonymous term.

Clinical and Radiologic Features. The nasopalatine duct cyst is discovered either incidentally upon radiographic examination or as a midline swelling of the anterior maxilla or incisive papilla (fig. 4-1). It may be associated with a discharge (1,2,9). Bony expansion is rare, however, Nortje and Farman (8) reported rapid growth of large (over 3.5 cm) nasopalatine duct cysts in adolescent South African blacks. Nasopalatine duct cysts accounted for 73 percent of nonodontogenic oral and jaw cysts in a survey by Daley et al. (3) of 40,000 consecutively accessioned oral biopsies. Anneroth et al. (2) reported that incisive canal cysts accounted for

4 percent of all oral cysts treated over an 8 year period. In a series of 334 cases documented by Swanson et al. (9), the mean patient age was 42.5 years, with a range of 9 to 84 years; 54.2 percent of the cysts occurred in males and 45.8 percent in females; and 93 percent of the affected individuals were white. Although variable in size, most were less than 2 cm. Surgical exploration and histologic examination may be necessary to distinguish a small nasopalatine duct cyst from an enlarged nasopalatine canal.

Radiographically, the cyst is a well-defined radiolucency which may be round, ovoid, or heart shaped (figs. 4-2, 4-3). If the cyst is located in the soft tissues of the incisive papilla and not within

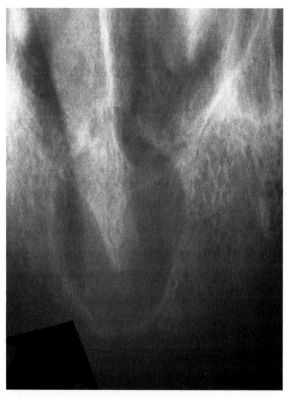

Figure 4-2
NASOPALATINE DUCT CYST
Occlusal radiograph shows a large well-defined radiolucency involving the nasopalatine duct.

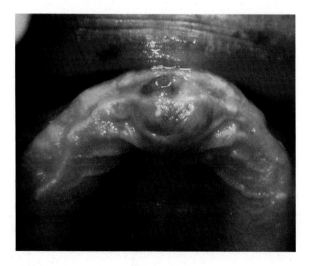

Figure 4-1
NASOPALATINE DUCT CYST
There is swelling of the anterior maxillary midline in this adult edentulous patient.

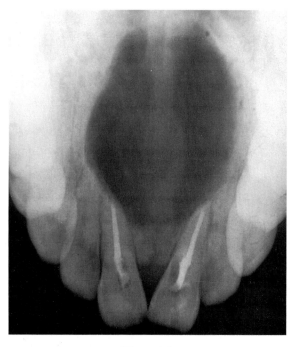

Figure 4-3
NASOPALATINE DUCT CYST
Occlusal radiograph shows a radiolucency between two endodontically treated maxillary central incisor teeth. Biopsy of this lesion revealed a nasopalatine duct cyst.

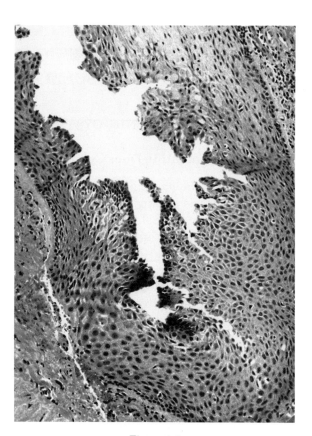

Figure 4-4
NASOPALATINE DUCT CYST
Metaplastic respiratory type epithelium lines a nasopalatine duct cyst.

the bony nasopalatine canal, the designation *cyst of the incisive (palatine) papilla* is applied. Periapical lesions such as radicular cysts, periapical granulomas, odontogenic keratocysts (7), and ameloblastomas associated with the central incisors can simulate nasopalatine duct cysts. A rare case of nasopalatine duct cyst associated with bilateral mesiodens was reported by Damm and colleagues (4).

Pathologic Findings. Epithelial remnants within the nasopalatine duct are thought to be the source of the cystic epithelium. Cysts form as a result of inflammation, trauma, or spontaneous proliferation of these remnants. Cysts in this anatomic location have been identified in human fetuses. Histologically, the nasopalatine duct cyst is lined by pseudostratified columnar ciliated epithelium, stratified squamous epithelium, columnar or cuboidal epithelium, or combinations of two or more of these types (fig. 4-4). Dendritic cells containing melanin pigment have been demonstrated in the epithelial lining of some (5). The wall of the cyst includes fibrous

connective tissue with veins, arteries, large nerves (fig. 4-5), minor mucous glands, adipose tissue, and sometimes a hyaline cartilage rest (fig. 4-6). Some of these structures are normally found in this anatomic location. Squamous metaplasia of respiratory epithelium may occur in association with chronic inflammation. Incisive canal cysts have been reported in two adult patients with severe periodontitis (6). There are isolated reports of carcinoma arising in nasopalatine duct cyst (10,11).

Treatment and Prognosis. Surgical enucleation is the recommended treatment. Removal of the neural elements of the canal results in anesthesia of the anterior palatal mucosa. A recurrence rate of 2 percent, occurring from 3 to 6 years after initial treatment, has been reported (9). Incomplete excision rather than an inherent biologic potential leads to recurrence.

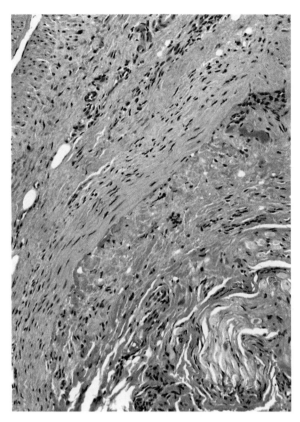

Figure 4-5
NASOPALATINE DUCT CYST
Peripheral nerve (lower right) and artery (upper left), which are common to the nasopalatine canal, are in the wall of a nasopalatine duct cyst.

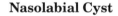

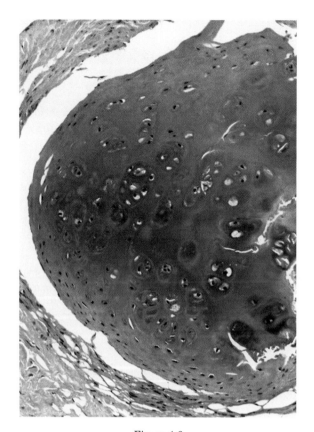

Figure 4-6
NASOPALATINE DUCT CYST
A cartilage rest is noted within the wall of a nasopalatine duct cyst.

Nasolabial Cyst

Definition. The nasolabial or nasoalveolar cyst is extraosseous and occurs slightly off the midline beneath the ala of the nose on the maxillary alveolar process.

Clinical and Radiologic Features. This rare nonodontogenic cyst usually presents as a unilateral, asymptomatic, fluctuant swelling of the maxillary vestibule and base of the nose (fig. 4-7) (12,14,20,22,24). The lesion is well defined and usually 1 to 3 cm in dimension; a 7 cm lesion has been reported by Cohen and Hertzanu (17). Secondarily inflamed nasolabial cysts should be differentiated from periodontal and endodontic inflammatory processes. A series of 26 cases reported by Kuriloff (19) demonstrated a female predilection, with most cases diagnosed in the fourth and fifth decades. An increased incidence in blacks has been reported. Approximately 10 percent of cases are bilateral (15). Radiographs may demonstrate bone rarefaction and deformity in the region of the anterior nasal fossa although most radiographs have no distinguishing features (16). At the time of surgical removal, a saucer-shaped cortical depression of the maxillary cortical bone is often identified.

Pathologic Findings. These cysts are most often lined by ciliated or nonciliated, pseudostratified columnar epithelium with mucous cells; foci of stratified squamous and simple cuboidal epithelia may also be present (fig. 4-8). Apocrine changes in the lining epithelium, with immunohistochemical staining for gross cystic disease fluid protein-15, has been reported in a nasolabial cyst by Lopez-Rios et al. (21). A case of malignant transformation of the epithelium has been reported (23). Inflammation of the connective tissue wall of the cyst is unusual but may

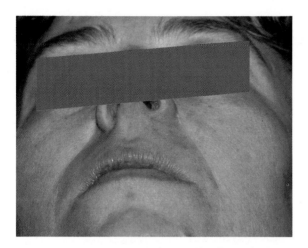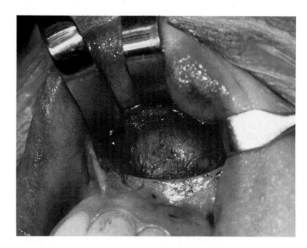

Figure 4-7
NASOLABIAL CYST
Left: Facial view shows filling-out of the nasolabial fold and slight displacement of the left ala of the nose.
Right: Intraoperative view of the cyst shown on the left. (Courtesy of Mark A. Cohen, Winnipeg, Canada.)

Figure 4-8
NASOLABIAL CYST
Photomicrograph demonstrates metaplastic cyst epithelium with mucous cells.

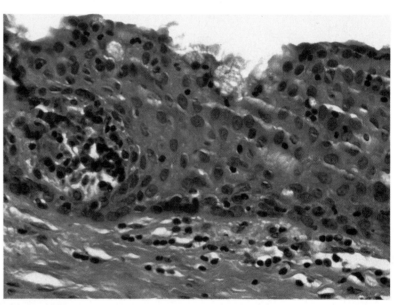

occur, particularly in those cysts that are painful at presentation. Calcium oxalate crystals within aspirated cyst fluid has been documented in one case (13).

Klestadt (18) suggested that the cystic process arose from epithelium entrapped at the point of fusion of the maxillary, medial nasal, and lateral nasal processes. Origin from the lower part of the nasolacrimal duct was proposed by Bruggeman (17), and was supported by Roed-Petersen (22).

Embryologic studies have not supported Klestadt's concept, so that origin from embryonic remnants of the nasolacrimal duct or the lower anterior portion of the mature duct epithelium is favored.

The nasolabial cyst needs to be distinguished from the glandular odontogenic cyst which also has prominent apocrine changes in the lining epithelium, mucous cells, and cilia. The latter is primarily an intraosseous cyst with features

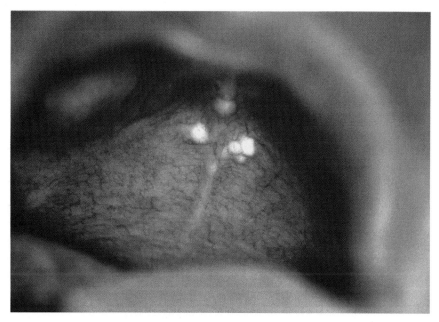

Figure 4-9
PALATAL CYST OF INFANTS
Newborn with multiple small white nodules of the hard palate.

characteristic of an odontogenic origin, specifically focal epithelial plaque-like thickenings that are noted also in the lateral periodontal, gingival, and botryoid odontogenic cysts. The clinical location differentiates a nasolabial cyst from a nasopalatine duct cyst.

Treatment and Prognosis. Surgical excision by an intraoral approach is recommended and recurrence is not expected.

Palatal Cyst of Infants

Definition. Midpalatal cysts of infants are small superficial microcysts of the midpalatal raphe, arising from epithelial inclusions along the fusion line of the palatal folds. They are also known eponymously as *Epstein pearls.*

Clinical Features. These developmental palatal midline cysts, which occur in newborn infants, are frequently multiple (fig. 4-9). They are also found at the junction of the hard and soft palates (25,26,28,29). The cysts are 1 to 3 mm white to yellow nodules. They involute or spontaneously rupture and are rarely identified after 3 months of age. Specimen submission for pathologic examination is rare. An evaluation of the oral mucosa of 420 Australian neonates revealed a 56 percent incidence of such cysts (29); an incidence of 88.7 percent was recorded in 541 Japanese newborns (26); and Monteleone and McLellan (27) found nodules in the midpalatal

area in 79 percent of black and 85 percent of white infants.

Pathologic Findings. Histologically, these cysts are located immediately below the epithelium of the mucosa and are lined by thin, stratified squamous epithelium with flattened basal cells and a parakeratinized surface (fig. 4-10). Keratin fills the cyst lumen, accounting for the white to yellow clinical presentation. These cysts are microscopically similar to gingival cysts of infants but are of different pathogenesis.

Treatment and Prognosis. No treatment is required as these cysts involute or rupture, with spillage of the contents shortly after discovery.

Surgical Ciliated Cyst

Definition. The surgical ciliated cyst occurs in the maxillary bone following trauma or surgery to the area of the maxillary sinus. *Postoperative cyst of the maxilla* is a synonymous term.

Clinical and Radiologic Features. This cyst results when a portion of the maxillary antral lining is detached, and persists and proliferates within maxillary bone. This may occur after trauma, extraction, or apical surgery of a tooth in close proximity to the sinus (33); a Caldwell-Luc procedure; or orthognathic surgery of the maxilla (31). The lesion is often discovered as an incidental radiographic finding or when pain and swelling occur. Radiographically, the

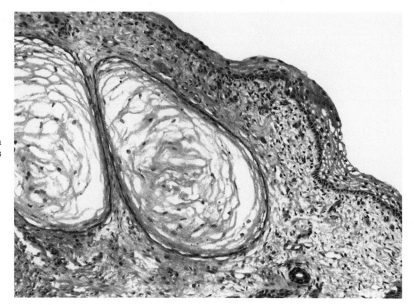

Figure 4-10
PALATAL CYST OF INFANTS
Small keratin-filled cysts beneath the palatal mucosa. A salivary duct is noted in the lower right corner.

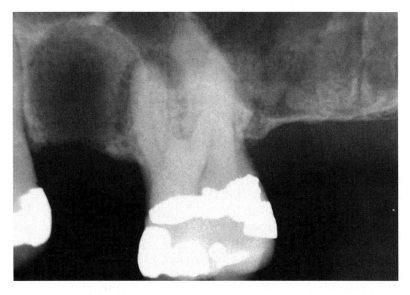

Figure 4-11
SURGICAL CILIATED CYST
A maxillary right first molar was extracted from a 51-year-old man 12 years previously. At the time of surgery, the palatal root was fractured. In the process of removing the root, it was displaced into the sinus. In attempting to extricate it via a Caldwell-Luc procedure, portions of the antral lining were curetted into the surgical site. Healing occurred without complication. The patient now presents with poorly localized pain in the right maxilla. The roentgenogram reveals a well-delineated radiolucent area encroaching upon the maxillary sinus. (Fig. 62, Fascicle 24, 2nd Series.)

cyst is as a well-defined unilocular radiolucency adjacent to the maxillary sinus (fig. 4-11). In Japan it has variably been reported as being common or extremely rare and as behaving in a more aggressive fashion than in cases reported from elsewhere (32). Yamamoto and Takagi (35) reported a peak incidence in the fourth and fifth decades with no sex predilection.

The surgical ciliated cyst is not related to the mucus impaction phenomenon. Mucus impaction occurs secondary to obstruction of the ostium of the sinus. Interference with mucin egress from the sinus results in its accumulation and possible expansion of the sinus, with associated bony erosion that clinically and radiographically simulates a malignant process. Antral pseudocyst (30), characterized by a dome-shaped inflammatory process affecting the sinus floor, is a common lesion and distinct from surgical ciliated cyst and mucus impaction of the maxillary sinus. True retention cyst of the seromucous glands of the antrum is rare (30).

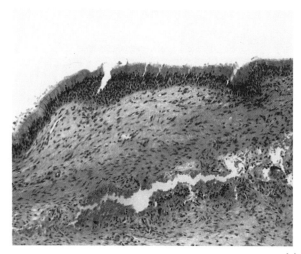

Figure 4-12
SURGICAL CILIATED CYST
Pseudostratified, ciliated, columnar epithelial lining of
the surgical ciliated cyst.

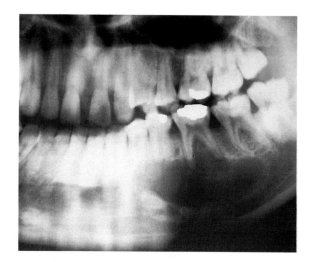

Figure 4-13
SOLITARY BONE CYST
Radiolucency involving the body of the mandible below
the first molar tooth.

Pathologic Findings. The surgical ciliated cyst is lined by pseudostratified columnar epithelium (fig. 4-12) with mucous cells that secrete mucin into the cyst lumen. A chronic inflammatory component is frequently present in the cyst wall and squamous metaplasia occurs in the adjacent cyst lining. The characteristic electrophoretic pattern of the gylcosaminoglycans aspirated from maxillary cysts, as reported by Smith et al. (34), may facilitate preoperative diagnosis.

Treatment and Prognosis. Surgical enucleation is the recommended treatment (33); large cysts have been treated with marsupialization (36). Recurrence may be expected in cysts that adhere to thin or perforated bony walls.

PSEUDOCYSTS

Solitary Bone Cyst

Definition. Solitary bone cyst is an intraosseous pseudocystic lesion lined by an attenuated fibrovascular membrane but lacking an epithelial lining. These cysts constitute about 2 percent of all jaw cysts (37). Synonymous terms include *traumatic bone cyst, hemorrhagic cyst, progressive bony cavity, simple bone cyst,* and *unicameral bone cyst.*

Clinical and Radiologic Features. Lucas (38) reported the first case of an intramandibular

traumatic cyst in the Western literature in 1929. By 1982, over 200 cases had been reported (38). The lesion is usually discovered incidentally during the first two decades of life (42). Males are affected slightly more frequently than females. The mandible is more often involved than the maxilla, with the molar and premolar regions the usual sites of occurrence; several cases have been reported within the condyle, however (42). Maxillary lesions are exceptionally rare.

The lesion is usually solitary, well demarcated, osteolytic, and nonexpansile (fig. 4-13). The nonexpansile nature of the lesion is explained by low intralesional pressure, although some expansion of the bone may be observed in about one third of cases. The margins of the lesion may be scalloped between vital teeth and there may also be tooth displacement (40). On T2-weighted magnetic resonance imaging (MRI) the fluid content may produce a high signal intensity (42). Traumatic bone cyst has been noted in association with florid osseous dysplasia (39,41).

Pathologic Findings. The pathogenesis of the lesion is not clearly understood. The preferred postulate is that the cyst forms following traumatic intraosseous hemorrhage, with subsequent lysis and resorption of the cellular content. It has also been postulated that it may be related to aneurysmal bone cyst and central giant cell reparative granuloma. The cyst contents are

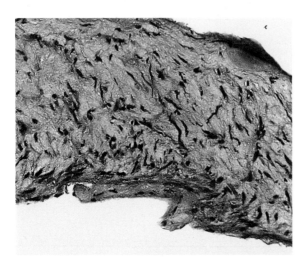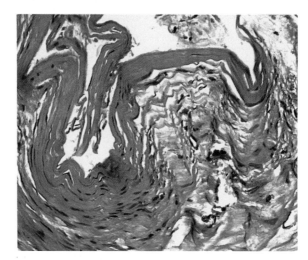

Figure 4-14
SOLITARY BONE CYST
Curettings composed of loose fibrous tissue removed from the periphery of a large "empty" cavity in the mandibular bone.

straw colored or blood tinged and the lining is an attenuated layer of loose fibrovascular tissue (fig. 4-14). Within this lining hemosiderin-laden macrophages, osteoclasts, and reactive woven bone may be seen.

Treatment and Prognosis. The exploratory diagnostic procedure is usually curative since the intralesional hemorrhage induced by the procedure excites formation of reparative granulation tissue. However, lesions over 5 cm may require placement of an intralesional graft. Recurrences have been documented but are infrequent (40).

OTHER DEFECTS

Lingual Mandibular Salivary Gland Defect

Definition. This is a developmental concavity occasionally found on the lingual surface of the mandible, which usually contains salivary gland, fat, or connective tissue. Synonymous terms such as *salivary gland cavity, concavity, depression, inclusion; latent bone cyst; static bone cyst;* and *Stafne defect* have also been used to describe this entity.

Clinical and Radiologic Features. In 1942, Stafne (52) described multiple examples of a radiographic abnormality which was located just anterior to the mandibular angle and usually below the mandibular canal. The lesions were round to oval radiolucencies between the angle of the mandible and the first molar tooth (figs. 4-15,

4-16). Rarely is clinical and radiographic evidence of buccal cortical expansion encountered. Most are unilateral, but bilateral (47) and multiple unilateral lesions have been documented as well as lesions in the alveolar bone of the mandible (fig. 4-17). A 0.3 percent incidence of these lesions has been found using panoramic radiographs (46). Surgical exploration most often reveals salivary gland tissue (fig. 4-18) which is in continuity with the submandibular salivary gland. The majority of these defects are identified in middle-aged or older men.

Since Stafne's description, a number of reports indicated that this phenomenon also occurs in the anterior portion of the mandible. Buchner and colleagues (45) have reported four such cases and reviewed 20 previously reported cases documented as anterior mandibular salivary gland defects. The demographic data on these anterior lesions are similar to that of posterior lesions (45). Most anterior lesions contain salivary tissue of the sublingual gland (45,49, 51,53). Barker (44) described a lesion of the ramus of the mandible containing parotid tissue. Ariji et al. (43) proposed a classification scheme based on outline and content of the defect as determined by computed tomography (CT) (fig. 4-19). Of 15 patients with 16 defects, they found that larger lesions that expanded the buccal cortical plate always contained salivary gland

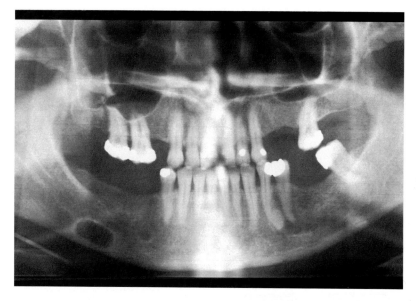

Figure 4-15
LINGUAL MANDIBULAR
SALIVARY GLAND DEFECT
Unilateral radiolucency below the mandibular canal in the body of the mandible.

Figure 4-16
LINGUAL MANDIBULAR
SALIVARY GLAND DEFECT
A radiolucent lesion with a well-defined sclerotic border is characteristic of lingual mandibular defect. Note the location below the mandibular canal.

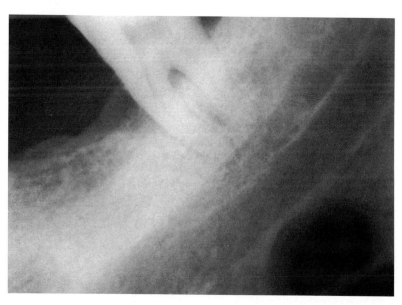

tissue whereas smaller lesions contained fat or soft tissue other than salivary gland.

These defects are likely developmental in origin but are only identified later in life. The variety of tissue within the defect suggests a multifactorial origin (43).

Idiopathic bone cavities of the mandibular posterior buccal surface have been identified in analyses of two major collections of skeletal abnormalities (50). Also, anterior buccal mandibular depressions have been identified in dry mandibles of a Bedouin tribe that lived 150 years ago;

these findings were more common in children (48). The etiology of these buccal mandibular defects remains speculative.

Treatment and Prognosis. Those lesions with a classic presentation can be diagnosed and followed radiographically. They may simulate other lesions such as odontogenic cysts or tumors, and lesions within the mandibular canal may require CT, MRI, or sialography for identification. Surgical exploration followed by histologic confirmation of normal gland, fat, or connective tissue allows for definitive diagnosis.

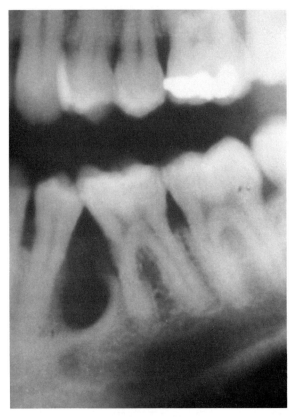

Figure 4-17
LINGUAL MANDIBULAR SALIVARY GLAND DEFECT
   The radiolucency involves the mandibular alveolar bone between the premolar and molar teeth. The clinical impression was lateral periodontal cyst; biopsy demonstrated salivary tissue similar to submandibular salivary gland.

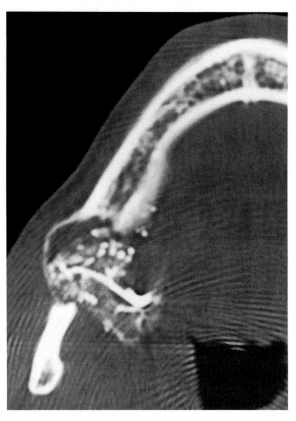

Figure 4-19
LINGUAL MANDIBULAR SALIVARY GLAND DEFECT
   An entrapped submandibular salivary gland is confirmed with computed tomography-sialography. (Fig. 4C from Ariji E, Fujiwara N, Tabata O, et al. Stafne's bone cavity, classification based on outline and content determined by computed tomography. Oral Surg Oral Med Oral Pathol 1993;76:378–80.)

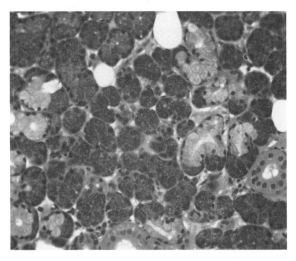

Figure 4-18
LINGUAL MANDIBULAR SALIVARY GLAND DEFECT
   Photomicrograph of salivary tissue removed from the radiolucent lesion depicted in figure 4-17.

Focal Bone Marrow Defect

   Definition. The focal bone marrow defect is an asymptomatic, radiolucent lesion of the jaws which contains normal hematopoietic and fatty bone marrow. *Osteoporotic bone marrow defect* is a synonymous term.

   Clinical Features. The focal bone marrow defect most commonly occurs in the posterior mandible, and less frequently in the maxillary tuberosity or other regions of the jaws (54–59,62,63). Patients are asymptomatic and the lesion is discovered during routine dental radiographs, most commonly in middle-aged females. Some patients present with pain in the region (57). Adjacent teeth are vital and a history of tooth extraction in the region is common.

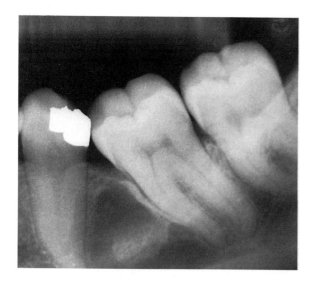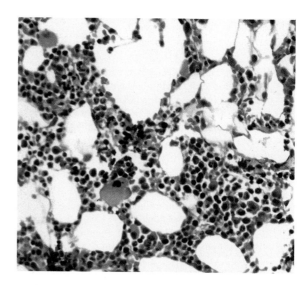

Figure 4-20
FOCAL BONE MARROW DEFECT
Left: Radiolucency between premolar and molar tooth. There was a history of extraction of the mandibular first molar many years previously. (Courtesy of Arthur S. Millier, Philadelphia, PA.)
Right: Photomicrograph of hematopoietic marrow from a suspicious radiolucency of the posterior mandible.

Radiologic Findings. The radiographic presentation is variable, with lesions being either well defined or diffuse with indistinct borders; an altered trabecular pattern is occasionally noted (fig. 4-20, left). CT has been reported as a means of making an accurate diagnosis (61). The radiographic features can simulate an inflammatory cyst or granuloma, Langerhans' cell histiocytosis, focal osteomyelitis, metastatic disease, solitary bone cyst, benign fibro-osseous lesion, lymphoma, leukemia, myeloma, intraosseous lipoma, or other pathologic processes (60).

The pathogenesis of this lesion is unknown. Remnants of embryonic bone marrow that persist into adulthood, bone marrow hyperplasia secondary to increased demand for hematopoiesis, and stimulatory effects on bone marrow secondary to extraction of adjacent teeth have been proposed (54,58). The unilateral nature of the lesion, its identification in adults, and its occurrence in areas without extraction detract from these suggested etiologies. Altered bone trabeculation of the jaws is well known in hereditary anemias, but is bilateral, more diffuse, and involves both maxilla and mandible.

Pathologic Findings. Histologically, hematopoietic bone marrow with red blood cells, myeloid cells, and megakaryocytes, or fatty bone marrow is encountered (fig. 4-20, right). Older patients may exhibit lymphoid hyperplasia of the marrow. A neoplastic process must be excluded. The presence of bone trabeculae within mature fat would favor a diagnosis of fatty bone marrow defect rather than intraosseous lipoma. Clinical correlation is also helpful in distinguishing these lesions.

Treatment and Prognosis. If the lesion is suspected radiographically and there are no significant symptoms or signs, periodic radiographic follow-up is all that is necessary. In cases in which the diagnosis is less certain, further imaging, such as CT, and biopsy may be indicated.

REFERENCES

Nasopalatine Duct Cyst

1. Allard Rh, van der Kwast WA, van der Waal I. Nasopalatine duct cyst. Review of the literature and report of 22 cases. Int J Oral Surg 1981;10:447–61.
2. Anneroth G, Hall G, Stuge U. Nasopalatine duct cyst. Int J Oral Maxillofac Surg 1986;15:572–80.
3. Daley TD, Wysocki GP, Pringle GA. Relative incidence of odontogenic tumors and oral and jaw cysts in a Canadian population. Oral Surg Oral Med Oral Pathol 1994;77:276–80.
4. Damm DD, Lu RJ, Rhoton RC. Concurrent nasopalatine duct cyst and bilateral mesiodens. Oral Surg Oral Med Oral Pathol 1988;65:264–5.
5. El–Bardaie A, Nikai H, Takata T. Pigmented nasopalatine duct cyst. Report of 2 cases. Int J Oral Maxillofac Surg 1989;18:138–9.
6. Mealey BL, Rasch MS, Braun JC, Fowler CB. Incisive canal cysts related to periodontal osseous defects: case reports. J Periodontal 1993;64:571–4.
7. Neville BW, Damm DD, Brock T. Odontogenic keratocysts of the midline maxillary region. J Oral Maxillofac Surg 1997;55:340–4.
8. Nortje CJ, Farman AG. Nasopalatine duct cyst. An aggressive condition in adolescent Negroes from South Africa? Int J Oral Surg 1978;7:65–72.
9. Swanson KS, Kaugars GE, Gunsolley JC. Nasopalatine duct cyst: an analysis of 334 cases. J Oral Maxillofac Surg 1991;49:268–71.
10. Takagi R, Ohashi Y, Suzuki M. Squamous cell carcinoma in the maxilla probably originating from a nasopalatine duct cyst. J Oral Maxillofac Surg 1996;54:112–5.
11. Takeda Y. Intra-osseous squamous cell carcinoma of the maxilla: probably arising from non-odontogenic epithelium. Br J Oral Maxillofac Surg 1991;29:392–4.

Nasolabial Cyst

12. Adams A, Lovelock DJ. Nasolabial cyst. Oral Surg Oral Med Oral Pathol 1985;60:118–9.
13. Aldred MJ, Surgar AW. Calcium oxalate crystals in a nasolabial cyst. J Oral Maxillofac Surg 1986;44:149–52.
14. Allard RH. Nasolabial cyst. Review of the literature and report of 7 cases. Int J Oral Surg 1982;11:351–9.
15. Barzilai M. Case report: bilateral nasoalveolar cysts. Clin Radiol 1994;49:140–1.
16. Chinellato LE, Damante JH. Contributions of radiographs to the diagnosis of naso-alveolar cyst. Oral Surg Oral Med Oral Pathol 1984;58:729–35.
17. Cohen MA, Hertzanu Y. Huge growth potential of the nasolabial cyst. Oral Surg Oral Med Oral Pathol 1985;59:441–5.
18. Klestadt WD. Nasal cyst and the facial cleft cyst theory. Ann Oto Rhino Laryngol 1953;62:84–92.
19. Kuriloff DB. The nasolabial cyst-nasal hamartoma. Otolaryngol Head Neck Surg 1987;96:268–72.
20. Graamans K, van Zanten ME. Nasolabial cyst: diagnosis mainly based on topography? Rhinology 1983;21:239–49.
21. Lopez-Rios F, Lassaletta-Atienza L, Domingo-Carrasco C, Martinez-Tello FJ. Nasolabial cyst: report of a case with extensive apocrine change. Oral Surg Oral Med Oral Pathol Radiol Endod 1997;84:404–6.
22. Roed-Petersen B. Nasolabial cysts. A presentation of five patients with a review of the literature. Br J Oral Surg 1969;7:84–95.
23. Walsh-Waring GP. Naso-alveolar cysts: aetiology, presentation, and treatment. J Laryngol Otol 1967;81:263–76.
24. Wesley RK, Scannel T, Nathan LE. Nasolabial cyst: presentation of a case with a review of the literature. J Oral Maxillofac Surg 1984;42:188–92.

Palatal Cyst of Infants

25. Cataldo E, Berkman MD. Cysts of the oral mucosa in newborns. Am J Dis Child 1968;116:44–8.
26. Ikemura K, Kahinoki Y, Nishio K, Suenaga Y. Cysts of the oral mucosa in newborns: a clinical observation. Sangyo Ika Daigaku Zasshi 1983;5:163–8.
27. Monteleone L, McLellan MS. Epstein's pearls (Bohn's nodules) of the palate. J Oral Surg 1964;22:301–4.
28. Moreillon MC, Schroeder HE. Numerical frequency of epithelial abnormalities, particularly microkeratocysts, in the developing human oral mucosa. Oral Surg Oral Med Oral Pathol 1982;53:44–55.
29. Rivers JK, Frederiksen, PC Dibdin C. A prevalence survey of dermatoses in the Australian neonate. J Am Acad Dermatol 1990;23:77–81.

Surgical Ciliated Cyst

30. Gardner DG, Gullane PJ. Mucoceles of the maxillary sinus. Oral Surg Oral Med Oral Pathol 1986;62:538–43.
31. Hayhurst DL, Moenning JE, Summerlin DJ, Bussard DA. Surgical ciliated cyst: a delayed complication of maxillary orthognathic surgery. J Oral Maxillofac Surg 1993;51:705–8.
32. Kaneshiro S, Nakajima T, Yoshikiawa Y, Iwasaki H, Tokiwa N. The postoperative maxillary cyst: report of 71 cases. J Oral Surg 1981;39:191–8.
33. Miller R, Longo J, Houston G. Surgical ciliated cyst of the maxilla. J Oral Maxillofac Surg 1988;46:310–2.
34. Smith G, Smith AJ, Basu MK, Rippin JW. The analysis of fluid aspirate gylcosaminoglycans in diagnosis of the postoperative maxillary cyst (surgical ciliated cyst). Oral Surg Oral Med Oral Pathol 1988;65:222–4.

35. Yamamoto H, Takagi M. Clinicopathologic study of the postoperative maxillary cyst. Oral Surg Oral Med Oral Pathol 1986;62:544–8.

36. Yoshikawa Y, Nakajima T, Kaneshiro S, Sakaguchi M. Effective treatment of the postoperative maxillary cyst by marsupialization. J Oral Maxillofac Surg 1982;40:487–91.

Solitary Bone Cyst

37. Cawson RA, Everson JW. Oral pathology and diagnosis. London: William Heinemann Med Books, 1987:5,13,14.

38. Gilman RH, Dingman RO. A solitary bone cyst of the mandibular condyle. Case report. Plast Reconstr Surg 1982;70:610–4.

39. Kaugars GE, Cale AE. Traumatic bone cyst. Oral Surg Oral Med Oral Pathol 1987;63:318–24.

40. Kuttenberger JJ, Farmand M, Stoss H. Recurrence of a solitary bony cyst of the mandibular condyle in a bone graft. A case report. Oral Surg Oral Med Oral Pathol 1992;74:550–6.

41. Melrose R, Abrams A, Mills B. Florid osseous dysplasia. Oral Surg Oral Med Oral Pathol 1976;41:62–82.

42. Tanaka H, Westesson PL, Emmings FG, Marashi AH. Simple bone cyst of the mandibular condyle: report of a case. J Oral Maxillofac Surg 1996;54:1454–8.

Lingual Mandibular Salivary Gland Defect

43. Ariji E, Fujiwara N, Tabata O, et al. Stafne's bone cavity: classification based on outline and content determined by computed tomography. Oral Surg Oral Med Oral Pathol 1993;76:375–80.

44. Barker GR. A radiolucency of the ascending ramus of the mandible associated with invested parotid salivary gland material and analogous with a Stafne bone cavity. Br J Oral Maxillofac Surg 1988;26:81–4.

45. Buchner A, Carpenter WM, Merrell PW, Leider A. Anterior lingual salivary defect: evaluation of twenty-four cases. Oral Surg Oral Med Oral Pathol 1991;71:131–6.

46. Correll RW, Jensen JL, Rhyne RR. Lingual cortical mandibular defects: a radiographic incidence study. Oral Surg Oral Med Oral Pathol 1980;50:287–91.

47. Fay JT, Berman F. Bilateral lingual mandibular salivary gland depression. Oral Surg Oral Med Oral Pathol 1978;45:654.

48. Finnegan M, Marcsik A. Anomaly or pathology: the Stafne defect as seen in archaeological material and modern clinical practice. J Hum Evol 1980;9:19–31.

49. Kaffe I, Littner MM, Arenburg B. The anterior buccal mandibular depression: physical and radiologic features. Oral Surg Oral Med Oral Pathol 1990;69:647–54.

50. Kocsis GK, Marcsik A, Mann RW. Idiopathic bone cavity on the posterior buccal surface of the mandible. Oral Surg Oral Med Oral Pathol 1992;73:123–6.

51. Miller AS, Winnick M. Salivary gland inclusion in the anterior mandible: report of a case with review of the literature on aberrant salivary gland tissue and neoplasms. Oral Surg Oral Med Oral Pathol 1971;31:790–7.

52. Stafne EC. Bone cavities situated near the angle of the mandible. J Am Dent Assoc 1942;29:1969–72.

53. Tominaga K, Kuga Y, Kubota K, Ohba T. Stafe's bone cavity in the anterior mandible: report of a case. Dentomaxillofac Radiol 1990;19:28–30.

Focal Bone Marrow Defect

54. Barker BF, Jensen JL, Howell FV. Focal osteoporotic bone marrow defects of the jaws: an analysis of 197 new cases. Oral Surg 1974;38:404–13.

55. Correll RW, Wescott WB. Asymptomatic, ill defined radiolucent area of the mandible. J Am Dent Assoc 1982;107:460–1.

56. Crawford BE, Weathers DR. Osteoporotic marrow defects of the jaws. J Oral Surg 1970;28:600–3.

57. Gordy FM, Crews KM, O Carroll MK. Focal osteoporotic bone marrow defect of the anterior maxilla. Oral Surg Oral Med Oral Pathol 1993;76:537–42.

58. Lipani CS, Natiella JR, Greene GW Jr. The hematopoietic defect of the jaws: a report of 16 cases. J Oral Pathol 1982;11:411–6.

59. Makek M, Lello GE. Focal osteoporotic bone marrow defects of the jaws. J Oral Surg 1986;44:268–73.

60. Miller W, Ausich J, Mcdaniel R, et al. Mandibular intraosseous lipoma. J Oral Maxillofac Surg 1982;40:594–6.

61. Sa'do B, Ozeki S, Higuchi Y, Nakayama E. Osteoporotic bone marrow defect of the mandible: report of a case diagnosed by computed tomography scanning. J Oral Maxillofac Surg 1992;50:80–2.

62. Schneider LC, Mesa ML, Fraenkel D. Osteoporotic bone marrow defect: radiographic features and pathogenic factors. Oral Surg Oral Med Oral Pathol 1988;65:127–9.

63. Standish SM, Shafer WG. Focal osteoporotic bone marrow defects of the jaws. J Oral Surg 1962;20:123–8.

5

BENIGN ODONTOGENIC TUMORS

EPITHELIAL TUMORS

Ameloblastoma

Definition. The ameloblastoma is a locally aggressive, epithelial odontogenic neoplasm having a close histologic resemblance to the enamel organ. This form of odontogenic neoplasm is "noninductive" in that it fails to induce any formed calcified product such as enamel, dentin, or other material.

General Considerations. As the most common odontogenic tumor, the ameloblastoma comprises 11 to 18 percent of noncystic lesions involving the oral and maxillofacial region (35). Of extraosseous or peripheral odontogenic tumors, the ameloblastoma is the most frequently occurring form, comprising 67 percent of cases (3). The absence of a formative product such as enamel or dentin or other calcified material is one of the distinguishing features of this class of odontogenic neoplasms. This tumor has intrigued clinicians and pathologists since its first description in the literature in 1868. Subsequently, several case studies and large series have been reported which have described a range of presentations, behavior, and management strategies. To this day, the origin of this lesion remains controversial. There is a lack of uniformity in classification and nomenclature and no standard approach with regard to treatment.

Classification. Classification schemes that have evolved over the years have resulted in five types of ameloblastoma: a unicystic variant, a solid or multicystic variant, an unusual desmoplastic variant, a peripheral variant, and a malignant form. The most common forms are the unicystic and multicystic, with the more recently designated unicystic type meriting separate consideration in view of its clinical behavior. There are no large published series of the malignant form due to the rarity of the neoplasm so that detailed analyses of prognosis and management are not available.

As a group, ameloblastomas are noted to occur chiefly in the third and fourth decades, however, a wide age range has been reported from the second through ninth decades, with no gender bias. The molar and ramus areas of the mandible are the favored sites of occurrence (over 80 percent of tumors).

Unicystic Ameloblastoma. The unicystic variant of the ameloblastoma was originally described by Robinson and Martinez in 1977 (23). It has been estimated that this variant accounts for approximately 5 percent of ameloblastomas (27). A confusing plethora of terminology has been used to describe this entity, including plexiform unicystic, intracystic, cystogenic, as well as unilocular and cystic ameloblastoma (1,7–9). From a clinical, radiographic, and pathologic standpoint, unicystic ameloblastoma is the most appropriate term. Theories of origin include the development of a cystic neoplasm from the outset; transformation of reduced enamel epithelial remnants or of a dental cyst lining, most commonly a dentigerous cyst, but also other odontogenic cysts such as the odontogenic keratocyst (2); cystic degeneration of a previously solid ameloblastoma; and multicystic change of individual islands of ameloblastoma which may coalesce to form a large cystic structure (2).

In contrast to the solid or multicystic ameloblastoma, the unicystic form occurs at a younger age (range, 10.6 to 23.8 years) and about 75 percent occur in the second and third decades (1, 11,13). Waldron and El-Mofty (34) noted that within their series of ameloblastomas, 9.7 percent were unicystic and occurred at an average age of 22 years versus 44 years for solid or multicystic lesions. The original series by Robinson and Martinez (23) had 27.7 years as mean age. Analyzing 57 cases, Ackermann et al. (1) found a mean age of 23.8 years, with 86 percent of lesions occurring between the second and fourth decades; there was a slight male predominance. While occasional cases have occurred in the maxilla, the majority are seen in the mandible, in particular within the molar and ramus areas (fig. 5-1). Of 43 cases of unicystic ameloblastoma, 77 percent located in the mandibular molar and ramus areas, 14 percent in the cuspid and premolar areas, and the remainder in the symphysis region (Table 5-1) (17,34).

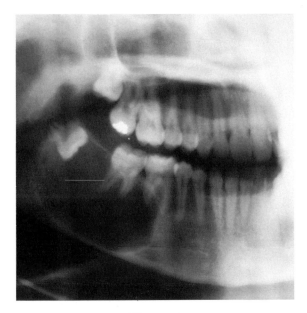

Figure 5-1
AMELOBLASTOMA

This panoramic radiograph demonstrates posterior displacement of an unerupted third molar situated at the superior pole of a discrete unilocular radiolucency. The lesion occupies the posterior body of the mandible and extends into the ramus.

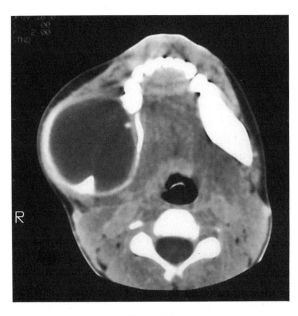

Figure 5-2
AMELOBLASTOMA

An axial CT of a unicystic ameloblastoma shows a circular radiolucent lesion with well-defined borders localized to the body of the mandible and extending posteriorly. At the distal aspect is an associated unerupted molar tooth.

Table 5-1

UNICYSTIC AMELOBLASTOMAS (MANDIBLE)

Location	Number Leider et al.	Waldron, El-Mofty	Total (%)
Molar/ramus	24	9	33 (77)
Cuspid/premolar	3	3	6 (14)
Symphysis	4	–	4 (9)

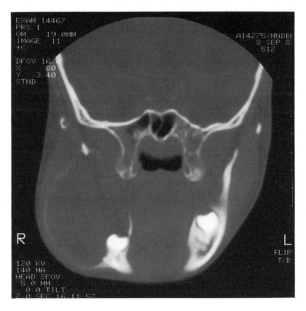

Figure 5-3
AMELOBLASTOMA

A coronal CT of this expansile unicystic ameloblastoma of the mandible demonstrates a thin bony shell, asymmetry, and extension to the tip of the coronoid process superiorly and the submandibular region inferiorly.

Radiographically, by definition, the lesion is unicystic, with an absence of pseudopartitioning or loculation within the purely radiolucent defect (figs. 5-2, 5-3). The majority of unicystic ameloblastomas occur in a dentigerous relationship (65 percent of cases [7,9,23]), particularly in younger patients (mean age in two series was 19.4 years [23] and 26.9 years [17]), while those not associated with impacted teeth occur approximately 8 years later.

Subsequent to the identification of this particular variant of ameloblastoma, three histopathologic subtypes were identified (1). The simplest

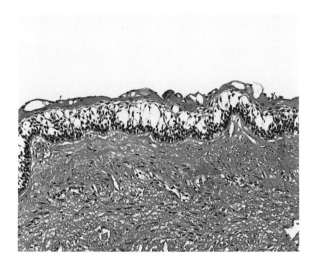

Figure 5-4
AMELOBLASTOMA
A lining type of unicystic ameloblastoma demonstrates a prominent epithelial basal cell layer with a slightly undulating margin beneath an expanded intermediate zone which is covered by parakeratinized type cells.

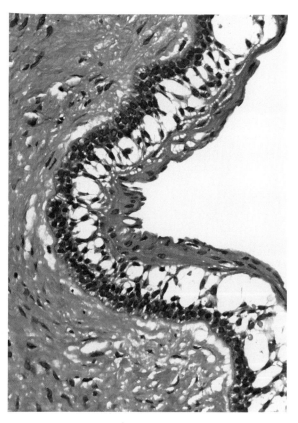

Figure 5-5
AMELOBLASTOMA
A detailed view of a lining type unicystic ameloblastoma features a hyperchromatic basal and parabasal cell lining in association with an expanded compartment of stellate cells upon which is superimposed parakeratinized squamous lining epithelium. The underlying connective tissue is moderately cellular and free of any invading or advancing epithelial proliferation.

is the *lining form,* characterized by a relatively thin lining epithelium within which all the diagnostic features are confined (figs. 5-4, 5-5). The supportive connective tissue wall or sac is uninvolved by the proliferating epithelial element. The lining may be totally or partially composed of ameloblastic epithelium with well-defined histologic features, as defined by Vickers and Gorlin in 1970 (32). These include hyperchromatic nuclei that exhibit so-called reverse polarity away from the basement membrane within columnar basal cells and which are amplified by the presence of subnuclear cytoplasmic vacuolization. There are widened parabasalar intercellular spaces and a zone of subepithelial hyalinization, representative of a thickened or reduplicated basal lamina and sometimes referred to as the "inductive effect," although no calcification occurs in this area. True induction is not present.

The second histologic subtype of the unilocular variant, *the luminal form,* is an epithelial proliferation which results in the formation of a nodule or mass along the luminal epithelial surface and which projects into the cyst lumen (figs. 5-6–5-8). The pattern of epithelial proliferation is essentially plexiform in nature in most cases and resembles that seen in the solid plexiform ameloblastoma; however, in many instances, the typical basal cell qualities seen in the lining form

are not present. These nodules may be small or may occupy a significant portion of the cyst lumen. Of importance is the absence of infiltration of the epithelial component into the fibrous wall of the cyst or adjacent tissue.

The third subtype, *the mural ameloblastoma,* contains infiltrative epithelial elements in the connective tissue wall which have plexiform or follicular microscopic features (figs. 5-9–5-11). The epithelial elements may or may not be connected to the epithelial lining of the cystic component and there is considerable variation in the amount of epithelial proliferation.

Incisional biopsies of large jaw cysts should be carefully examined for the presence of ameloblastomatous change. Likewise, enucleated

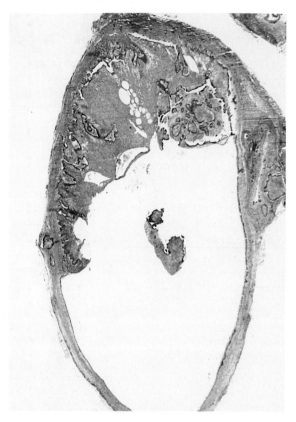

Figure 5-6
AMELOBLASTOMA

A luminal type of unicystic ameloblastoma composed of a crescent-shaped proliferation extends into the cystic lumen which is lined elsewhere by a thin epithelial layer.

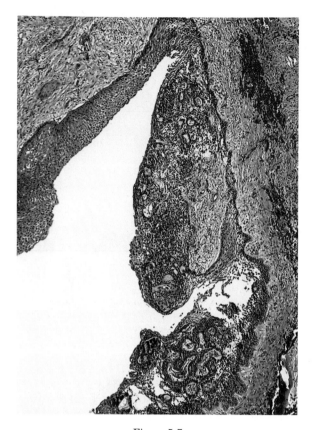

Figure 5-7
AMELOBLASTOMA

A closer view of a luminal ameloblastoma of the unicystic type shows transition from the attenuated squamous lining to the nodular proliferation into the cyst lumen in the absence of proliferation into the surrounding connective tissue layer.

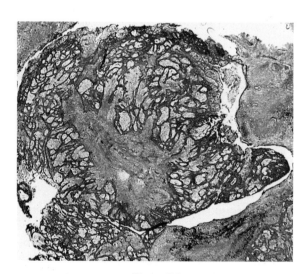

Figure 5-8
AMELOBLASTOMA

A medium-power view of a unicystic ameloblastoma with a predominantly plexiform pattern of growth.

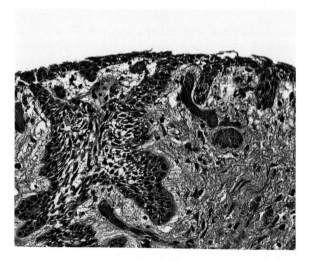

Figure 5-9
AMELOBLASTOMA

Early invasion of the connective tissue layer of a unicystic ameloblastoma by an ameloblastomatous proliferation.

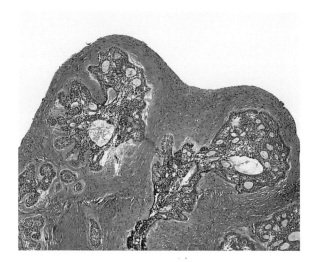

Figure 5-10
AMELOBLASTOMA
Multicentric nodules of ameloblastoma display a follicular pattern with solid and multicystic internal qualities. This proliferation is within the connective tissue wall of a mural type of ameloblastoma.

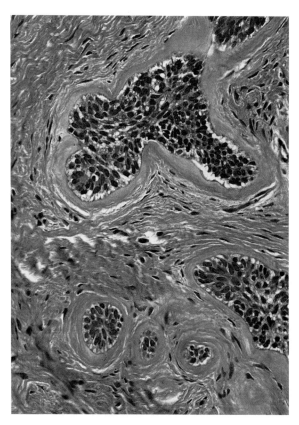

Figure 5-11
AMELOBLASTOMA
A detailed view of an odontogenic epithelial island with a suggestion of a peripheral columnar layer enveloped by a densely collagenous fibroblastic stroma.

specimens should be thoroughly sectioned to rule out mural or transmural extension.

The majority of unicystic ameloblastomas, in particular the luminal and intraluminal forms, may be treated as dentigerous cysts, by simple enucleation and careful follow-up. In cases with a significant mural ameloblastomatous component local resection or thorough curettage is preferable. In either case the patients must be carefully followed for many years. A recurrence of the mural subtype at 5 years has been reported, emphasizing the need for an increased level of vigilance for this subtype (29). Overall recurrence rates of 10 to 25 percent have been reported after simple enucleation or curettage (17,23,30).

Infiltrating ("Solid") Ameloblastoma. While the unicystic and multicystic forms of this tumor share some clinical and microscopic features, there are significant differences in terms of behavior, management, and prognosis. In general, the locally aggressive reputation of ameloblastoma is attributable to this particular form. Most investigators believe that ameloblastoma is a locally aggressive benign neoplasm, while some have characterized it as a neoplasm of low-grade malignancy (10,14,18,21,28).

As with the unicystic ameloblastoma, a wide age range is noted with most occurring during the third and fourth decades, with a mean age in the mid-fourth decade. Analysis of several large series indicates that the mandible, in particular in the molar-ramus area, is the most common site of occurrence accounting for over 80 percent of such tumors (14,18,22,28). These lesions are rare in childhood. There does not appear to be a gender predilection.

Peripheral Ameloblastoma. The peripheral or soft tissue counterpart of the central or intraosseous ameloblastoma is a rare entity. It usually presents as a nontender swelling or smooth surfaced mass on the gingiva (fig. 5-12); it may present in an extragingival location (36).

Histogenetically, it is considered to be derived from remnants of the dental lamina that are in a supraperiosteal location. The oral epithelial basal cell layer has also been considered a possible site of origin. Immunohistochemical studies

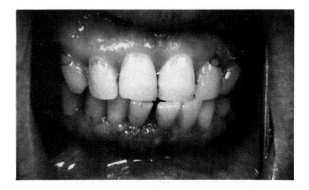

Figure 5-12
AMELOBLASTOMA
This peripheral ameloblastoma presents along the labial aspect of the mandibular incisor region as a polypoid swelling with no associated bone destruction.

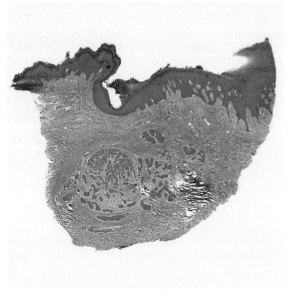

Figure 5-13
AMELOBLASTOMA
A survey view of this wedge resection shows the peripheral ameloblastoma to be situated in the submucosal region of the gingiva, which is covered by intact orthokeratinized stratified squamous epithelium.

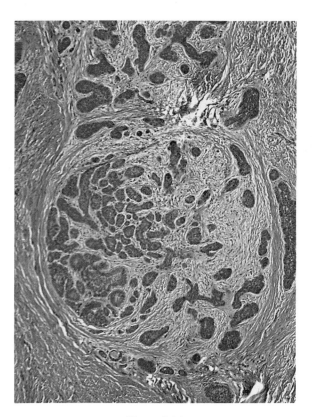

Figure 5-14
AMELOBLASTOMA
Scattered islands and nests of odontogenic epithelium with a follicular pattern are associated with peripherally collagenized stroma within this peripheral ameloblastoma.

have demonstrated similarities to cutaneous basal cell carcinoma but not to intraosseous ameloblastoma (33).

This lesion does not exhibit aggressive behavior and usually does not invade underlying bone (figs. 5-13–5-15). Recurrences are infrequent after local excision (3). A diagnosis of peripheral ameloblastoma based on superficial or incisional

biopsy specimens should be made only after ensuring that they do not represent extension of a central infiltrating tumor.

Malignant Ameloblastoma. There has been controversy concerning the biologic nature of ameloblastoma since its original description in the 19th century. The 1992 World Health Organization (WHO) classification (15) defines malignant ameloblastoma as "a neoplasm in which the pattern of an ameloblastoma and cytologic features of malignancy are shown by the growth in the jaws and/or by any metastatic growth. Tumors meeting these criteria may arise as a result of malignant change in a preexisting ameloblastoma, or possibly as a primary malignant ameloblastoma not preceded by an ordinary ameloblastoma." It places the malignant ameloblastoma under the broader category of odontogenic carcinoma. This grouping also includes primary intraosseous carcinoma, malignant variants of other odontogenic

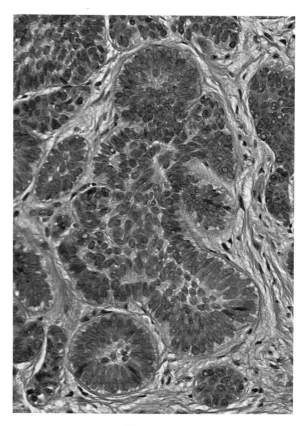

Figure 5-15
AMELOBLASTOMA
A higher power view of a peripheral ameloblastoma shows the typical tall, columnar, peripheral palisaded layer enclosing a stellate reticulum type zone which is analogous in structure to its more aggressive intrabony counterpart.

epithelial tumors, and malignant transformation in previously existing odontogenic cysts (see specific chapters). *Ameloblastic carcinoma* consists essentially of cytologically malignant cells in the primary, recurrent, or metastatic foci, yet which retain their overall odontogenic (ameloblastic) quality.

The definition of malignant ameloblastoma therefore includes the presence of cytologic features of malignancy. However, there are tumors with essentially benign histologic features at the primary site but with metastases demonstrating identical histologic features to those of the primary tumor; the WHO definition does include such. Laughlin (16) has shown that the lung is the most frequent site for metastases (75 percent), followed by the cervical lymph nodes and spine (15 percent), and other sites making up the bal-

ance. The male to female ratio for malignant ameloblastoma is approximately 1.5 to 1, with 80 percent of the lesions located in the mandible and 20 percent in the maxilla. Patient ages range from 5 to 60 years, with a mean of 30.5 years. The interval between the initial treatment of the primary lesion and the development of metastases varies from 2 to 24 years, with a mean of 11 years. The mean survival period following a diagnosis of metastasis is 2 years, with long-term survival periods also noted. Slootweg and Muller (28) reviewed 31 cases with histologically confirmed metastases from the literature and an additional 14 cases in which the primary tumors were histologically malignant but in which metastasis did not occur or in which clinically or radiographically suspected metastases had not been histologically verified. In 20 of these 31 cases, the primary tumor and metastases were composed of well-differentiated ameloblastoma with no histologic features of malignancy. Therefore, all infiltrative ameloblastomas have the potential to metastasize, albeit exceptionally. In the presence of cytologic features of malignancy, a diagnosis of ameloblastic carcinoma should be made (28).

Corio et al. (4) reported an additional eight cases of ameloblastic carcinoma. All eight lesions were aggressive, rapidly growing, and painful, and demonstrated perforation of bony cortices with extension into soft tissues. These authors defined ameloblastic carcinoma as a lesion arising from various potential sources including ameloblastoma, odontogenic cysts, and epithelial odontogenic rests. Only one case demonstrated regional metastases.

The definition of malignant ameloblastoma remains controversial: the degree of cellular atypia and mitotic activity required to establish such a diagnosis is not well defined. As the sine qua non of malignancy remains the ability of a lesion to metastasize, it is evident from the literature that a significant number of biologically malignant ameloblastomas are histologically indistinguishable from their benign counterparts.

Recently, Gold (10) stated that while some metastases are clearly recognizable histologically as ameloblastoma, others exhibit such atypical patterns that they may not be recognizable as ameloblastomas. He noted that ameloblastomas may pursue an aggressive clinical course without metastasizing and may demonstrate great variation in histologic features. Thus, the behavior of ameloblastoma is by no means predictable by histologic parameters alone. In order to distinguish metastasizing ameloblastomas with benign features from those with malignant histologic features, Elzay (5) proposed a modification of the WHO classification to separate malignant ameloblastomas from ameloblastic carcinoma. Attempts at placing ameloblastomas within an aggressive or benign category may not possible. Gold, while in the minority, considers ameloblastoma to be a low-grade malignant basaloid tumor with a range of clinical presentations and histopathologic and behavioral patterns.

Sinonasal Ameloblastoma. An additional variant, the sinonasal ameloblastoma, has recently been described by Schafer and colleagues (24). A mean age of 61 years, with a range from 45 to 81 years, and a male predominance have been noted. Presenting signs and symptoms include nasal obstruction, epistaxis, and sinusitis. Opacification is noted on CT scan and plain films. Of conceptual and anatomic significance is the absence of an origin from or continuity with alveolar bone. The lesion is thought to arise from the totipotential cells of the sinonasal surface epithelium. Microscopically, a plexiform variant is seen in the majority of cases. The treatment of choice is surgical ranging from local excision, if complete removal can be assured, to partial maxillectomy. While recurrences may occur, no metastases or tumor-related deaths have been reported.

Clinical Features. Ameloblastomas tend to be associated with unerupted or impacted teeth, in particular mandibular third molars. Patients are generally asymptomatic and the lesions are often discovered during routine dental or radiographic examination and less commonly present as an asymptomatic jaw expansion or facial deformity. Tooth movement or developing malocclusion may be an early or initial presenting sign. As undiagnosed or untreated tumors progress they can loosen or displace teeth as well as expand the cortices. Long-term neglect of such expansile lesions often results in extreme thinning of the inferior cortex of the mandible, with a potential for pathologic fracture. Inferior alveolar nerve paraesthesia is a very uncommon clinical presentation, even with large tumors.

The molar and maxillary sinus regions of the maxilla are the most commonly affected sites.

Tsaknis and Nelson (31) noted that nearly 90 percent of ameloblastomas of the maxilla occur in the posterior segment, while nearly half involve the maxillary sinus.

Clinical presentation of maxillary ameloblastoma differs from the mandibular counterpart since the anatomic nature of the maxilla allows for considerable expansion and growth prior to development of bony deformity or other signs of tumor growth such as proptosis or elevation of orbital contents. Other clinical signs include buccal expansion, nasal obstruction, malocclusion, facial asymmetry, or poor healing of extraction sites. Initial manifestations of maxillary ameloblastoma may result from extensive and destructive tumor growth into the orbit, base of skull, and parasellar structures (24,25,31).

Radiologic Findings. While no pathognomonic radiographic feature of ameloblastoma exists, there are several findings that tend to characterize ameloblastomas as a group. The lesions are well defined, purely radiolucent, and usually demonstrate a hyperostotic border. While a minority of ameloblastomas present as a unilocular process, the majority are partitioned or loculated, with a broad range of compartmental sizes from those with a honeycomb pattern to others with broadly scalloped borders (figs. 5-16–5-23). Early lesions may resemble a dentigerous cyst or other forms of odontogenic circumcoronal pathology. In advanced lesions, normally dense cortical bone may assume a thin, barely perceptible level of thickness and perforate and extend into soft tissue. By combining computed tomography (CT) and scintigraphy, finer details of bone marrow invasion are achievable (26).

The recently described desmoplastic form (see Histopathologic Findings) is radiographically and clinically dissimilar to the more common ameloblastomas (12,20). The radiographic pattern is a mixed radiolucent and radiopaque one, with ill-defined margins reminiscent of a fibro-osseous process. The distribution of the lesion favors the anterior segments of the jaws, particularly the maxilla. The majority of mandibular desmoplastic ameloblastomas are located in the premolar or anterior regions.

Histopathologic Findings. One or more patterns of the histologic subtypes may occur in any particular tumor. The most common patterns are the follicular and plexiform, with variable

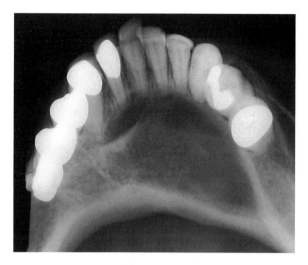

Figure 5-16
AMELOBLASTOMA
An expansile, well-defined radiolucent lesion of the anterior mandible crosses the midline. The predominant expansion is labial or buccal, with a thin but intact cortical rim.

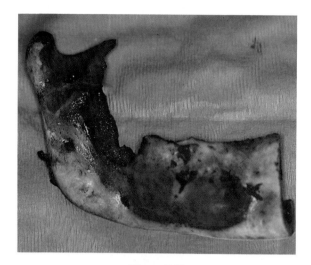

Figure 5-17
AMELOBLASTOMA
A multilobulated solid form of ameloblastoma occupies much of the body of the mandible and extends into the ramus and subcondylar regions, elevating the floor of the sigmoid notch.

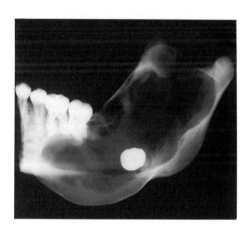
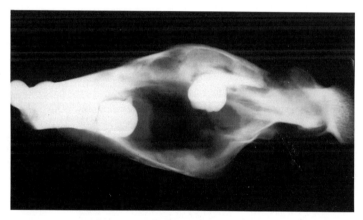

Figure 5-18
AMELOBLASTOMA
Radiographs of a disarticulated mandibular ameloblastoma demonstrate a fusiform enlargement of the inferior border of the mandible and scalloped margins along the posterior border of the ramus with extension anteriorly toward the symphysis region. There is expansion of the ramus as well as superior extension into the coronoid process. Buccal and lingual expansion are seen in the superior view while an erupted molar tooth is seen toward the inferior aspect of the specimen.

degrees of cystic change. Cellular variations also occur within either of the two major patterns.

The most common pattern, the follicular, closely resembles the enamel organ: islands of odontogenic epithelium are bordered by palisaded and polarized columnar cells. These surround a central population of variably spaced stellate-shaped cells reminiscent of the stellate reticulum of the enamel organ. The size of the islands varies from relatively

small and solid to larger with variable degrees of cystic change or degeneration (figs. 5-24, 5-28).

The plexiform variant is composed of anastomosing strands and cords of cells with a minimal stellate reticulum-like component; in some areas a more solid epithelial pattern predominates. The bordering cells are columnar and have hyperchromatic nuclei that are polarized away from the basement membrane (reverse polarity). The stroma

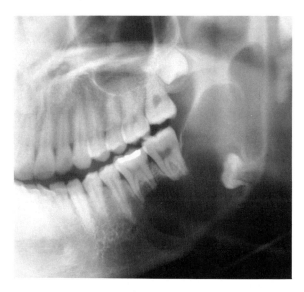

Figure 5-19
AMELOBLASTOMA

A multilocular radiolucency in the posterior mandible extends from the mid-body to the subcondylar region. An impacted third molar is seen at the angle of the mandible. There is a moderate degree of associated root resorption and combined lingual and buccal thinning with perforation.

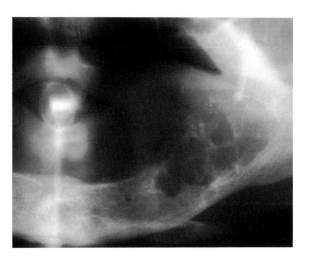

Figure 5-20
AMELOBLASTOMA

This radiolucent lesion in the endentulous mandible demonstrates a subtle multilocular pattern. There is associated intraoral swelling and alveolar ridge expansion.

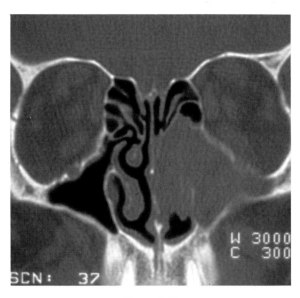

Figure 5-22
AMELOBLASTOMA

The coronal reconstruction of this maxillary ameloblastoma demonstrates extension of the process beyond the maxillary sinus and erosion of the medial wall. The nasal fossa is compromised because the process extends to the vomer, nasal septum, and superiorly into the ethmoid sinus.

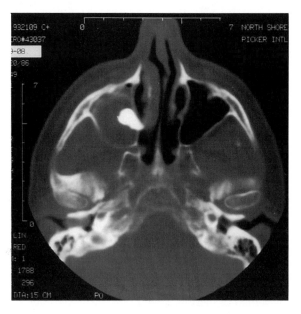

Figure 5-21
AMELOBLASTOMA

This axial CT features an impacted maxillary molar at the mid-portion of the maxillary sinus in association with a cystic process that displaces the posterior wall of the maxillary sinus laterally and toward the skull base.

in plexiform and follicular ameloblastomas varies from delicately fibrillar to well collagenized, and is moderately vascular (figs. 5-26, 5-27).

Cellular variations of either the plexiform or follicular types include the acanthomatous variant, in which variable degrees of squamous metaplasia occur. Keratin pearl formation may even be noted within the stellate reticulum component (fig. 5-25). The less common granular cell variant is composed of few to large numbers of epithelial cells with coarsely granular eosinophilic cytoplasm (figs. 5-29, 5-30). These granules correspond to an abundance of lysosomes. An unusual variant, the basal cell form (figs. 5-31, 5-32), has a minimal stellate reticulum type component and a greater degree of cellular isomorphism involving broad sheets with a less well-developed peripheral columnar component which is not as regimented or as palisaded as that seen in the more common plexiform and follicular variants. A recently described variant, the desmoplastic, demonstrates a highly collagenized stroma which is

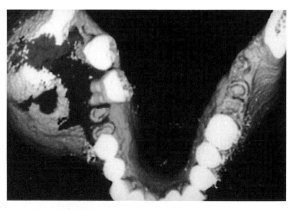

Figure 5-23
AMELOBLASTOMA
A three-dimensional reconstructed CT of a mandibular ameloblastoma shows a predominantly buccal or lateral growth component that displaces the molar dentition toward the midline.

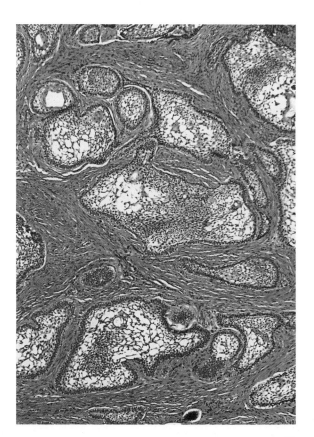 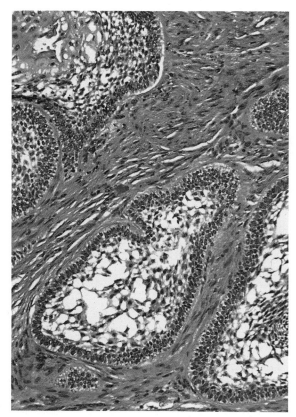

Figure 5-24
AMELOBLASTOMA
A follicular ameloblastoma with islands of odontogenic epithelial proliferation is associated with a mature collagenous stroma. Follicular islands of odontogenic epithelium are bordered by columnar and palisaded ameloblastic cells with polarized hyperchromatic nuclei. Enclosed within is a stellate reticulum-like component with unevenly dispersed polygonal to fusiform cells.

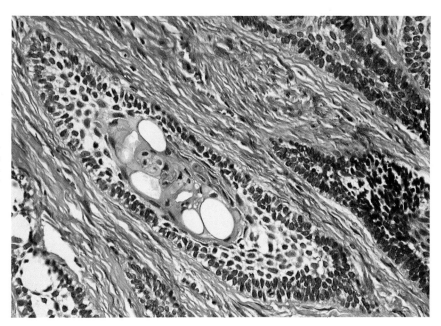

Figure 5-25
AMELOBLASTOMA
Acanthomatous or squamous differentiation within the stellate reticulum component of this follicular ameloblastoma is a commonly encountered feature.

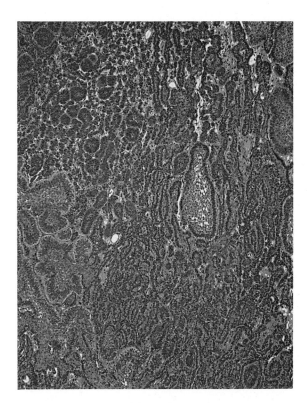

Figure 5-26
AMELOBLASTOMA

A low-power view of a predominantly plexiform ameloblastoma with complex interweaving cords of ameloblastic epithelium within a moderately collagenized background stroma. Scattered at the periphery and within the plexiform component are well-defined follicular elements.

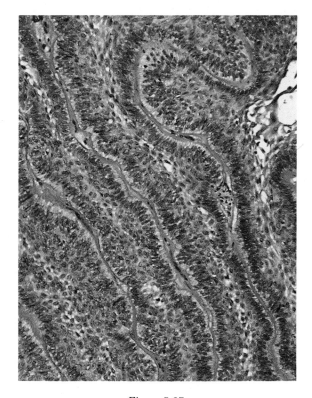

Figure 5-27
AMELOBLASTOMA

Parallel ribbons of plexiform ameloblastoma show the typical palisaded, columnar peripheral layer enclosing a limited stellate reticulum-like component.

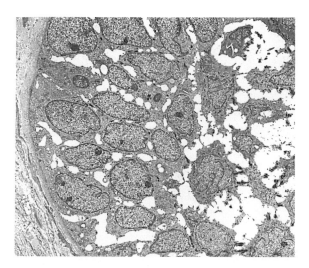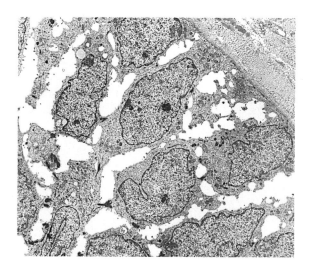

Figure 5-28
AMELOBLASTOMA

Electron micrographs of a follicular ameloblastoma demonstrate the juxtaposition of columnar epithelial cells resting on a thickened basal lamina. Widened intercellular spaces are seen, corresponding to the stellate reticulum component, with well-formed desmosomes evident in many areas.

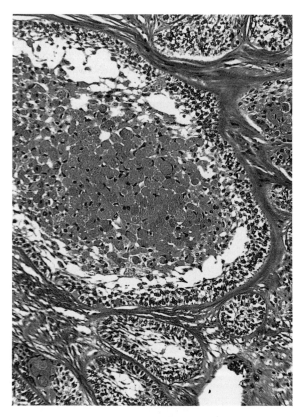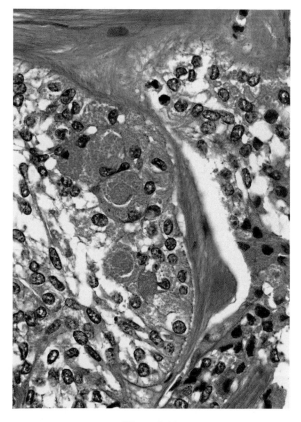

Figure 5-29
AMELOBLASTOMA

Within this follicular pattern is a dense cluster of enlarged, stellate reticulum type cells containing granular eosinophilic cytoplasm, typical of the granular cell ameloblastoma.

Figure 5-30
AMELOBLASTOMA

A higher power view of a granular cell ameloblastoma shows transformation from stellate to rounded cells with granular eosinophilic cytoplasm.

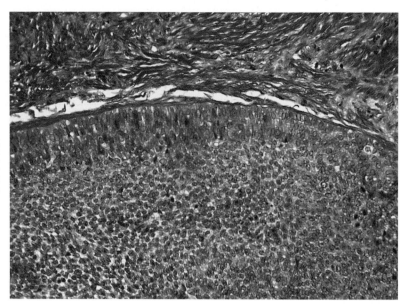

Figure 5-31
AMELOBLASTOMA
A basaloid ameloblastoma features a minimally discernible peripheral columnar layer in association with tightly aggregated cells to form a sheet-like array with little distinction between peripherally and centrally placed cells.

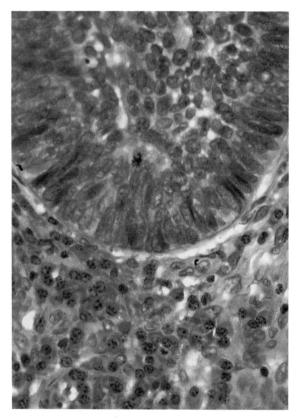

Figure 5-32
AMELOBLASTOMA
This basaloid ameloblastoma shows a slightly more open but densely basophilic central component in the epithelial island while peripherally degenerative ameloblasts are seen as hyperchromatic slender elements. A mitotic figure is at the periphery of the island.

poorly cellular and cytologically bland (6,34). Epithelial islands are widely scattered within the stroma and are bordered by cuboidal cells. Rarely do columnar cells demonstrate typical ameloblastic qualities (figs. 5-31, 5-33, 5-34).

Other histologic variants have been noted including papilliferous, clear cell, and keratoameloblastomatous types. There is no apparent clinical or behavioral specificity.

Treatment and Prognosis. Treatment is dependent upon location, size, and surgical philosophy. Some surgeons favor a conservative approach consisting of curettage of surrounding bone ("peripheral ostectomy"); others tend to resect such lesions with a margin of radiographically normal bone. Resections may take the form of marginal mandibulectomies, partial maxillectomies, or true through and through resection in cases involving the mandible with a partial hemimaxillectomy for larger maxillary lesions.

The medullary bone is more frequently infiltrated by this tumor, while cortical bone is spared but often thinned. When cortical erosion occurs, the periosteum tends to form a barrier. When tumor extends beyond the periosteum, no encapsulation is noted and the tumor impinges on submucosal tissue. Muller and Slootweg (19), therefore, suggest a 1 cm resection margin of spongy bone while cortical bone need be resected only sparingly. Where bone is perforated, resection of the overlying alveolar or oral mucosa is recommended.

In the case of small, histologically well-circumscribed lesions surrounded by a mature fibrous connective tissue capsule, enucleation followed by curettage is generally curative. In the case of lining or luminal unicystic ameloblastomas, particularly in the young, this conservative form of therapy is preferred. In cases with extreme cortical attenuation, however, regardless of histologic subtype, resection followed by reconstruction may be the only option. Maxillary ameloblastomas require a more aggressive approach as a consequence of their more posterior location and the complex anatomy of the antrum and its superior margin. For relatively small lesions within the body of the mandible where the cortical plates remain, thorough curettage may be adequate.

Calcifying Epithelial Odontogenic Tumor

Definition. This rare odontogenic tumor was described and defined by Pindborg (46,47). It accounts for less than 1 percent of odontogenic tumors (50), and only 150 cases have been described in the literature (41,43,48,49). It is a histologically distinctive, benign, slow-growing neoplasm but may be locally invasive. While most cases arise within bone, they may also occur within peripheral soft tissue (38,48). Calcification within this tumor is characteristic, however, noncalcifying variants have been reported (53).

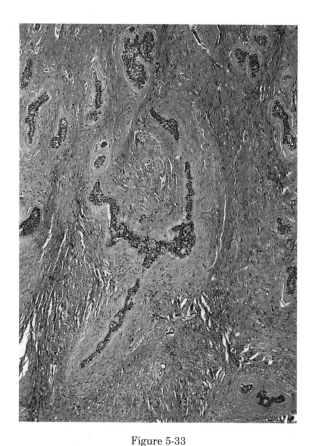

Figure 5-33
AMELOBLASTOMA
A desmoplastic ameloblastoma is characterized by dense accumulations of poorly cellular collagen with dispersed islands of ameloblastic epithelium.

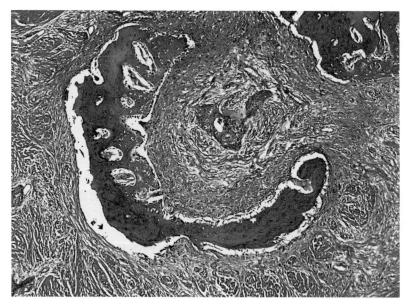

Figure 5-34
AMELOBLASTOMA
Individual islands of ameloblastic epithelium are surrounded by collagenized stroma which in turn is partially surrounded by reactive bone rimmed by osteoblasts.

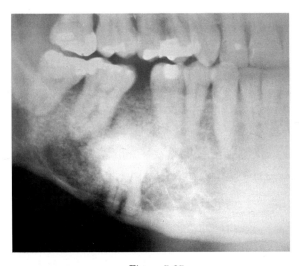

Figure 5-35
CALCIFYING EPITHELIAL ODONTOGENIC TUMOR
A panoramic radiograph demonstrates a central dense opacification in association with an inferiorly displaced first molar. The diffuse nature of the process is noted anteriorly, while more posteriorly is a reasonably well-defined periphery.

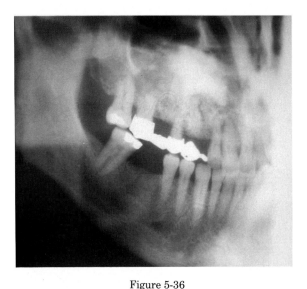

Figure 5-36
CALCIFYING EPITHELIAL ODONTOGENIC TUMOR
A diffusely opacified maxillary alteration is appreciated above the premolar dentition which extends superiorly, raising the floor of the maxillary sinus. The borders are diffuse and ill defined.

Clinical and Radiologic Features. The peak incidence is between 20 and 60 years of age, with essentially equal frequency within each decade. There is a bimodal pattern of frequency, with an early peak in the third decade and a later peak in the fifth decade (49). There is no gender

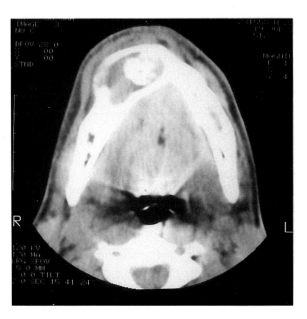

Figure 5-37
CALCIFYING EPITHELIAL ODONTOGENIC TUMOR
An axial CT scan shows a well-defined mixed radiolucency/radiopacity in the symphysis region of the mandible with labial and lingual expansion.

predilection. Mandibular cases outnumber maxillary cases by a 2 to 1 ratio, with the molar region predominating over the premolar region. The anterior segment of the jaws demonstrates a predilection for peripheral extraosseous cases. Clinically, a slowly enlarging, expansile, painless mass is seen, generally within the posterior portion of the affected jaw.

Radiographically, in over slightly half of all cases, the process has at its epicenter the crown of a mature unerupted tooth (fig. 5-35). The earliest phases demonstrate a radiolucent area mimicking an odontogenic cyst of developmental origin or possibly an ameloblastoma. Over time, the radiographic margins may gradually shift from well defined to more diffuse and, as maturation proceeds, form radiopaque foci which increase in size and density and often obscure the associated tooth and bony margins of the lesion. Variable degrees of multiloculation may be found, which range from a "honeycomb" to a "driven snow" appearance (figs. 5-36–5-38).

Microscopic Findings. Histologically, in its classic form, sheets or strands of variably sized, polyhedral epithelial cells with well-defined borders and distinct intercellular bridges are seen

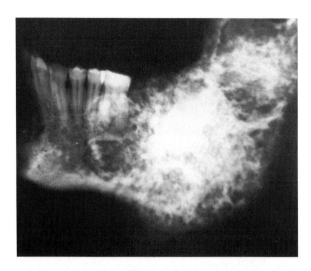

Figure 5-38
CALCIFYING EPITHELIAL ODONTOGENIC TUMOR

A gross specimen demonstrates a massive, expansile, predominantly radiopaque tumor extending from the coronoid and condylar processes into the body of the ramus and anteriorly to the premolar area. Small loculations characterize the periphery of the lesion, while an essentially homogeneous opacification forms the epicenter.

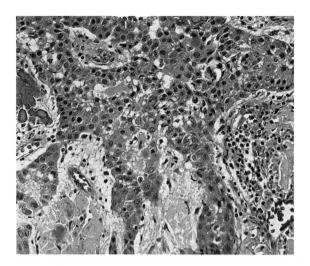

Figure 5-39
CALCIFYING EPITHELIAL ODONTOGENIC TUMOR

Sheaths of polyhedral epithelial cells with densely staining nuclei and focal mineralization are seen.

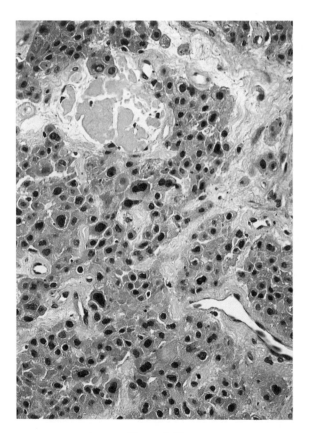

Figure 5-40
CALCIFYING EPITHELIAL ODONTOGENIC TUMOR

Nuclear hyperchromatism and pleomorphism are evident in association with a minimally cellular stroma and focal areas of acellular amyloid type material.

(fig. 5-39). Nuclear pleomorphism ranges from mild to moderate, with mitotic figures rarely being encountered (fig. 5-40). The nuclei may be slightly lobulated and may include mononucleated and multinucleated giant forms that have prominent nucleoli. Variation in histologic patterns include lesions with clear cell features and pseudoglandular architecture, which are associated with older patients, as well as the more classic calcifying epithelial odontogenic tumor (CEOT). The clear cell variant constitutes 6 percent of all CEOTs reported (42,51). Rounded, eosinophilic, homogeneous deposits within sheets of tumor cells are commonly noted and are often calcified (fig. 5-41). A pattern of calcification in a concentric, droplet-like fashion, often showing appositional basophilic concentric rings (Liesegang rings), is common but not always present (fig. 5-42).

CEOTs may be similar to salivary gland neoplasms, with cribriform features containing eosinophilic "amyloid-like" material (figs. 5-43, 5-44). Special stains, including thioflavin-T (UV illumination) (fig. 5-45) and Congo red (polarized light) identify this "amyloid-like" homogeneous material as having a reaction similar to that of typical amyloid, although the exact nature of the odontogenically-derived material is controversial.

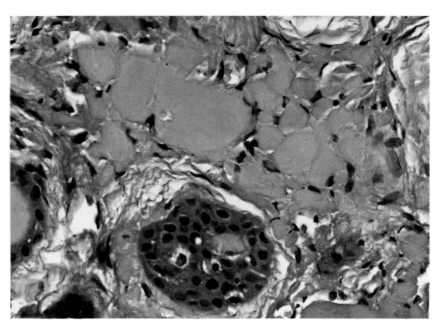

Figure 5-41
CALCIFYING EPITHELIAL
ODONTOGENIC TUMOR
An island of polyhedral epithelial cells with nuclear pleomorphism is surrounded by globular
deposits of hyaline pink material
characterized as amyloid.

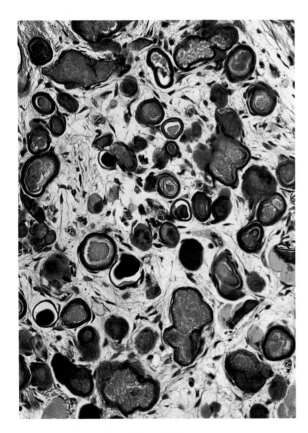

Figure 5-42
CALCIFYING EPITHELIAL ODONTOGENIC TUMOR
Droplet type calcifications with concentric lamellar appositional rings (Lisengang) represent one form of calcification noted within this tumor.

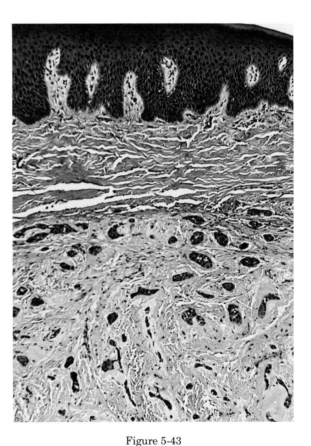

Figure 5-43
CALCIFYING EPITHELIAL ODONTOGENIC TUMOR
A peripheral calcifying epithelial odontogenic tumor
shows a sharply marginated superior surface as it ap-
proaches the lamina propria.

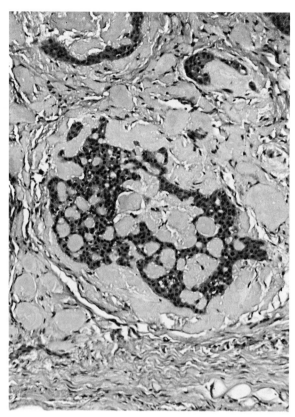

Figure 5-44
CALCIFYING EPITHELIAL ODONTOGENIC TUMOR
Amyloid masses enclose the proliferative epithelial element, which in turn encloses other droplets of forming amyloid.

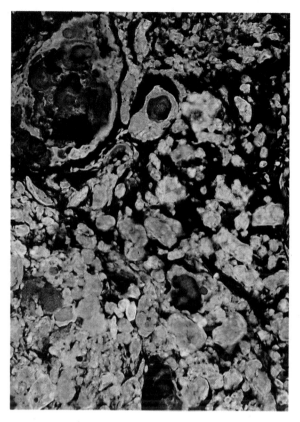

Figure 5-45
CALCIFYING EPITHELIAL ODONTOGENIC TUMOR
A thioflavin T stain highlights the globular nature of the amyloid deposits.

Whether it represents a degradation product of the epithelial component or an active secretory product remains a question. In areas where epithelial degeneration is noted these deposits persist and coalesce to form a wide variety of shapes which may mineralize (fig. 5-46). Evaluation of amino acids within the amyloid demonstrates qualities similar to enamel tuft protein, immunogenic amyloid, and variable region immunoglobulin light chains (40).

Immunohistochemically, the profile of the epithelial component includes positivity for cytokeratins, epithelial membrane antigen, *Ulex europeaus,* and peanut agglutinin as well as blood group antigen expression. Histochemically, the spherical acellular bodies are positive for a non-AA amyloid and nonkeratin or basal lamina-like structures. Occasional S-100–positive cells may be noted (40).

In about 6 percent of cases, the CEOT may be seen in a composite relationship with the adenomatoid odontogenic tumor (37,39,45,52,54).

Ultrastructural observations indicate complex lateral infoldings of cellular processes similar to those noted in the stratum intermedium of the enamel organ. This substantiates Pindborg's view (46) that this tumor bears a close resemblance to this component of the odontogenic apparatus. This concept is supported by ultrastructural localization of alkaline phosphatase within this lesion (44).

Differential Diagnosis. From the clinical and radiographic perspective, several entities must be considered. In the early developmental stages, prior to the formation of significant levels of intralesional mineralization, ameloblastoma, central giant cell granuloma, odontogenic keratocyst, odontogenic myxoma, odontogenic fibroma, and ameloblastic fibroma need to be considered.

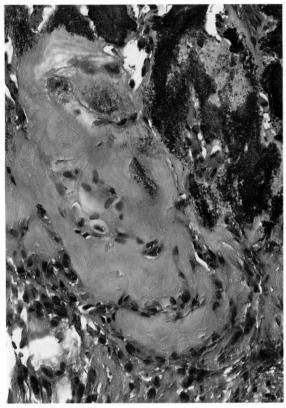

Figure 5-46
CALCIFYING EPITHELIAL ODONTOGENIC TUMOR
A juxtaposition of amyloid with dystrophic type mineralization in a granular rather than droplet-like pattern represents a second form of mineralization noted within this tumor.

As the lesion matures and increasing levels of mineralization are present, ameloblastic fibroodontoma, ossifying fibroma (cemento-ossifying fibroma), and adenomatoid odontogenic tumor are to be considered. The differential diagnosis of the peripheral soft tissue counterpart of the intraosseous lesion includes ameloblastoma, peripheral giant cell granuloma, peripheral odontogenic fibroma, and the so-called odontogenic hamartoma. The clear cell variant needs to be distinguished from metastatic renal cell carcinoma, acinic cell carcinoma, mucoepidermoid carcinoma, and glycogen-rich adenocarcinoma (51). Microscopically, however, the classic CEOT is quite distinctive.

Treatment and Prognosis. In view of the locally aggressive nature of this lesion definitive therapy must include resection of the entire mass, with tumor-free surgical margins and long-term

follow-up. The clear cell variant has been described by some as demonstrating more aggressive clinical features, suggesting that en bloc resection be performed with long-term follow-up (42,51). Recurrence rates of 14 percent have been documented (42); a 22 percent rate of recurrence has been noted with the clear cell variant (42).

Adenomatoid Odontogenic Tumor

Definition. The adenomatoid odontogenic tumor (AOT) is an uncommon, benign, usually cystic tumor of odontogenic epithelial origin but which has an inductive effect on adjacent mesenchyme, resulting in the production of an amyloid-like material (62). The most distinctive feature of the epithelial component is the presence of duct-like spaces lined by cuboidal to columnar cells within the odontogenic cell rests, which accounts for the descriptive terminology "adenomatoid."

Clinical Features. The earliest account of this lesion was by Ghosh in 1934 (61) who described it as an adamantinoma of the upper jaw. Subsequently, three maxillary cases were reported as cystic neoplasms which arose in relation to developmental cysts (71). Early designations of this lesion included the term "adenoameloblastoma" which resulted in inappropriate aggressive treatment given an absence of any behavioral relationship to ameloblastoma.

AOT tends to predominate in the anterior dental arch, is characteristically slow growing, and is uncommon beyond 30 years of age. Females are affected nearly twice as often as males. A racial predisposition favoring Asians and blacks may be present (55,73). While a soft tissue or peripheral counterpart exists, over 97 percent occur within bone. Nearly three fourths of these are noted in a follicular relationship to an impacted or unerupted tooth (figs. 5-47, 5-48). The mean age of patients with the central variant is 17 years, and 24 years for those with the extrafollicular or peripheral variant. Sixty percent of those lesions associated with embedded teeth occur in the four canine teeth (57,66).

Radiologic Findings. Radiographically, the AOT is a well-defined, unilocular lesion surrounding the crown of an unerupted or impacted tooth. Small radiopaque foci may be distributed within the radiolucent lesion. Root divergence may be seen when the lesion is located in the

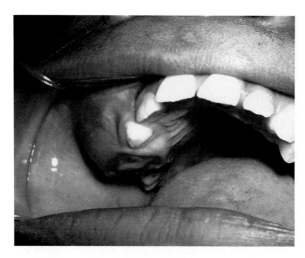

Figure 5-47
ADENOMATOID ODONTOGENIC TUMOR
This 11-year-old female had delayed eruption of the maxillary posterior dentition in association with an expansile mass of the alveolar process. (Figures 5-47 and 5-48 are from the same patient.)

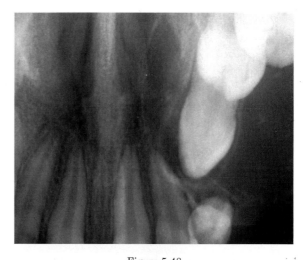

Figure 5-48
ADENOMATOID ODONTOGENIC TUMOR
A radiograph shows several impacted teeth in association with a radiolucent lesion which has expanded the buccal and palatal cortices. Scattered dot-like calcifications are within the dominantly lucent lesion.

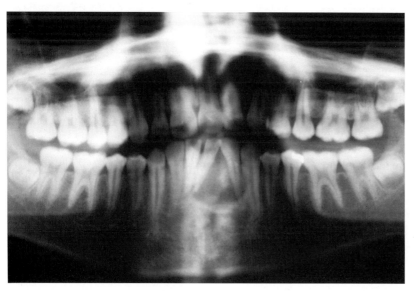

Figure 5-49
ADENOMATOID
ODONTOGENIC TUMOR
A mixed radiolucent and radiopaque lesion, which is well delimited, separates the mandibular canine and central incisors. Diffuse and focal calcifications are seen within the interior portion of the lesion.

anterior segment of the dental arch between teeth (figs. 5-49, 5-50), often in a so-called globulomaxillary cyst-like arrangement. Root resorption is uncommon. In the follicular type of AOT, the lesion may be differentiated from a dentigerous cyst by the presence of apical extension along the root plane beyond the cemento-enamel junction.

The extrafollicular variant, or those within bone but without direct relationship to an impacted or unerupted tooth (figs. 5-50, 5-51), tend to be located within the alveolar segment of the jaws between the roots of unerupted teeth, similar in presentation to a lateral periodontal cyst. The internal aspect of the radiolucency may contain faint, multiple, opaque foci which, over time, increase in size and density. The pattern of calcification is generally flocculent or "snowflake"-like in appearance. A panoramic radiograph may not demonstrate the radiopacities when the degree of calcification is minimal (59); intraoral

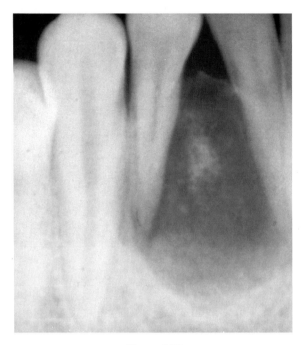

Figure 5-50
ADENOMATOID ODONTOGENIC TUMOR
The radiograph at surgery shows a well-demarcated cystic lesion separating the roots of the lateral and central incisor teeth. (Figures 5-50 and 5-51 are from the same patient.)

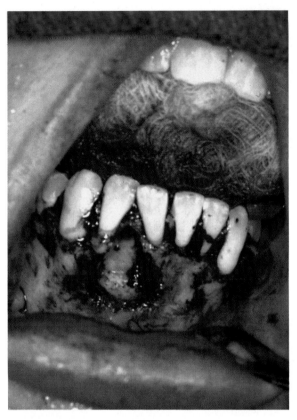

Figure 5-51
ADENOMATOID ODONTOGENIC TUMOR
An expansile lesion with discrete lateral and inferior margins in the anterior portion of the mandible displaces the mandibular lateral and central incisors.

radiographs may be more helpful in this respect and can aid in formulating a differential radiographic diagnosis.

Histogenesis. The origin of the AOT remains uncertain. The central lesion may originate from the postsecretory ameloblast subsequent to amelogenesis; however, the stratum intermedium, the reduced enamel epithelium, and the inner enamel epithelium at the preameloblastic stage are possible precursor structures (67,70). In the case of the extraosseous AOT, the basal cell layer of the overlying oral epithelium may be the source of the lesion (73). Dental lamina remnants within the gingival soft tissues may retain the potential for neoplastic differentiation as in other peripheral odontogenic tumors.

Gross Findings. A well-defined soft tissue mass surrounding the crown of an unerupted tooth is encased by a thick fibrous capsule (fig. 5-52). On section, a cystic cavity is partially or completely filled with solid tissue. Depending upon the degree of mineralization, a gritty consistency may be noted. The outer surface of the connective tissue sac is generally smooth.

Microscopic Findings. The connective tissue wall forms a well-defined capsule surrounding the epithelial component of the lesion, which grows in an intraluminal fashion (fig. 5-53). The degree of epithelial proliferation may be extensive, causing complete filling of the lumen and formation of intraluminal excrescences or excrescences adjacent to the crown of the associated tooth.

The epithelial component is comprised of a dual cell population. Spindle-shaped and polyhedral cells form large aggregates with a swirling pattern and exhibit an overall nodular quality at low-power examination (figs. 5-54–5-56). A second cell type is more cuboidal in nature, and a columnar cell population may be noted around microcystic or duct-like spaces, producing the gland-like pattern characteristic of this lesion (fig. 5-57). The nodular aggregates of cells tend to be solid in configuration with a minimal stromal component

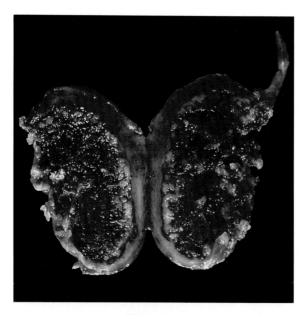

Figure 5-52
ADENOMATOID ODONTOGENIC TUMOR
A cystic mass with a slightly uneven external surface was easily removed from the surrounding mandibular bone. Note the intraluminal proliferation and nodular growth features.

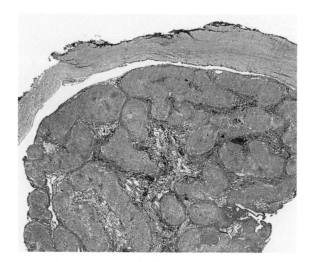

Figure 5-53
ADENOMATOID ODONTOGENIC TUMOR
A survey view of the lesion depicted in figure 5-52 shows intracystic proliferation of tissue, with a sharp demarcation between tumor and the connective tissue supporting wall.

(fig. 5-60). Within the nodules, small nests or rosettes may be noted, often surrounding small, eosinophilic, amorphous nodules which are periodic acid–Schiff (PAS) positive and diastase resistant. The characteristic duct-like spaces are generally lined by a single row of cuboidal to columnar cells with foamy cytoplasm and central to basally placed oval nuclei with vesicular or stippled chromatin. In some cases a gradual continuum from rosette structures to well-formed duct-like spaces is evident, suggesting that the duct-like spaces result from central breakdown or expansion of previously solid rosettes of epithelial cells. Toward the periphery of the lesion and at the junction of the epithelium and capsular connective tissue, arborizing trabeculae of odontogenic epithelium may be noted. These strands tend to be one to two cell layers in thickness and parallel but do not penetrate the collagen fibers within the cyst wall.

The eosinophilic masses mentioned above are amphophilic to basophilic and may be laminated with a variable degree of mineralization (figs. 5-58, 5-59). The eosinophilic material has variously been interpreted as calcified amyloid (60) or enamel proteins (63,64,68). Ultrastructural study has

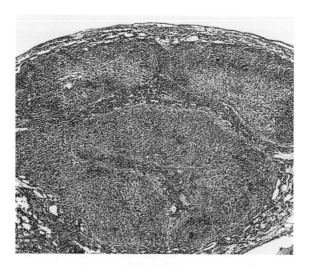

Figure 5-54
ADENOMATOID ODONTOGENIC TUMOR
Typical nodular intracystic growth patterns are surrounded in part by strands and trabeculae of epithelial cells.

shown it to have a fibrillar to granular quality (69) but without the substructure of amyloid (63). In addition to being PAS positive, the material also demonstrates other histochemical qualities consistent with enamel matrix material. (63) Also, the presence of pigment in the form of melanin has been reported in this tumor (72). This has been attributed to the neural crest

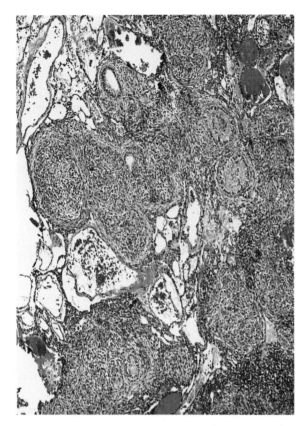

Figure 5-55
ADENOMATOID ODONTOGENIC TUMOR
Nodular aggregates of cells within an intraluminal location suggest early duct-like proliferation.

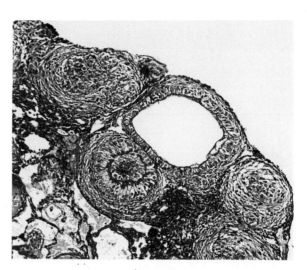

Figure 5-56
ADENOMATOID ODONTOGENIC TUMOR
Nodular duct-like and calcified structures extend into a cyst lumen.

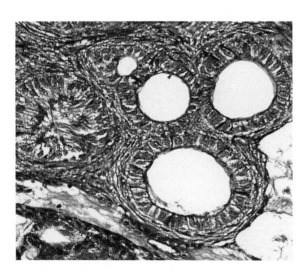

Figure 5-57
ADENOMATOID ODONTOGENIC TUMOR
Gland-like spaces are surrounded by cuboidal to columnar cells, which in turn are surrounded by a spindle cell population. Eosinophilic hyaline droplet material can be seen in a separate nodular aggregate.

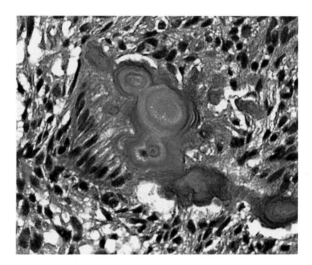

Figure 5-58
ADENOMATOID ODONTOGENIC TUMOR
Annular calcification juxtaposes spindle and columnar epithelial cells.

influence on the development of odontogenic tissues. There is no relationship between the presence of melanocytes and the behavior of this lesion.

There are reports of AOT coexisting with calcifying epithelial odontogenic tumor (56,58,65). The coexistence of these lesions has been attributed to an enamel organ origin, since preameloblasts and stratum intermedium participate in the histogenesis of both lesions. Okada and colleagues

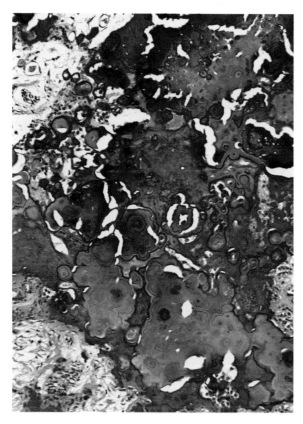

Figure 5-59
ADENOMATOID ODONTOGENIC TUMOR
Calcification is dystrophic in nature and uneven in its distribution.

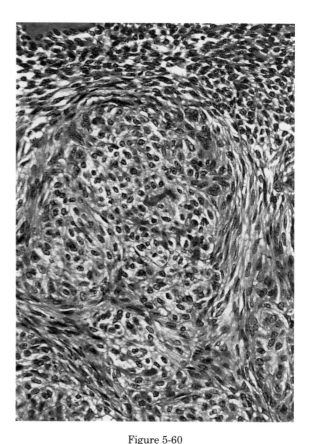

Figure 5-60
ADENOMATOID ODONTOGENIC TUMOR
Predominantly, spindle cells swirl in varied directions with no evidence of gland-like differentiation.

(65) have reported immunohistochemical similarities between these lesions, thus also supporting a similar histogenesis.

Treatment and Prognosis. The character of the thick connective tissue capsule allows for easy enucleation of the lesion. The risk of recurrence is extremely low: in a review of nearly 500 cases, Philipsen (66) noted multiple recurrences with intracranial extension in only one case. This well-documented case was reported in the Japanese neurosurgical literature and quoted elsewhere (66). In appropriate circumstances, it may be possible to preserve the involved tooth by enucleating of the cystic lesion.

Squamous Odontogenic Tumor

Definition. This is a benign neoplasm or hamartoma originating from epithelial rests of Malassez of the periodontal membrane. It occurs in juxtaposition to tooth roots, is composed of discrete nests and cords of bland, stratified, squamous epithelium, and may contain foci of mineralization.

Clinical and Radiologic Features. The squamous odontogenic tumor is a lesion of periodontal membrane origin, specifically the epithelial rests of Malassez, and was first described by Pullon et al. in 1975 (78). It is uncertain whether the lesion is a benign neoplasm or a hamartoma. It is almost exclusively of intraosseous origin, with less than five cases reported in a peripheral location. When noted to occur exclusively in soft tissue, a dental lamina origin has been postulated (76); such an origin can conceivably explain the case reported by van der Waal et al. (80) which arose in an edentulous segment of the jaw.

The most frequent presentation is that of a localized loosening of teeth in the absence of adjacent or generalized, periodontal disease-associated bone loss. The lesion occurs over a broad age

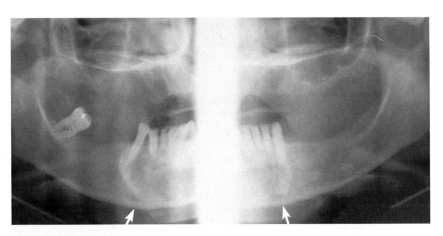

Figure 5-61
SQUAMOUS
ODONTOGENIC TUMOR
A vague radiolucency is noted in the anterior portion of the mandible and extends from canine to canine with the superior margin being the alveolar crest and inferior margin the inferior cortex.

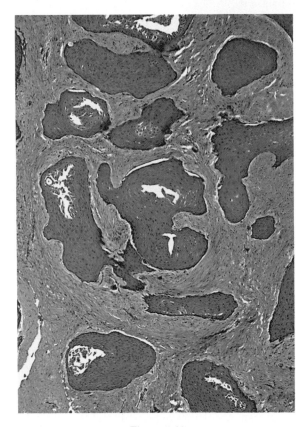

Figure 5-62
SQUAMOUS ODONTOGENIC TUMOR
Islands of squamous epithelium are discretely scattered through a dense, modestly cellular connective tissue stroma.

the alveolar segment of bone directly involving and surrounding the tooth root. Margins tend to be well corticated (fig. 5-61), although occasionally, a more ill-defined margin may mimic periodontal disease, the major radiographic differential diagnosis. Lesions arising in multiple quadrants have been reported (77) as well as multicentric familial lesions (75).

Microscopic Findings. Bland squamous epithelium in the form of discrete islands (fig. 5-62) or anastomosing strands is surrounded by mature fibrous connective tissue of moderate vascularity. Plump ovoid to spindle-shaped, evenly spaced fibroblasts are separated by fibrillar collagen. The squamous epithelial component demonstrates a characteristic flattened, smoothly contoured connective tissue interface. There is no stellate reticulum, peripheral columnar cell layer with palisaded nuclei, or any other features reminiscent of ameloblastoma (fig. 5-63). The squamous cells show no atypia and have well-defined intercellular bridges. Individual cell keratinization is uncommon. Calcified areas may be found, frequently in juxtaposition to mature keratin. These tend to appear more bone-like than cementum-like in nature. Central epithelial cell degeneration within larger epithelial islands is often noted (fig. 5-64). Less frequently, spherical, eosinophilic masses that stain strongly with PAS may be seen. Odontogenic cysts of inflammatory or developmental origin may contain proliferations of cells forming discrete squamous islands (79). In such instances, a microscopic appearance similar to that of the squamous odontogenic tumor may be noted but is less dominant than in that lesion (82).

spectrum, with a predilection for the anterior portion of the maxilla and the posterior portion of the mandible. Maxillary lesions tend to be more aggressive than their mandibular counterparts (74). Radiographically, there is a semilunar or triangular, well-defined radiolucency within

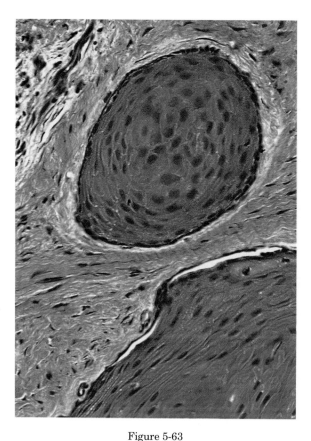

Figure 5-63
SQUAMOUS ODONTOGENIC TUMOR
An island of squamous epithelium with flattened peripheral cells and more plump central cells is characteristic of this lesion. The stroma consists of fibroblasts separated by bands of collagen.

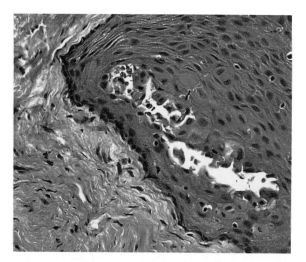

Figure 5-64
SQUAMOUS ODONTOGENIC TUMOR
A medium-power view demonstrates early cystic degeneration within a squamous island.

Differential Diagnosis. The most important differential diagnosis is ameloblastoma with acanthomatous features and desmoplastic ameloblastoma. Primary intraosseous carcinoma and odontogenic carcinoma must also be considered; however, these display cytologically malignant features in contrast to the bland features of squamous odontogenic tumor. Ameloblastoma can be distinguished by the presence of peripheral palisaded columnar cells in which nuclei reverse polarity away from the basement membrane and a stellate reticulum component with acanthomatous change within the cellular islands.

Consideration must also be given to desmoplastic ameloblastoma with fibro-osseous type radiographic changes. The centrally placed epithelial cells tend to be polygonal to spindle shaped. Unlike squamous odontogenic tumor, desmo-

plastic ameloblastoma invades between bone trabeculae and occasionally, active new bone forms about the margins of the lesion. Occasional tumor islands within desmoplastic ameloblastoma may show the typical structure of a follicular ameloblastoma with peripheral polarized columnar cells and stellate reticulum (81).

Treatment and Prognosis. Extraction of the involved tooth or teeth in conjunction with conservative surgical removal of the lesion is the treatment of choice. In the rare case of clinically more aggressive behavior, as with some maxillary lesions, a wider surgical resection margin and close follow-up is recommended. Peripheral or extraosseous lesions require simple excision with a thin rim of clinically uninvolved tissue. Multicentric presentation may occur, albeit uncommonly, and should be a consideration during evaluation and follow-up.

Odontogenic Ghost Cell Tumor

Definition. The odontogenic ghost cell tumor is a rare, locally aggressive odontogenic neoplasm arising de novo or from a preexisting calcifying odontogenic cyst (89). It is so named because of the presence of keratinized ghost cells occurring in association with an ameloblastomatous type epithelial component and a calcifying odontogenic cyst (92). The term *odontogenic ghost*

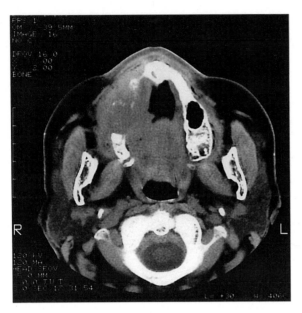

Figure 5-65
ODONTOGENIC GHOST CELL TUMOR
An expansile and destructive lesion of the maxilla obliterates the buccal and palatal components, and extends into buccal soft tissues and superiorly into the maxillary sinus.

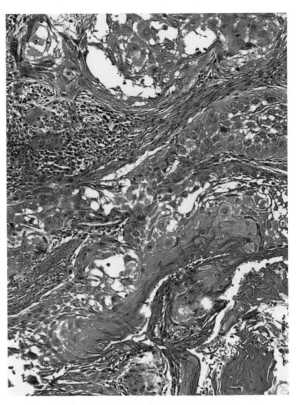

Figure 5-66
ODONTOGENIC GHOST CELL TUMOR
A medium-power photomicrograph shows keratinizing ghost cells in association with polygonal epithelial cells that contain centrally placed vesicular nuclei and prominent nucleoli.

cell carcinoma has been applied to the frankly malignant counterpart.

Clinical Features. A rare lesion, the odontogenic ghost cell tumor arises across a wide age spectrum (second to seventh decades) and is usually noted as an intraosseous process, although three cases have originated in an extraosseous location (93). Raubenheimer's review (93) documented a total of 10 central and peripheral cases in the English literature, with an additional 2 malignant cases (84,90) and a single intraosseous case (83) reported since that time.

Clinical presentation may include a nonhealing extraction site (91), jawbone expansion (86), painful swelling, ulcerated mass, and asymptomatic swelling (85). The clinical course is generally an aggressive one, with multiple recurrences and distant metastases (86,90). Such an aggressive quality has led some to consider this a variant of ameloblastoma (84,87,91,93,94).

Extraosseous lesions behave in a less aggressive fashion, although mucosal infiltration is common (93). Greater experience needs to be garnered, however, prior to establishing prognostic conclusions since only three peripheral cases have been reported (93).

Radiologic Findings. An irregular and destructive, variably mixed, radiolucent-radiopaque lesion is noted. The tumor may cross the midline, may be expansile, and may infiltrate into adjacent sites including the antrum and nasal and ethmoid sinuses (fig. 5-65) (86,91). Complete opacification of the maxillary sinus may be noted, while poorly demarcated features secondary to buccal and lingual cortical destruction have been seen (85).

Microscopic Findings. The epithelial component resembles an ameloblastoma occurring in association with a calcifying odontogenic cyst (figs. 5-66, 5-67). Additionally, pale-staining ghost cells, some of which demonstrate variable dystrophic mineralization, are noted. Cytologic atypia may be present within the epithelial component focally or diffusely. More specifically, the epithelial component is characterized by the presence of large, pleomorphic, polygonal cells

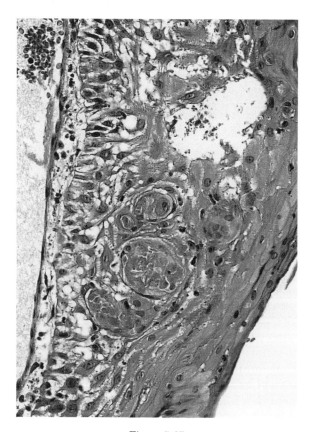

Figure 5-67
ODONTOGENIC GHOST CELL TUMOR
A peripheral columnar cell population is adjacent to rounded masses of keratinizing ghost cells.

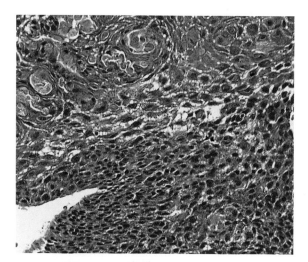

Figure 5-68
ODONTOGENIC GHOST CELL TUMOR
Spindled epithelial cells separate nests of ghost cells from malignant epithelial cells characterized by enlarged hyperchromatic nuclei and a small focus of necrosis.

with central vesicular to hyperchromatic nuclei (fig. 5-68). Dentinoid material may be present (88,95), while ghost cell keratinization is a consistent finding. Necrosis is variable.

Treatment and Prognosis. From the few cases reported to arise within the jaws, it appears that resection with wide margins should be performed. Partial maxillectomy or mandibulectomy in association with a metastatic disease evaluation is advised. Metastases have been documented in 2 of 10 intraosseous cases (86,90). Wide local excision of peripheral lesions is advised, followed by careful long-term assessment.

MESENCHYMAL TUMORS

Odontogenic Myxoma

Definition. The odontogenic myxoma is a relatively uncommon odontogenic tumor of mesenchymal/ectomesenchymal origin (109), with a relatively high recurrence rate and microscopic features similar to those of the soft tissue myxoma (114). Controversy exists as to whether intraosseous myxomas occur in extragnathic locations (97,98,114a).

Histogenesis. This tumor is considered to originate from undifferentiated odontogenic mesenchyme of the dental papilla of the developing tooth (figs. 5-69–5-71). The dental papilla is an ectomesenchymal derivative of the neural crest (107). Histochemical and immunohistochemical investigations of the odontogenic myxoma suggest an origin from fibroblasts, histiocytic elements, or myofibroblastic cells (111).

Clinical Features. The odontogenic myxoma usually develops in tooth-bearing areas, although it may arise within oral soft tissues (105). Most myxomas are diagnosed in the second or third decades of life, while children and those in the sixth decade and beyond are seldom affected (106). Several series failed to demonstrate a gender predilection (96,99,102) although a study by Barros et al. (96) noted over 60 percent of cases in females. The most frequently involved sites are the tooth-bearing areas of the mandible or maxilla. The rate of growth is generally slow and the patient is usually asymptomatic. The lesion may be found incidentally on routine oral

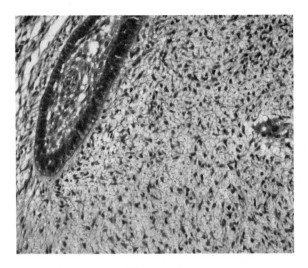

Figure 5-69
DENTAL PAPILLA
The dental papilla of a developing tooth in utero is highly cellular and represents the pulpal precursor.

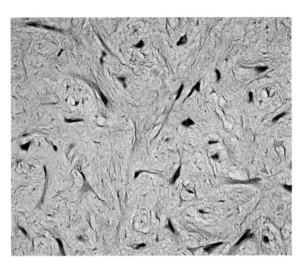

Figure 5-71
DENTAL PAPILLA
Swirling spindle to stellate fibroblastic cells within this dental papilla mimic those within the odontogenic myxoma.

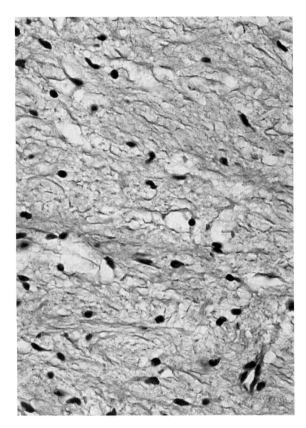

Figure 5-70
DENTAL PAPILLA
This dental papilla was present in the mandible of a 3-year-old child. It represented a developing permanent tooth bud papilla. The degree of cellularity is similar to the odontogenic myxoma.

or panoramic radiographic evaluation or it may present as an expansion of the affected jaw segment (fig. 5-72). Spreading, migration, and loosening of teeth within the affected area are commonly noted (100,113).

Radiologic Findings. Radiographically, the odontogenic myxoma may present as a unilocular or multilocular radiolucent lesion (figs. 5-73–5-76). It may be well defined with sclerotic margins or ill-defined with diffuse margins (96,108). When evaluating a multilocular radiolucency of this type, the differential diagnosis should include ameloblastoma, odontogenic keratocyst, aneurysmal bone cyst, central or intraosseous hemangioma, central giant cell granuloma, cherubism, and metastatic cancer (101). Careful evaluation of the radiolucency often reveals fine trabeculations, a feature useful in differentiating this lesion from central giant cell granuloma (108). Multilocular odontogenic myxomas tend to be larger than their unicystic counterparts.The tumor often causes root displacement rather than root resorption. Cortical expansion is commonly noted, while perforation into surrounding soft tissues is rare.

Gross Findings. The margins of the odontogenic myxoma may be lobulated and well defined in some cases. In more gelatinous lesions the margins are usually ill-defined. On cut section, the surface may be homogeneous and translucent,

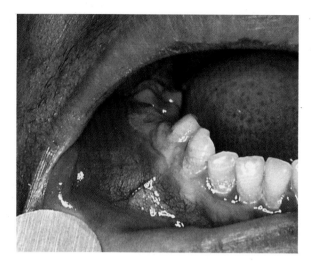

Figure 5-72
ODONTOGENIC MYXOMA
An expansile lesion has obliterated the mucobuccal fold and occupies the body of the mandible.

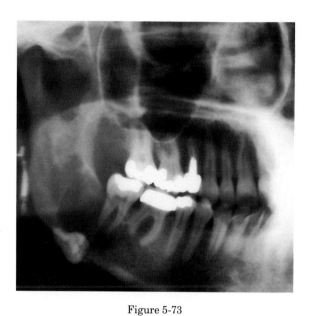

Figure 5-73
ODONTOGENIC MYXOMA
A well-defined radiolucency associated with an un-erupted third molar tooth is situated at the angle of the mandible. The entirely lucent lesion extends superiorly to the mid-portion of the ramus and anteriorly to the mesial aspect of the first molar.

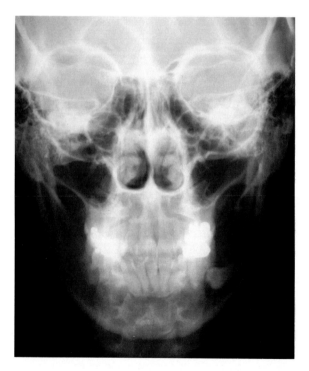

Figure 5-74
ODONTOGENIC MYXOMA
A posterior-anterior view of a mandibular odontogenic myxoma demonstrates a fully formed molar tooth within the radiolucent lesion.

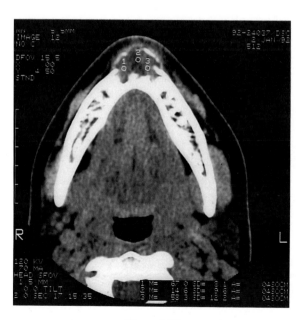

Figure 5-75
ODONTOGENIC MYXOMA
An axial CT scan demonstrates a paramedian, expansile radiolucency. Delicate, ill-defined osseous striations may be noted within the radiolucent defect.

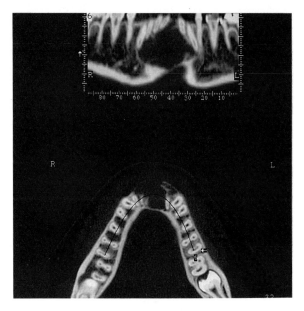

Figure 5-76
ODONTOGENIC MYXOMA

An axial and coronal reconstructed CT shows this odontogenic myxoma to be splaying the incisor and canine roots. Well-demarcated margins are evident on the coronal reconstructed image.

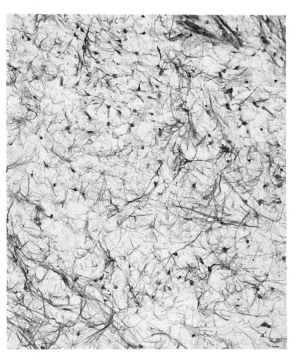

Figure 5-78
ODONTOGENIC MYXOMA

A poorly cellular odontogenic myxoma has widely separated stellate cellular elements. Long cytoplasmic tendrils and collagen fibers comprise much of the tissue.

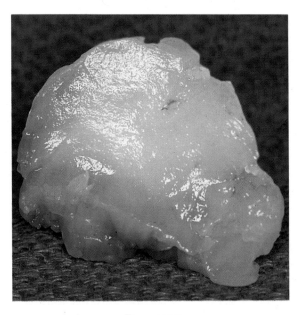

Figure 5-77
ODONTOGENIC MYXOMA

On cut section this odontogenic myxoma demonstrates a typically homogeneous, slightly translucent texture and smooth margins.

and retain its shape (fig. 5-77) while lesions of a more gelatinous nature collapse or become fragmented. More heavily collagenous lesions tend to be firm and cohesive.

Microscopic Findings. Bipolar and stellate cells are loosely and evenly arranged in a myxoid to slightly fibrous stroma (figs. 5-78, 5-79). Collagen fibers of variable density are present and their distribution is uniform within any particular lesion (106). Most cells are slender and elongated, with branching cytoplasmic processes extending away from centrally placed nuclei. Capillaries may be prominent in the lesion. Nests of odontogenic epithelium may be present in variable amounts (fig. 5-80) or may be absent. Nuclei tend to be rounded when cut in cross section and fusiform in longitudinal section (fig. 5-81). The stroma is rich in acid mucopolysaccharides, particularly chondroitin sulfate and hyaluronic acid; the latter accounts for nearly 75 percent of glycosaminoglycans present (110). This imparts to the lesion qualities similar to those of the

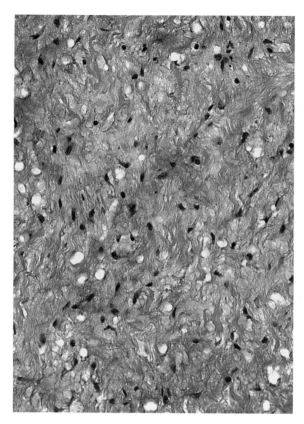

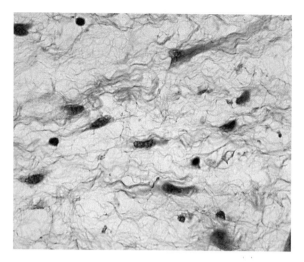

Figure 5-80
ODONTOGENIC MYXOMA
A high-power view reveals delicate fibrillar qualities of the
stroma, within which are uniformly dispersed fibroblastic cells.

Figure 5-79
ODONTOGENIC MYXOMA
In contrast to figure 5-78, this odontogenic myxoma is
more cellular, with an intervening amphophilic hyaluronic
acid-rich stroma.

chondromyxoid fibroma and the dental follicle.
Positivity for S-100 protein, vimentin, neuron-
specific enolase, glial fibrillary acidic protein,
desmin, and factor VIII–related protein antigen
have been described in the tumor cells by
Lombardi et al (104); however, Takahashi et al.
(111) were unable to document positivity for neu-
ron-specific enolase, S-100 alpha and beta units,
and factor VIII–related antigen.

Both dental follicles and dental papillae are
structural components of odontogenesis. The
dental papilla may become separated from the
corresponding developing tooth during surgery
and may be included within a surgical specimen
separate from any formed tooth elements. This
structure is the formative dental pulp whose
histologic features include a myxoid element
that may be rimmed by palisaded odontoblasts.

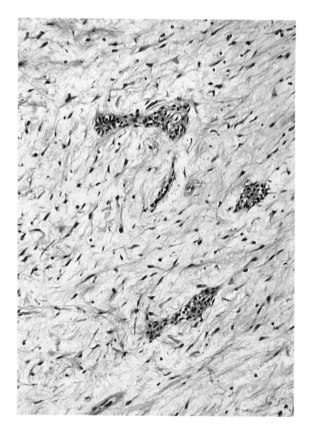

Figure 5-81
ODONTOGENIC MYXOMA
Occasionally, well-defined islands or strands of odontogenic epithelium may be present within the myxoma, however,
this is not a diagnostic criterion.

The odontoblasts manufacture the matrix for dentin formation and may be associated with premineralized eosinophilic dentinoid, a histologic feature that distinguishes it from odontogenic myxoma.

Of importance is the distinction of odontogenic myxoma from myxomatous dental papilla. Kim and Ellis (103) quote a nearly 6 percent incidence of overdiagnosis of odontogenic myxoma in material submitted from the dental papilla. In this study, 20 percent of dental follicles were misdiagnosed, with the most common misdiagnosis being the odontogenic myxoma. Additional distinguishing features include columnar ameloblastic epithelium, cuboidal cells, and squamous epithelium within the papilla. The myxomatous dental follicle, on the other hand, is generally more highly collagenized than the dental papilla and has lining odontogenic epithelium, odontogenic epithelial rests, and, often, foci of calcification. A myxoid component within follicular tissues is present in about 75 percent of cases; however, the myxoid material is focally deposited rather than diffuse and uniform (103). Additional entities to consider in a microscopic differential diagnosis include myxomatous degeneration of an intramandibular neurofibroma (111) and metastatic Wilms' tumor with myxoid features.

Treatment and Prognosis. Treatment is influenced by the nonencapsulated nature of odontogenic myxomas and their gelatinous quality. Small lesions may be curetted while larger lesions, in particular those with ill-defined radiographic margins, may require local resection. The less common, large, multilocular, expansile lesions may require en bloc resection and subsequent reconstruction (99). Finally, careful evaluation of bony margins should be undertaken. If myxoid-appearing areas are present within bone marrow, stains for mucopolysaccharides should be performed in order to establish the presence of tumor within this marginal tissue. The patient should be followed for a lengthy period of several years.

Sinonasal Myxoma

A rare myxomatous lesion of nonodontogenic origin which arises in the maxilla of children has been termed the sinonasal myxoma (98). The proximity of the sinonasal structures to the odontogenic apparatus notwithstanding, the sinonasal

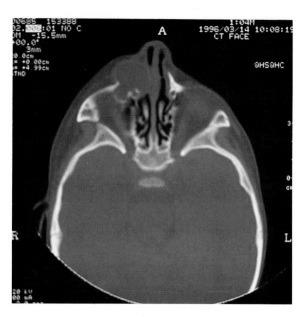

Figure 5-82
SINONASAL MYXOMA

An 18-month-old child has a mid-face asymmetry that represents a sinonasal myxoma. A well-defined mass in the anterior maxillary sinus region extends superiorly and surrounds the nasolacrimal duct.

myxoma has as its epicenter the sinonasal tract, with no suggestion of an odontogenic origin from a clinical or radiographic perspective (fig. 5-82). The anterior component of the maxillary sinus is the usual site of origin of this lesion, which is grossly and histologically similar to the odontogenic myxoma. The lesion is friable and gelatinous to mucoid in nature, and may be difficult to remove completely. It has a potential for local destructive growth and recurrence.

Histologically, the most important differential diagnosis is embryonal rhabdomyosarcoma. Other differential diagnoses include inflammatory nasal polyp with stromal atypia, heterotopic central nervous system tissue or so-called glioma, myxoid chondrosarcoma, chordoma, benign mixed tumor, inspissated mucus, mucocele, and low-grade fibrosarcoma. The loose stroma contains abundant, uniformly distributed, stellate-shaped cells with ample cytoplasm which contain bland-appearing nuclei and slender elongated cytoplasmic processes. Necrosis, inflammation, and cellular atypia are absent.

Treatment requires excision with adequate margins because of the potential for recurrence.

Odontogenic Fibroma

Definition. The odontogenic fibroma is a rare, benign, mesenchymal odontogenic neoplasm composed of a spectrum of fibrous, myxoid, and collagenized tissue and the presence or absence of odontogenic epithelial nests or cords. A rare peripheral or extragnathic variant has also been described.

Clinical and Radiologic Features. There is a wide age range of occurrence for the intraosseous form of this lesion (first through ninth decades), with a female predilection. The highest frequency is within the maxilla anterior to the molar dentition (123,125). When found in the mandibular arch, lesions are more frequently noted posterior to the first molars (fig. 5-83) and may occasionally be associated with an unerupted third molar tooth. Lesions in the anterior maxillary region may present as a palatal cortical depression rather than an expansion. An exception to the usual female dominance and maxillary predilection is the series of Gunhan et al. (122) in which 13 of 18 cases were found in the mandible and 55 percent were in males. The tumor is slow growing with a limited tendency to recur after surgical enucleation (119,133).

Recently, a rare juxtaposition of central giant cell granuloma and central odontogenic fibroma-like lesion has been reported. Features included a wide age range, jaw expansion, occasional cortical perforation, and a unilocular or multilocular radiographic pattern (115,130).

Radiographically, most odontogenic fibromas present as unilocular lesions with well-defined, thinly corticated, hyperostotic margins (fig. 5-84). Less frequently, they present as multilocular lesions and rarely as a mixed radiolucent-radiopaque process with ill-defined, blending, diffuse borders (125). Root divergence and separation as well as resorption may be noted. When located in the maxilla, the odontogenic fibroma favors the anterior segment, while mandibular lesions are more commonly noted in the molar and premolar regions. Larger lesions may produce bony expansion without cortical erosion or perforation. Root resorption may occasionally be noted as may root divergence or separation between teeth.

The peripheral variant of odontogenic fibroma is generally solitary and uncommon. Rarely, it may be multiple and must be differentiated from

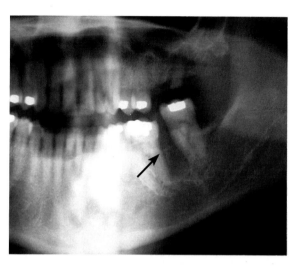

Figure 5-83
ODONTOGENIC FIBROMA
A radiolucency is located between the mandibular first and second molar teeth. The superior margins are ill defined and the inferior margin is thinly corticated. There is slight separation between these teeth, and the second molar tooth is supraerupted.

the more commonly occurring peripheral ossifying fibroma (117,126). Age of onset varies widely (11 to 76 years), with a slight male predilection. Mandible and maxilla are equally involved, with the attached gingiva most commonly affected (see below) (120).

Gross Findings. This is a well-defined, encapsulated, firm mass with a solid white appearance. On cut section, a homogeneous, glistening quality is appreciated. The mass may be smooth to lobulated along the external surface, with a definite cleavage plane between it and surrounding bone, permitting enucleation.

Microscopic Findings. A wide variation in histopathologic features has caused confusion in interpretation and nosologic complexity. Controversy exists with regard to separation of a single entity into various histologic types, although the most recent WHO odontogenic tumor classification (1992) does not recognize subsets of this entity (128). While a so-called simple form and a WHO variant have been described (121), this separation serves no useful purpose. The lesion exhibits a wide spectrum of appearances, ranging from a predominantly myxoid and fibroblastic tumor to a densely hyalinized lesion. It may be moderately cellular to relatively acellular, with or without the presence of calcification. Odontogenic epithelium

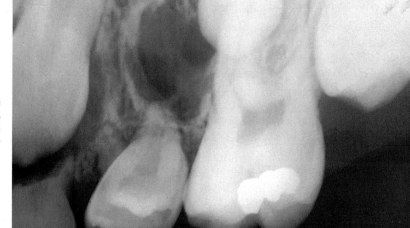

Figure 5-84
ODONTOGENIC FIBROMA

An odontogenic fibroma in the maxilla is characterized by a thin corticated periphery and a central lucency with an ill-defined loculated quality.

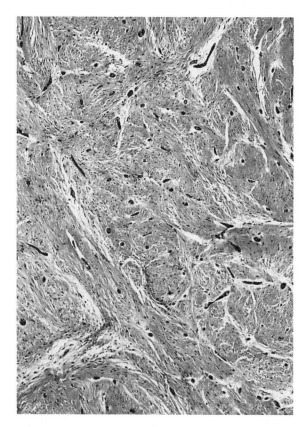

Figure 5-85
ODONTOGENIC FIBROMA

Whorled clusters of fibroblastic elements with ample amounts of collagen characterize the background stroma of this odontogenic fibroma. Uniformly scattered thin strands, small rosettes, and clusters of odontogenic epithelium are seen.

may be absent, scanty, and inactive appearing, or easily discernible, forming cords and nests throughout the lesion. On occasion, follicular odontogenic epithelial structures may be found.

The least histologically complex ("simple") form of this entity consists of a well-defined and circumscribed mass of fusiform to stellate-shaped fibroblasts arranged in a slightly whorled to storiform pattern, with a stromal background of eosinophilic, finely to slightly coarse, fibrillar collagen with ample amounts of protoglycan material (figs. 5-85, 5-86). Individual cells are uniformly distributed, with evenly stained nuclei demonstrating a spindled to ovoid shape. While usually fibrous in nature the intercellular matrix may be myxoid. The amount of odontogenic epithelium is widely variable, ranging from none to a uniformly distributed pattern of small nests or thin, elongated strands. There is no formation of stellate reticulum or mesenchymal "induction" by the odontogenic epithelial component. Calcification of the dystrophic type may be noted within the stroma and, less commonly, cementum or dentin-like substance may be present.

Histologic variants include a granular cell form and a variant with a giant cell granuloma component. The latter may represent a "collision effect" resulting from simultaneous development of a giant cell granuloma and an odontogenic fibroma. Alternatively, the odontogenic fibroma

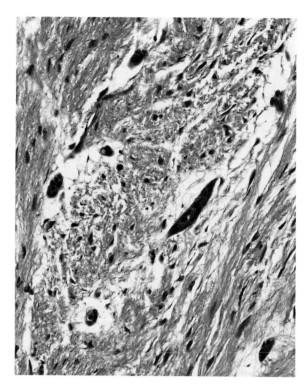

Figure 5-86
ODONTOGENIC FIBROMA
A higher power view of the stroma shows fibroblastic cells aligned in parallel bands in association with parallel arrays of small odontogenic epithelial clusters.

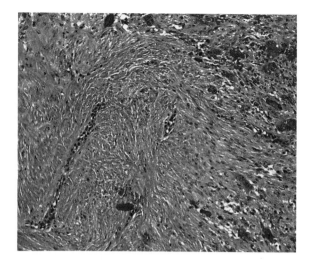

Figure 5-87
ODONTOGENIC FIBROMA
A low-power view of a hybrid odontogenic fibroma and central giant cell granuloma with hemorrhagic background, spindle-shaped cells, and scattered multinucleate giant cells. The odontogenic fibroma component consists of thin strands of odontogenic epithelium surrounded by a well-collagenized and moderately cellular fibroblastic background.

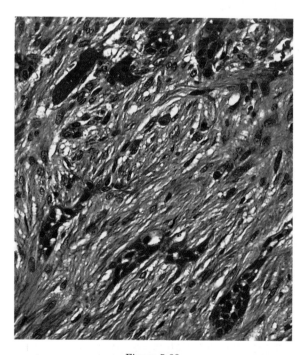

Figure 5-88
ODONTOGENIC FIBROMA
A higher power view of the juxtaposed central giant cell granuloma and odontogenic fibroma, with multinucleate giant cells in close association with the small odontogenic epithelial cell islands. The stromal component within the giant cell lesion has a vacuolated appearance while that of the odontogenic fibroma is more dense.

may induce a giant cell granuloma–like response in a manner similar to the association between other primary bone neoplasms and aneurysmal bone cysts (figs. 5-87, 5-88) (115,124,129). This hybrid lesion also affects patients of a wide age range; the radiographic features are similar to those of giant cell granuloma. Unlike pure odontogenic fibroma, the lesion may perforate bone and has a higher risk of recurrence (120).

The rare *granular cell odontogenic fibroma* had previously been considered to be an ameloblastic fibroma variant (132). From a clinical and radiographic perspective it is no different than the usual odontogenic fibroma. The granular cell component is composed of round, large cells with a delicately granular, lightly basophilic cytoplasm and evenly stained, small eccentric nuclei (fig. 5-89). Immunoperoxidase stains for prekeratin and S-100 protein within the granular cells are negative. Ultrastructurally, however, the granular cells contain lysosome-like organelles which are identical to those noted in the soft

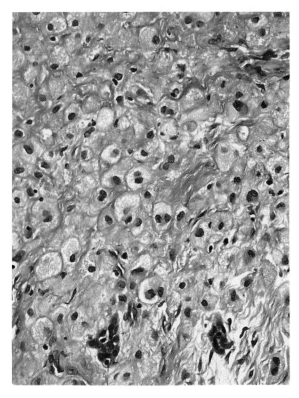

Figure 5-89
ODONTOGENIC FIBROMA

An odontogenic fibroma with granular cell features is characterized by enlarged stromal cells with delicately granular cytoplasm. Small clusters of odontogenic epithelium are also seen within the stromal tissue.

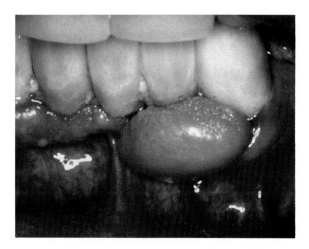

Figure 5-90
PERIPHERAL ODONTOGENIC FIBROMA

This peripheral odontogenic fibroma manifests as a firm, pale, broadly based gingival mass which involves the mandibular attached gingiva.

Peripheral Odontogenic Fibroma

The peripheral odontogenic fibroma is the extraosseous counterpart of the central odontogenic fibroma. This lesion is uncommon and has been included in previous classifications under the terms odontogenic epithelial hamartoma and peripheral ameloblastic fibrodentinoma. We consider all such lesions as examples of peripheral odontogenic fibroma.

The clinical presentation is that of a sessile, firm, painless mass of the attached gingiva (fig. 5-90) which may simulate fibrous hyperplasia, fibroma, peripheral giant cell granuloma, peripheral ossifying fibroma, or pyogenic granuloma. A mean size of 1 cm has been noted, with a range from 0.3 to 2.0 cm (116). The duration of such lesions is variable, ranging from a few months to several years, with a mean of 1.4 years. The attached gingiva over the facial aspect of the mandibular arch is the favored site. Radiographically, there are scattered calcifications, however, the underlying alveolar bone is unaffected. Multifocal cases have been reported and a single case was associated with cutaneous and ocular lesions, raising the possibility of an as yet undefined syndrome (120). Histologically, the lesion is identical to the central odontogenic fibroma.

Osteoid trabeculae may be noted within the peripheral lesion, necessitating distinction from

tissue granular cell myoblastoma (134). The epithelial component lies within lobules of granular cells in the form of small nests composed of cuboidal to low columnar cells with eccentric, round to ovoid nuclei. Larger aggregates of epithelial cells may show a stellate, reticulum-like appearance; they are negative with mucicarmine or PAS staining techniques.

From a histologic standpoint the differential diagnosis may include an enlarged or hyperplastic dental follicle (127), central desmoplastic fibroma (131), or infantile myofibromatosis (124),

Treatment and Prognosis. Enucleation followed by curettage is usually adequate given the physical characteristics and marginal qualities of this lesion, even though true encapsulation is absent. Recurrences are uncommon. In the unusual case in which a giant cell granuloma is also present, an increased risk of recurrence following curettage has been noted (130).

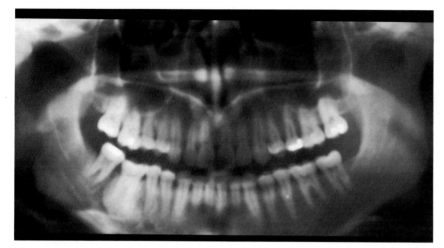

Figure 5-91
CEMENTOBLASTOMA
A panoramic film demonstrates the presence of a densely opacified mass juxtaposed to the roots of the mandibular left first molar tooth. A well-delineated, circumferential peripheral radiolucency can be appreciated.

peripheral ossifying fibroma, a reactive process involving the gingiva (117). The distinguishing feature is the presence of odontogenic epithelium in the odontogenic fibroma, and its absence in ossifying fibroma. The connective tissue component within the peripheral ossifying fibroma tends to be more cellular than within the peripheral odontogenic fibroma.

Conservative, local surgical excision is the treatment of choice.

Cementoblastoma

Definition. The cementoblastoma is a rare benign neoplasm of cementoblastic origin occurring in juxtaposition to the roots of the teeth. It is composed of a fibrovascular stroma that separates spicules or masses of mineralized matrix resembling cementum, rimmed by plump cementoblasts. Histologically, the lesion appears identical to osteoblastoma and comprises approximately 4 percent of cementum-containing lesions (135).

Clinical Features. Most cases of benign cementoblastoma are found within the mandible, usually within the posterior segment of the alveolus. A slight female predilection has been noted (143), with most cases occurring in patients in the third decade. Pain is a presenting feature in many cases. Larger lesions may expand the affected area. Nearly all cases affect erupted permanent teeth, although involvement of the deciduous dentition has been reported (137,145) as well as occurrence in relation to unerupted teeth (138,140).

Radiographic and pathologic correlation is crucial in establishing the diagnosis. A rounded mass of radiopaque tissue with a narrow radiolucent rim, in intimate association with a tooth root, is typical (figs. 5-91, 5-92). Variable degrees of associated root resorption may be seen, although the root may be obscured by the density of the mass. An occlusal film may be useful in defining the expansile nature of the lesion.

Gross Findings. A mass of cementum-like tissue is fused to the root of the tooth as a round, hard swelling with contoured peripheral margins (fig. 5-92B,C).

Pathologic Findings. Dense masses of cementum-like tissue with prominent basophilic incremental lines, irregular lacunae, and cellular fibrovascular stroma are characteristic (fig. 5-93). An attenuated, cellular, fibrous connective tissue margin is present, corresponding to the radiolucent rim. Plump cementoblasts with large nuclei line the surface of the calcified tissue in a linear pattern (fig. 5-94). Cementocytes within the lacunae are also large but smaller than the marginally located cementoblasts (fig. 5-95). Peripheral features include a prominent, often dilated, vasculature and a spoke-like or radially oriented array of bony spicules at the stromal/calcified tissue interface. Resorption of root surface cementum by osteoclast type giant cells may be seen.

The cementoblastoma histologically resembles osteoblastoma or osteoid osteoma (142,144), however, osteoblastoma does not develop in relationship to a tooth root (141). Distinguishing

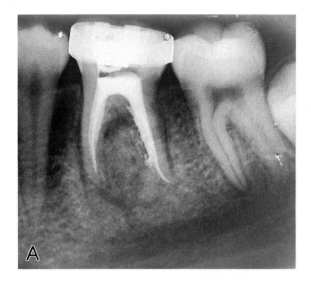

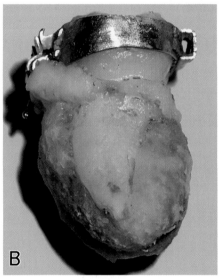

Figure 5-92
CEMENTOBLASTOMA

A: A dense radiopaque mass is contiguous with the roots of the mandibular first molar.

B: The gross specimen of the extracted first molar demonstrates the nodular calcified mass which is fused to the roots.

C: A survey view of the decalcified histologic section shows root resorption in association with the cemental mass.

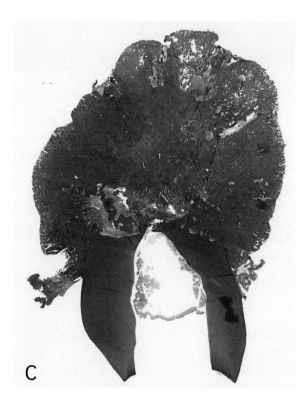

cementoblastoma from osteoblastoma is difficult and requires demonstration of fusion with and even resorption of the involved tooth root.

Cemental tissue may be distinguished from bone by specific patterns of collagen within the unmineralized matrix material. With polarized light, the collagenous component of the cementum demonstrates a random and irregular arrangement (fig. 5-96), while the mineralized phase consists of low crystalline hydroxyapatite (139).

Treatment and Prognosis. Management of the cementoblastoma is surgical, including removal of the affected tooth and the associated mass. On occasion, retention of the tooth may be possible through prior endodontic therapy, fol-

lowed by surgical removal of the lesion in association with partial root amputation (136). Recurrence does not develop if the mass is totally removed; incomplete excision, however, will usually be followed by recurrence.

MIXED TUMORS

Ameloblastic Fibroma/Fibro-odontoma

Definition. Ameloblastic fibroma and the closely related fibro-odontoma are benign, mixed epithelial-mesenchymal odontogenic neoplasms in which the mesenchymal compartment resembles the connective tissue of the dental papilla

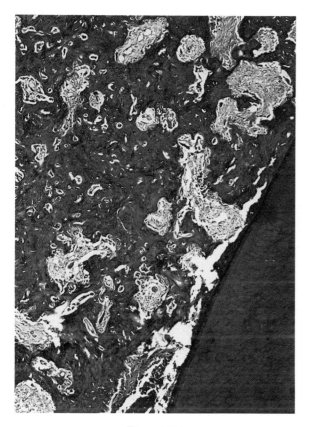

Figure 5-93
CEMENTOBLASTOMA
A low-power photomicrograph shows the relationship between the tooth root, periodontal ligament space, and cementoblastoma composed of fused islands of cementum and cellular stroma.

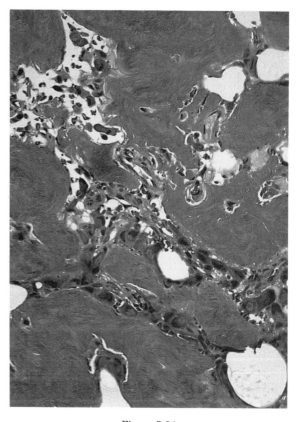

Figure 5-94
CEMENTOBLASTOMA
A high-power view shows nodular masses of cementum lined by plump cementoblasts.

while the epithelial component, composed of islands of cells with stellate reticulum, resembles early enamel organ development. Separation of ameloblastic fibroma from ameloblastic fibro-odontoma is dependent on the presence of inductive change, with formulation of mineralized dental hard tissue products in the latter.

Clinical and Radiologic Features. The ameloblastic fibroma represents only 2 percent of odontogenic tumors (152). Although a mixed odontogenic tumor, some classification schemes have placed this entity within the group of odontogenic tumors demonstrating the so-called inductive effect. The mean age of occurrence is 14 years, with an essentially equal distribution among males and females (155). Over 80 percent are found within the mandible and 88 percent within the posterior regions (155). Trodahl (156) noted that the most common presentation was

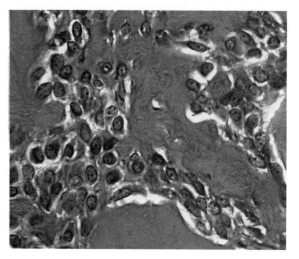

Figure 5-95
CEMENTOBLASTOMA
A high-power view shows rimming of cemental masses by cementoblasts.

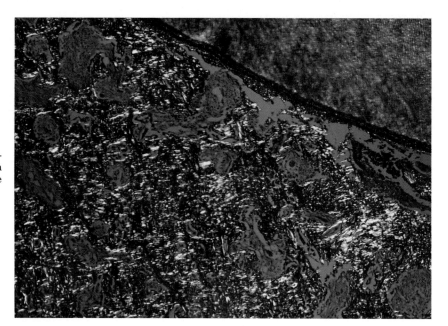

Figure 5-96
CEMENTOBLASTOMA
Polarized light shows a complex array of collagen fibers within the premineralized portion of the lesion.

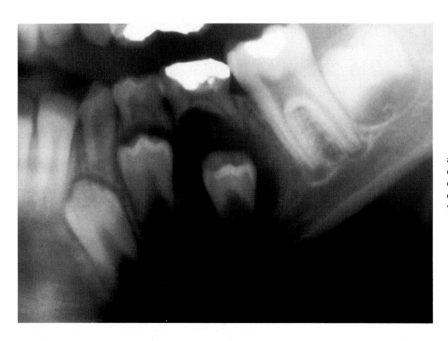

Figure 5-97
AMELOBLASTIC FIBROMA
A well-defined radiolucency is associated with unerupted mandibular premolar teeth. The second premolar tooth is at the epicenter of the lesion, which has a well-defined margin.

that of a swelling of the involved segment of jaw; one or more teeth may be absent.

The original description by Cahn and Blum (146) suggested that ameloblastic fibromas mature to odontomas. However, recurrent or residual tumor shows no evidence of such maturation, while ameloblastic fibroma has been reported beyond the period of odontogenesis. In other words, ameloblastic fibroma should predominate in young people and ameloblastic fibro-odontoma and finally the complex odontoma in older individuals. However, analysis has shown that these tumors occur within the same age group. The male to female ratio is 1.6 to 1 for ameloblastic fibroma and 1 to 2 for complex odontoma (147).

Radiographically, ameloblastic fibroma produces a well-defined radiolucency (fig. 5-97). This may be unilocular or multilocular, and is

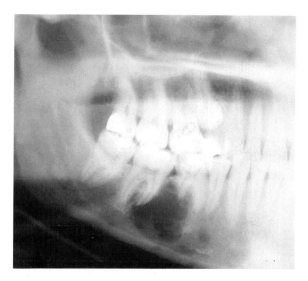

Figure 5-98
AMELOBLASTIC FIBROMA
A young adult has a sharply delimited radiolucency within the body of the mandible, extending from the alveolar crest to the inferior cortex. The margins are corticated and well defined with no associated impacted or unerupted tooth.

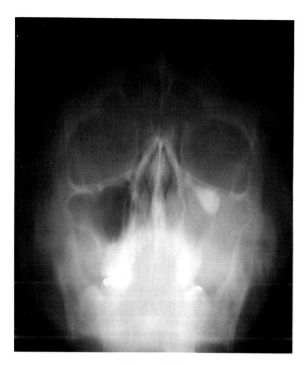

Figure 5-99
AMELOBLASTIC FIBROMA
A maxillary ameloblastic fibroma in an adolescent female demonstrates a superiorly displaced molar tooth in association with an opacified maxillary sinus and a considerable degree of buccal expansion. Margins are ill defined and the sinus is obliterated.

frequently associated with an unerupted tooth or located in an area where a tooth has failed to develop (150). The borders of the lesion are well defined with a thin, hyperostotic margin. Cortical expansion may be noted (fig. 5-98). When involving the maxilla, the sinus may appear opacified, with ill-defined margins (fig. 5-99).

The ameloblastic fibro-odontoma is considered to be a variant of ameloblastic fibroma from a clinical, radiographic, and histologic perspective. The mean age range is from 8.1 to 11.5 years, with the majority of patients under 10 years, while the male-female ratio ranges from 3 to 1 to a slight male predominance (150,155). Sixty-two percent of cases are found in the mandible, of which 54 percent occur in the posterior portion. In the maxilla, there is a nearly equal distribution in anterior and posterior segments (155).

Radiographically, the ameloblastic fibro-odontoma exhibits a unilocular or multilocular radiolucent appearance with well-defined, hyperostotic borders (fig. 5-100). Within the radiolucency, multiple radiopacities are present and these correspond to the odontoma component of the lesion. They manifest the same radiodensity as tooth structure and may appear as multiple, individual, small radiopacities or as a fused mass of dental

hard tissues (fig. 5-101). Often, an unerupted tooth is present within the lesion, either centrally or at one of the margins (fig. 5-102). Less commonly, only a small amount of calcifying dentin and enamel matrix may be noted within the radiolucent lesion. In some cases, the lesion may be predominantly radiopaque, with a lobulated to rounded peripheral margin and only a thin radiolucent rim at the periphery adjacent to the hyperostotic bony margin.

Gross Findings. Ameloblastic fibroma appears white to tan, with a translucent quality. Margins are well defined and smooth. The ameloblastic fibro-odontoma, on the other hand, is variable in texture, with the mineralized component ranging from gritty to predominantly nodular in areas of the odontoma component (fig. 5-103).

Microscopic Findings. Histologically, the ameloblastic fibroma is dominated by an immature connective tissue background reminiscent of the dental papilla. Within this background are

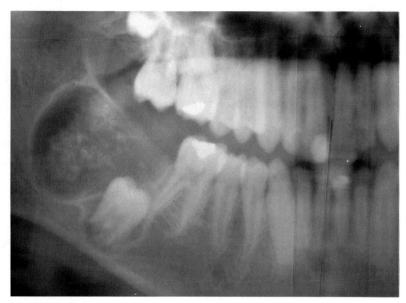

Figure 5-100
AMELOBLASTIC
FIBRO-ODONTOMA
An ameloblastic fibro-odontoma is adjacent to an impacted mandibular second molar. Granular opacities are uniformly distributed, while the periphery of the lesion is well corticated and clearly defined.

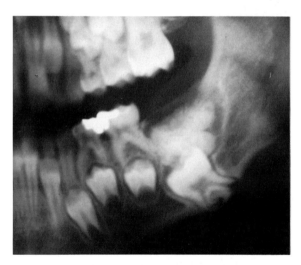

Figure 5-101
AMELOBLASTIC FIBRO-ODONTOMA
An unerupted mandibular first molar is displaced inferiorly, while the lobulate radiopaque mass representing the odontoma component of this lesion appears contiguous with the crown. The margins are well defined and corticated.

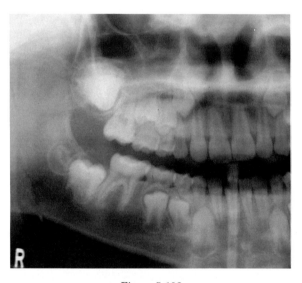

Figure 5-102
AMELOBLASTIC FIBRO-ODONTOMA
A maxillary ameloblastic fibro-odontoma is associated with an unerupted second molar tooth. The circular lesion has a hyperostotic margin. A dense opacity anteriorly is contiguous with the unerupted tooth.

islands and cords of cuboidal to columnar epithelial cells (fig. 5-104). The islands are reminiscent of the early stages of enamel organ development, including a central component with stellate reticulum type morphology (figs. 5-105, 5-106). At the interface between the epithelial and mesenchymal components, a well-defined basement membrane is evident; adjacent seams of hyaline, acel-

lular, eosinophilic material suggest induction of the adjacent mesenchyme. The mesenchymal or dental papilla-like element is composed of uniformly dispersed, bipolar to stellate-shaped cells with a delicate intercellular fibrillar and granular amorphous matrix. Both mesenchymal and epithelial cells are cytologically bland and no calcified material is produced.

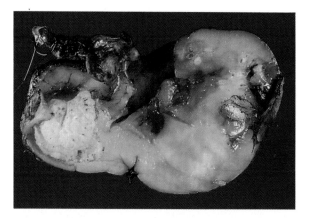

Figure 5-103
AMELOBLASTOMA FIBROMA

A gross specimen of an ameloblastic fibroma demonstrates the lobular configuration. Its internal heterogeneity includes a translucent soft tissue component and gnarled masses of enamel, dentin, and other tooth structures.

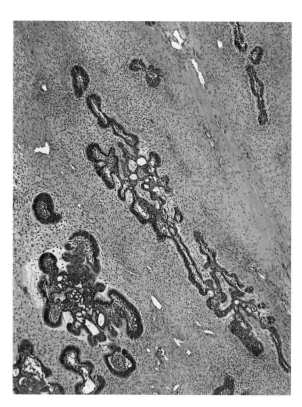

Figure 5-104
AMELOBLASTIC FIBROMA

An ameloblastic fibroma at low power consists of a uniform cellular mesenchymal background within which numerous small to larger islands and cords of odontogenic epithelium are scattered. Vascular features are readily demonstrated.

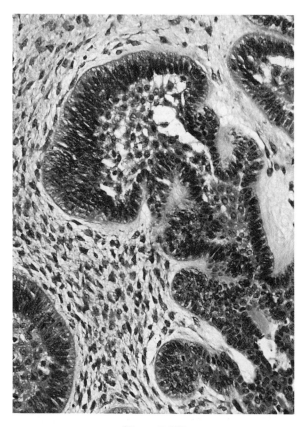

Figure 5-105
AMELOBLASTIC FIBROMA

The cellular matrix reminiscent of dental papilla supports a proliferating epithelial component characterized by a peripheral, tall columnar palisaded layer within which are stellate reticulum type cells. (Figures 5-105 and 5-106 are from the same patient.)

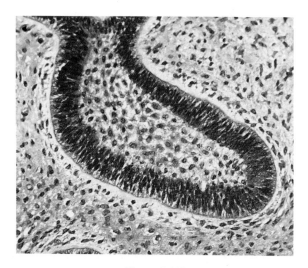

Figure 5-106
AMELOBLASTIC FIBROMA

A higher power view shows a discrete ameloblastic epithelial island with a well-defined basement membrane separating the island from the cellular mesenchyme. Stellate reticulum component is surrounded by a peripheral bordering layer.

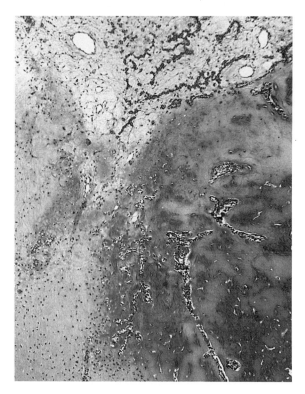

Figure 5-107
AMELOBLASTIC FIBROMA
An ameloblastic fibroma is characterized by a cellular mesenchymal stroma and cords of epithelial cells, some of which are surrounded by an eosinophilic osteodentin matrix. Such lesions have been designated as ameloblastic fibrodentinoma.

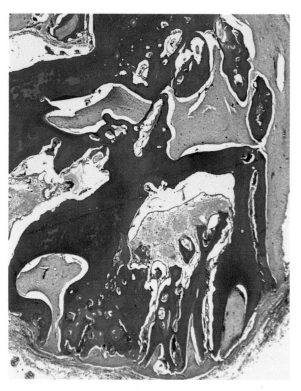

Figure 5-108
AMELOBLASTIC FIBRO-ODONTOMA
An ameloblastic fibro-odontoma at low power is characterized by a lobulated periphery and irregular masses of dentin and enamel matrix.

When dentin or osteodentin-like material is produced (fig. 5-107), the terms *ameloblastic fibrodentinoma* and *immature dentinoma* have been used (151,154). The dentinoid material in the area of hyalinization surrounding the epithelial islands is a result of aborted inductive change (157). Gardner (148) and Hansen and Ficarra (149) state that there is no difference in biologic behavior between ameloblastic fibroma and ameloblastic fibrodentinoma, and that all such lesions should be referred to as ameloblastic fibroma with a qualifying description regarding the presence of hyalinization or dentin-like material.

The ameloblastic fibro-odontoma contains enamel, enamel matrix, dentin, and cementum. The structure and arrangement of these mineralized elements may be haphazard or recognizable grossly or microscopically as teeth (figs. 5-108–5-110). When teeth or tooth-like structures are present, pulpal elements may be seen (fig. 5-111). Separation of ameloblastic fibroma

from ameloblastic fibro-odontoma is dependent on the presence of mineralized dental hard tissue products.

Histologic variants include lesions with granular cells and ghost cells. Controversy exists concerning the histogenesis of the granular cell variant of ameloblastic fibroma, with recent reports favoring a relationship to the central odontogenic fibroma with granular cell features (158). This is supported by the fact that vimentin has been demonstrated within the granular cells of the so-called ameloblastic fibroma (153). Ghost cells within an ameloblastic fibroma are a rare phenomenon and have no associated prognostic significance (152).

Treatment and Prognosis. Treatment consists of an excisional biopsy by way of enucleation. Where an unerupted tooth with eruptive potential is present, the tooth may be spared. Recurrence is unusual and the innocuous behavior of these tumors does not justify more aggressive

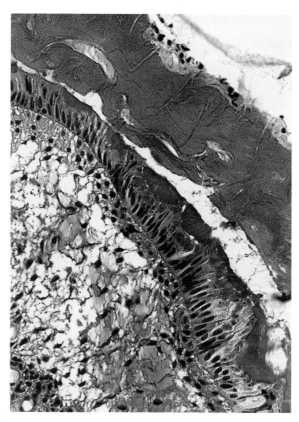

Figure 5-109
AMELOBLASTIC FIBRO-ODONTOMA
The ameloblastic fibro-odontoma shows an intimate association between the epithelial component and osteodentin. The formed element in this example is haphazard and consists of enamel matrix as well as dentin-like material.

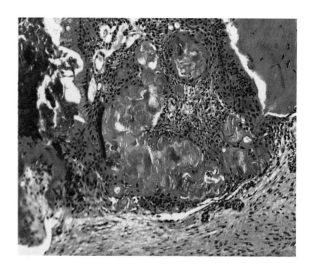

Figure 5-110
AMELOBLASTIC FIBRO-ODONTOMA
Sheets of odontogenic epithelium surround amorphous masses of enamel matrix-type material. Peripheral to this are sheets of osteodentin, an additional product manufactured within the lesion.

management. In the event of a recurrence, the resection may be more extensive and include a margin of normal bone.

Odontoma

Definition. Compound and complex odontomas are hamartomatous rather than neoplastic lesions composed of developed teeth or tooth-like masses derived from epithelial and mesenchymal odontogenic tissue. The term "compound" refers to the formation of recognizable tooth and the term "complex" to haphazardly arranged tooth elements. The WHO has continued to place these lesions into the neoplastic category (165); they account for between 18 and 65 percent of such tumors (162,170).

Clinical and Radiologic Features. The greatest prevalence is within the second decade

of life, with the median age at diagnosis ranging from 14 to 16 years (160,164), but they may be discovered at any age. There is an equal sex incidence and the most common location is the anterior portion of the maxilla. There is a predilection for complex odontomas to occur in the posterior segments of the jaws (160). Symptoms are usually absent. Occasionally, the lesion may become sufficiently large to produce bony expansion. Altered patterns of tooth eruption or impaction may occur (164). Rarely, odontomas erupt into the oral cavity or are located in oral soft tissues (161, 166,168). Extraoral and extragnathic odontomas unassociated with a teratoma are extremely rare. Such cases have been reported in the retrotympanic region and middle ear (159,169).

Radiographically, densely opaque masses in the presence or absence of an impacted or supernumerary tooth are characteristic (figs. 5-112, 5-113). A surrounding lucent zone of variable width is present, corresponding to a cystic component or a connective tissue capsule. Recognizable but stunted tooth-like forms may be seen. Margins may be smooth and bosselated or irregular and fissured. Peripheral to the limiting lucent rim, is a thin layer of dense cortical bone or a hyperostotic margin (fig. 5-114). When associated with impacted teeth, the odontoma is usually deep to the

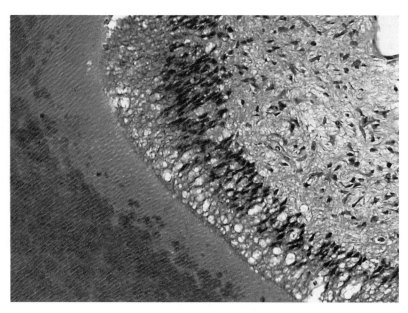

Figure 5-111
AMELOBLASTIC
FIBRO-ODONTOMA

In the odontoma component, pulpal tissue with an odontoblastic layer is seen immediately juxtaposed to a predentin matrix which blends into a calcospherite type of mineralization. The calcospherites ultimately fuse to form mature dentin.

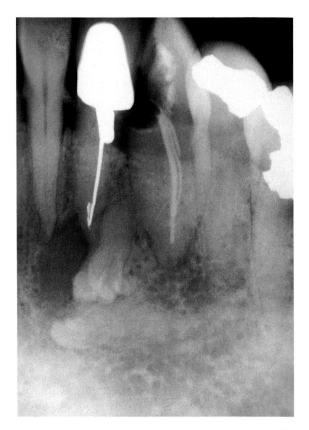

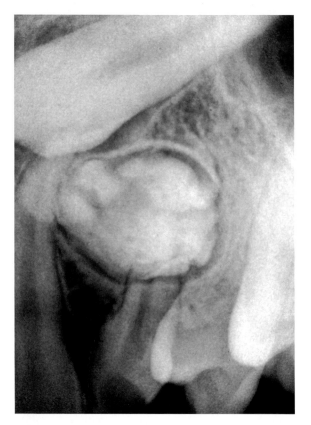

Figure 5-112
ODONTOMA

Left: A periapical radiograph demonstrates an ovoid radiolucency with two tooth-like elements situated laterally and inferiorly.

Right: A nodular radiopacity noted on this periapical film shows variable densities in association with a radiolucent halo and a well-corticated peripheral margin.

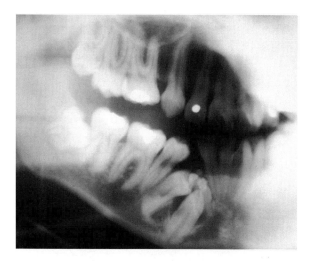

Figure 5-113
ODONTOMA
A densely opaque, well-defined lesion within the symphysis of the mandible characterizes this compound odontoma.

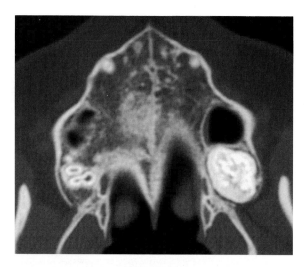

Figure 5-114
ODONTOMA
A CT scan of a complex odontoma of the posterior maxilla shows a thin radiolucent rim bordered by a hyperostotic margin. The odontoma component is exceedingly radiodense.

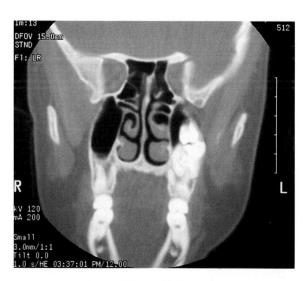

Figure 5-115
ODONTOMA
A coronal CT scan demonstrates a close association between the roots of an erupted maxillary first molar and a lobulated opacity representative of the odontoma. Superior to the odontoma is a displaced maxillary left second molar tooth extending toward the orbital floor.

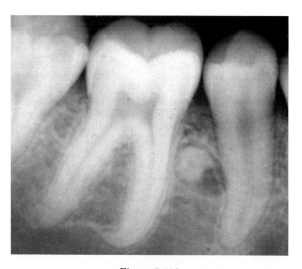

Figure 5-116
ODONTOMA
A small odontoma of the mandible is located between the second premolar and first molar teeth. It measured approximately 3 mm in diameter and was composed chiefly of dentin-like material.

opaque mass (fig. 5-115). Smaller odontomas may be situated between the roots of erupted teeth or superimposed upon them (fig. 5-116).

Microscopic Findings. Compound odontomas are characterized by a loose myxoid stroma within which are scattered multiple, single-rooted teeth or tooth-like structures. There is an organized relationship between enamel, dentin, and pulpal elements (fig. 5-117). Odontogenic epithelium is often of the reduced enamel type, with a double-layered cuboidal cell population lining the connective tissue component. Pulpal tissue with a well-defined tall columnar odontoblastic layer occupies the coronal and radicular

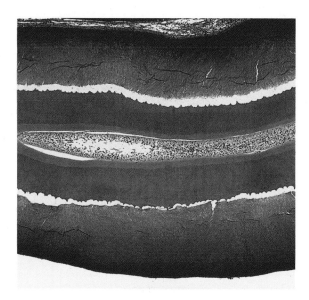

Figure 5-117
ODONTOMA

A compound odontoma with an orderly pattern of enamel, dentin, and pulpal tissue, each in their usual anatomic relationship.

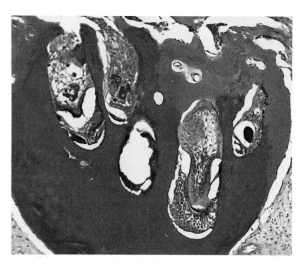

Figure 5-119
ODONTOMA

A complex odontoma composed predominantly of dentin encloses enamel matrix, droplet-like mineralizations characteristic of cementum, and reduced enamel epithelium with residual areas of stellate reticulum.

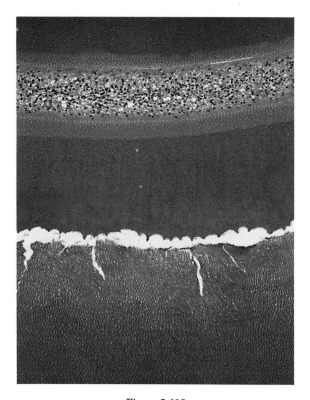

Figure 5-118
ODONTOMA

A compound odontoma with a well-defined pulpal component adjacent to predentin, dentin, and enamel matrix.

components of the formed teeth or tooth-like elements (fig. 5-118).

Aggregates of enamel matrix, enamel, tubular dentin, and pulpal tissue arranged in a haphazard array characterize the complex odontoma (fig. 5-119). Little or no resemblance to formed teeth exists. Masses of dentin enclose arcades of enamel matrix (fig. 5-120) and formed enamel with pulpal tissue is peripheral to or surrounded by dentinal structures.

Up to 20 percent of cases have variations in epithelial cell morphology, including ghost cell patterns with keratinization and calcification similar to the calcifying odontogenic cyst (167); these are of no prognostic significance. Odontomas may form within the wall of a calcifying odontogenic cyst in 24 to 33 percent of cases (160, 163). In the rare case, an ameloblastoma may coexist with an odontoma, forming the odontoameloblastoma.

Treatment and Prognosis. Conservative surgical excision is recommended. Recurrence has not been reported (160).

Odontoameloblastoma

Definition. This is a rare composite tumor composed of a typical ameloblastoma and an odontoma type component or one that shows evidence of induction. This entity includes

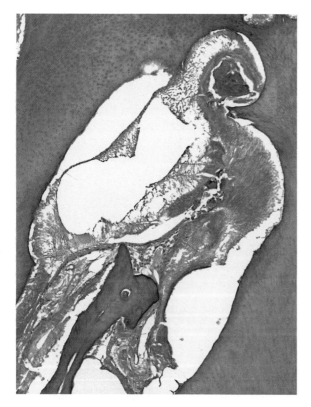

Figure 5-120
ODONTOMA
Enamel matrix is surrounded by dentin. Focal areas of cementum type material are also seen in juxtaposition to the enamel with no normal anatomic relationship as in a tooth.

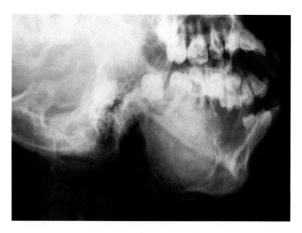

Figure 5-121
ODONTOAMELOBLASTOMA
This radiograph shows a large, expansile, loculated radiolucency and radiopacity involving the mandibular molar and ramus region of the mandible. Note the superior enlargement of the jaw and the anterior expansion of the ramus, suggesting aggressive behavior of the tumor. (Fig. 106 from Fascicle 24, 2nd Series.)

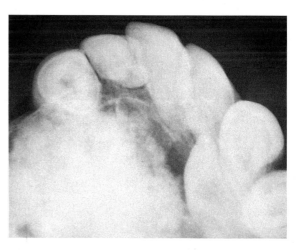

Figure 5-122
ODONTOAMELOBLASTOMA
A dense opacification is seen in the anterior portion of the mandible with a slightly loculated peripheral radiolucent component, causing resorption of the roots of the associated erupted teeth.

ameloblastoma with induction of dentin or dentinoid material as well as fully formed odontoma elements with a complex array of enamel, dentin, pulp, and cementum. There is controversy as to whether odontoameloblastoma is a discrete entity or a variant of an ameloblastic fibro-odontoma (175).

Clinical and Radiologic Features. The paucity of reported cases precludes a broad description of the clinical and radiographic features of this lesion. The analysis of 12 cases by Kaugars and Zussmann (173) showed an essentially even distribution between the mandible and maxilla, with nearly 75 percent occurring within the first two decades of life (average age, 18.5 years) (174). There was a tendency for occurrence posterior to the canine teeth (67 percent) and most patients presented clinically with a mass or swelling.

Radiographically, the predominant finding is a dense radiopacity separated from a well-defined corticated margin by a lucent rim. The central radiopacity corresponds to the odontoma component of this entity (figs. 5-121–5-123).

Histologic Findings. The ameloblastoma component is usually of the plexiform or follicular type and is admixed with dental tissue consisting of complex masses of enamel, dentin, and cementum, as in compound or complex odontomas (figs. 5-124, 5-125).

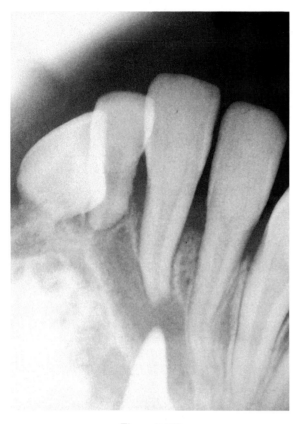

Figure 5-123
ODONTOAMELOBLASTOMA
Root resorption is noted at the periphery of the multi-loculated soft tissue component of this odontoameloblastoma, with the odontoma component well defined and opaque.

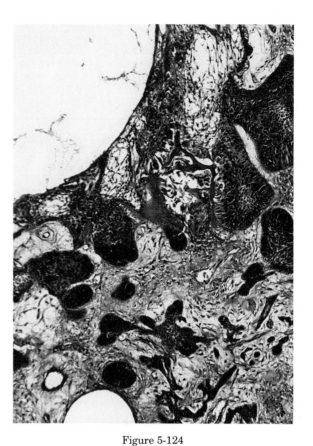

Figure 5-124
ODONTOAMELOBLASTOMA
Islands of ameloblastoma in association with eosinophilic matrix product within a loose, delicate stroma.

Figure 5-125
ODONTOAMELOBLASTOMA
A premineralized product is juxtaposed to an ameloblastic epithelial cord.

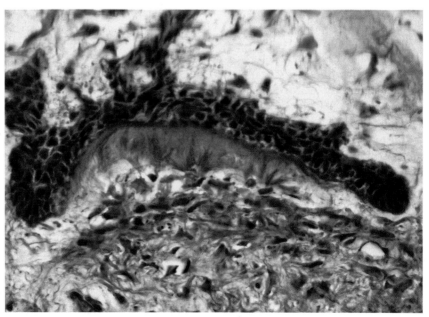

Treatment and Prognosis. This lesion possesses the same biologic potential as ameloblastoma since multiple recurrences have been reported after local curettage alone (171,172). Treatment is therefore excision in the form of a marginal or block resection, with long-term follow-up.

REFERENCES

Ameloblastoma

1. Ackermann GL, Altini M, Shear M. The unicystic ameloblastoma: a clinicopathologic study of 57 cases. J Oral Pathol 1988;17:541–6.
2. Browne RM. Investigative pathology of the odontogenic cysts. Boca Raton, FL: CRC Press, 1991:12.
3. Buchner A, Sciubba JJ. Peripheral epithelial odontogenic tumors: a review. Oral Surg Oral Med Oral Pathol 1987;63:688–97.
4. Corio RL, Goldblatt LI, Edwards PA, Hartman KS. Ameloblastic carcinoma: a clinicopathologic study and assessment of eight cases. Oral Surg Oral Med Oral Pathol 1987;64:570–6.
5. Elzay RP. Primary intraosseous carcinoma of the jaws: review and update of odontogenic carcinomas. Oral Surg 1982;54:299–303.
6. Eversole LR, Leider AS, Hansen L. Ameloblastoma with pronounced desmoplasia. J Oral Maxillofac Surg 1984;42:735–40.
7. Eversole LR, Leider AS, Strub D. Radiographic characteristics of cystogenic ameloblastoma. Oral Surg Oral Med Oral Pathol 1984;57:572–7.
8. Gardner DG. Plexiform unicystic ameloblastoma: a diagnostic problem in dentigerous cysts. Cancer 1981;47:1358–63.
9. Gardner DG, Corio RL. Plexiform unicystic ameloblastoma. A variant of ameloblastoma with a low recurrence rate after enucleation. Cancer 1984;53:1730–5.
10. Gold L. Biologic behavior of ameloblastoma. Oral Maxillofac Surg Clin 1991;3:21–71.
11. Kaffe I, Buchner A, Taicher S. Radiologic features of desmoplastic variant of ameloblastoma. Oral Surg Oral Med Oral Pathol 1993;76:525–9..
12. Kahn MA. Ameloblastomas in young persons: a clinicopathologic analysis and etiologic investigation. Oral Surg Oral Med Oral Pathol 1989;67:706–15
13. Keszler A, Dominguez FV. Ameloblastoma in childhood. J Oral Maxillofac Surg 1986;44:609–13.
14. Kramer IR. Ameloblastoma: a clinicopathologic appraisal. Br J Oral Surg 1963;1:13–21.
15. Kramer IR, Pindborg JJ, Shear M. Histologic typing of odontogenic tumors. 2nd ed. Berlin: Springer-Verlag, 1992.
16. Laughlin EH. Metastasizing ameloblastoma. Cancer 1989;64:776–80.
17. Leider AS, Eversole LR, Barkin ME. Cystic ameloblastoma: clinicopathologic analysis. Oral Surg Oral Med Oral Pathol 1985;60:624–30.
18. Mehlisch DR, Dahlin DC, Masson, JK. Ameloblastoma. A clinicopathologic study. J Oral Surg 1972;30:9–22.
19. Muller H, Slootweg PJ. The growth characteristics of multilocular ameloblastomas. A histological investigation with some inferences with regard to operative procedures. J Maxillofac Surg 1985;13:224–30.
20. Philipsen HP, Ormiston IW, Reichart PA. The desmo- and osteoplastic ameloblastoma. Histopathologic variant or clinicopathologic entity? Int J Oral Maxillofac Surg 1992;21:352–7.
21. Pindborg JJ, Kramer IR. Histologic typing of odontogenic tumours, jaw cysts and allied lesions. International Classification of Tumours, No. 5. Geneva: World Health Organization, 1971:24, 35.
22. Regezi JA, Kerr DA, Courtney RM. Odontogenic tumors: analysis of 706 cases. J Oral Surg 1978;36:771–8.
23. Robinson L, Martinez MG. Unicystic ameloblastoma: a prognostically distinct entity. Cancer 1977;40:2278–85.
24. Schafer DR, Thompson LD, Smith BC, Wenig BM. Primary ameloblastoma of the sinonasal tract: a clinicopathologic study of 24 cases. Cancer 1998;82;667–74.
25. Sehdev MK, Huvos AG, Strong EW. Ameloblastoma of maxilla and mandible. Cancer 1974;33:324–33.
26. Shibuya H, Hanafusa K, Shagdarsuren M, Okada N, Suzukis S. The use of CT and scintigraphy in diagnosing a cystic ameloblastoma of the jaw. Clin Nucl Med 1994;19:15–8.
27. Shteyer A, Lustmann J, Lewin-Epstein J. The mural ameloblastoma: a review of the literature. J Oral Surg 1978;36:866–72.
28. Slootweg PJ, Muller H. Malignant ameloblastoma or ameloblastic carcinoma. Oral Surg Oral Med Oral Pathol 1984;57:168–76.
29. Small IA, Waldron CA. Ameloblastomas of the jaws. Oral Surg 1955;8:281–7.
30. Thompson IO, Ferreira R, Van Wyk CW. Recurrent unicystic ameloblastoma of the maxilla. Br J Oral Maxillofac Surg 1993;30:180–2.
31. Tsaknis PJ, Nelson JF. The maxillary ameloblastoma: an analysis of 24 cases. J Oral Surg 1980;38:336–42.
32. Vickers RA, Gorlin RJ. Ameloblastoma: delineation of early histopathologic features of neoplasia. Cancer 1970;26:699–710.
33. Vigneswaran N, Whitaker SB, Budnick SD, Waldron CA. Expression patterns of epithelial differentiation antigens and lectin binding sites in ameloblastomas: a comparison with basal cell carcinomas. Hum Pathol 1993;24:49–57.
34. Waldron CA, El-Mofty SK. A histopathologic study of 116 ameloblastomas with special reference to the desmoplastic variant. Oral Surg Oral Med Oral Pathol 1987;63:441–51.
35. Williams TP. The ameloblastoma. A review of the literature. Selected Readings in Oral and Maxillofacial Surgery 1992;2:1–17.
36. Woo SB, Smith-Williams JE, Sciubba JJ, Lipper S. Peripheral ameloblastoma of the buccal mucosa. Oral Surg Oral Med Oral Pathol 1987;63:78–84.

Calcifying Epithelial Odontogenic Tumor

37. Bingham RA, Adrian JC. Combined epithelial odontogenic tumor-adenomatoid odontogenic tumor and calcifying epithelial odontogenic tumor: report of a case. J Oral Maxillofac Surg 1986;44:574–7.
38. Buchner A, Sciubba JJ. Peripheral epithelial odontogenic tumors. Oral Surg Oral Med Oral Pathol 1987;63:688–97.
39. Damm DD, White DK, Drummond JF, Poindexter JB, Henry BB. Combined epithelial odontogenic tumor: adenomatoid odontogenic tumor and calcifying epithelial odontogenic tumor. Oral Surg 1983;55:487–96.
40. Franklin CD, Martin MV, Clark A, Smith CJ, Hindle MO. An investigation into the origin and nature of "amyloid" in a calcifying epithelial odontogenic tumor. J Oral Pathol 1981;10:417–29.
41. Franklin CD, Pindborg JJ. The calcifying epithelial odontogenic tumor. A review and analysis of 113 cases. Oral Surg 1976;42:753–65.
42. Hicks MJ, Flaitz CM, Wong ME, McDaniel RK, Cagle PT. Clear cell variant of calcifying epithelial odontogenic tumor: case report and review of the literature. Head Neck 1994;16:272–7.
43. Krolls SO, Pindborg JJ. Calcifying epithelial odontogenic tumor. A survey of 23 cases and discussion of histomorphologic variations. Arch Pathol 1974;98:206–10.
44. Morimoto C, Tsujimoto M, Shimaoka S, Shirasa R, Takasu J. Ultrastructural localization of alkaline phosphatase in the calcifying epithelial odontogenic tumor. Oral Surg Oral Med Oral Pathol 1983;56:409–14.
45. Okada Y, Mochizuki K, Sigimura M, Noda Y, Mori M. Odontogenic tumor with combined characteristics of adenomatoid odontogenic and calcifying epithelial odontogenic tumors. Pathol Res Pract 1987;182:647–57.
46. Pindborg JJ. Calcifying epithelial odontogenic tumors. APMIS 1955;111(Suppl):71.
47. Pindborg JJ. A calcifying epithelial odontogenic tumor. Cancer 1958;11:838–43.
48. Pindborg JJ. The calcifying epithelial odontogenic tumor. Review of the literature and report of one extraosseous case. Acta Odontol Scand 1966;24:419–30.
49. Pindborg JJ, Vedtofte P, Reibel J, Praetorius F. The calcifying epithelial odontogenic tumor. A review of recent literature and report of a case. APMIS 1991;23(Suppl):152–7.
50. Regezi JA, Kerr DA, Courtney RM. Odontogenic tumors: analysis of 706 cases. J Oral Surg 1978;36:771–8.
51. Schmidt-Westhausen A, Philipsen HP, Reichart PA. Clear cell calcifying epithelial odontogenic tumor. A case report. Int J Oral Maxillofac Surg 1992;21:47–9.
52. Siar CH, Ng KH. The combined epithelial odontogenic tumor in Malaysians. Br J Oral Maxillofac Surg 1991;29:106–9.
53. Takata T, Ogawa I, Miyauchi M, Ijuhin N, Mikai H, Fujita M. Non-calcifying Pindborg tumor with Langerhans cells. J Oral Pathol Med 1993;22:378–83.
54. Takeda Y, Kudo K. Adenomatoid odontogenic tumor associated with calcifying epithelial odontogenic tumor. Int J Oral Maxillofac Surg 1986;15:469–73.

Adenomatoid Odontogenic Tumor

55. Aldred MJ, Gray AR. A pigmented adenomatoid odontogenic tumor. Oral Surg Oral Med Oral Pathol 1990;70:86–9.
56. Bingham RA, Adrian JC. Combined epithelial odontogenic tumor—adenomatoid odontogenic tumor and calcifying epithelial odontogenic tumor. J Oral Maxillofac Surg 1986;44:574–7.
57. Courtney RM, Kerr DA. The odontogenic adenomatoid tumor. A comprehensive study of 20 new cases. Oral Surg Oral Med Oral Pathol 1975;39:424–35.
58. Damm D, White DK, Drummond JF, Poindexter JB, Henry BB. Combined epithelial odontogenic tumor: adenomatoid odontogenic tumor and calcifying epithelial odontogenic tumor. Oral Surg Oral Med Oral Pathol 1983;55:487–96.
59. Dare A, Yamaguchi A, Yoshiki S, Okano T. Limitation of panoramic radiography in diagnosing adenomatoid odontogenic tumors. Oral Surg Oral Med Oral Pathol 1994;77:662–8.
60. El Labban NG. The nature of the eosinophilic and laminated masses in the adenomatoid odontogenic tumor: a histochemical and ultrastructural study. J Oral Pathol Med 1992;21:75–81.
61. Ghosh LS. Adamantinoma of the upper jaw. Am J Pathol 1934;10:773–89.
62. Kramer IR, Pindborg JJ, Shear M. Histologic typing of odontogenic tumors, 2nd ed. Berlin: Springer-Verlag, 1992.
63. Mori M, Makino M, Imai K. The histochemical nature of homogeneous amorphous materials in odontogenic epithelial tumors. J Oral Surg 1980;2:96–102.
64. Moro I, Okamura N, Okuda S, Komiyama K, Umemura S. The eosinophilic and amyloid-like materials in adenomatoid odontogenic tumor. J Oral Pathol 1982;11:138–50.
65. Okada Y, Mochizuki K, Sugimura M, Noda Y, Mori M. Odontogenic tumor with combined characteristics of adenomatoid odontogenic and calcifying odontogenic tumors. Pathol Res Pract 1987;182:647–57.
66. Philipsen HP, Reichart PA, Zhang KH, Nikai AH, Yu QX. Adenomatoid odontogenic tumor: biologic profile based on 499 cases. J Oral Pathol Med 1991;20:149–58.
67. Poulsen TC, Greer RO. Adenomatoid odontogenic tumor: clinicopathologic and ultrastructural concepts. J Oral Maxillofac Surg 1983;41:818–24.
68. Saku T, Okabe H, Shimokawa H. Immunohistochemical demonstration of enamel proteins in odontogenic tumors. J Oral Pathol Med 1992;21:113–9.
69. Schlosnagel DC, Someren A. The ultrastructure of the adenomatoid odontogenic tumor. Oral Surg Oral Med Oral Pathol 1981;52:154–61.
70. Smith RR, Olson JL, Hutchins GM, Crawley WA, Levin LS. Adenomatoid odontogenic tumor: ultrastructural demonstration of two cell types and amyloid. Cancer 1979;43:505–11.
71. Stafne EC. Epithelial tumors associated with developmental cysts of the maxilla: report of these cases. Oral Surg Oral Med Oral Pathol 1948;1:887–94.
72. Warter A, George-Diolombi G, Chazal M, Ango A. Melanin in a dentigerous cyst and associated adenomatoid odontogenic tumor. Cancer 1990;66:786–8.
73. Yazdi I, Nowparast B. Extraosseous adenomatoid odontogenic tumor with special reference to the probability of the basal-cell layer of oral epithelium as a potential source of origin. Report of a case. Oral Surg Oral Med Oral Pathol 1974;37:249–56.

Squamous Odontogenic Tumor

74. Goldblatt LI, Brannon RB, Ellis GL. Squamous odontogenic tumor. Report of five cases and review of the literature. Oral Surg Oral Med Oral Pathol 1982;54:187–96.

75. Leider AS, Jonker LA, Cook HE. Multicentric familial squamous odontogenic tumor. Oral Surg Oral Med Oral Pathol 1989;68:175–81.

76. McClatchey KD. Tumors of the dental lamina: a selective review. Semin Diagn Pathol 1987;4:200–4.

77. Mills WP, Davila MA, Beuttenmuller EA, Koudelka BM. Squamous odontogenic tumor. Report of a case with lesions in three quadrants. Oral Surg Oral Med Oral Pathol 1986;61:557–63.

78. Pullon PA, Shafer WG, Elzay RP, Kerr DA, Corio RL. Squamous odontogenic tumor. Oral Surg 1975;40:616–30.

79. Simon JH, Jensen JL. Squamous odontogenic cyst-like proliferation in periapical cysts. J Endod 1985;11:446–8.

80. van der Waal I, De Rijcke TH. Possible squamous odontogenic tumor: report of a case. J Oral Surg 1980;38:460–2.

81. Waldron CA, El-Mofty SK. A histopathologic study of 116 ameloblastomas with special reference to the desmoplastic variant. Oral Surg Oral Med Oral Pathol 1987;63:441–51.

82. Wright JM. Squamous odontogenic tumorlike proliferation in odontogenic cysts. Oral Surg Oral Med Oral Pathol 1979;47:354–8.

Odontogenic Ghost Cell Tumor

83. Alcalde RE, Sasaki A, Misaki M, Matsumura T. Odontogenic ghost cell carcinoma: report of a case and review of the literature. J Oral Maxillofac Surg 1996;54:108–11.

84. Dubiel-Bigaj M, Olszewski E, Stachura J. The malignant form of calcifying odontogenic cyst. A case report. Patol Pol 1993;44:39–41.

85. Ellis GL, Shmookler BM. Aggressive (malignant?) epithelial odontogenic ghost cell tumor. Oral Surg Oral Med Oral Pathol 1986;61:471–8.

86. Grodjesk JE, Dolinski HB, Schneider LC, Dolinski EH, Doyle JL. Odontogenic ghost cell carcinoma. Oral Surg Oral Med Oral Pathol 1987;63:576–81.

87. Gunhan O, Mocan A, Can C, Kisnisci R, Aksy AY, Finci R. Epithelial odontogenic ghost cell tumor: report of a peripheral solid variant and review of the literature. Ann Dent 1991;50:8–11, 48.

88. Hirshberg A, Dayan D, Horowitz I. Dentinogenic ghost cell tumor. Int J Oral Maxillofac Surg 1987;16:620–5.

89. Ikemura K, Horie A, Toishiro H, Nandate M. Simultaneous occurrence of a calcifying odontogenic cyst and its malignant transformation. Cancer 1985;56:2861–4.

90. Kao SY, Pong BY, Li WY, Gallagher GT, Chang RC. Maxillary odontogenic carcinoma with distant metastases to axillary skin, brain and lung: case report. Int J Oral Maxillofac Surg 1995;24:229–32.

91. McCoy BP, O'Carroll MK, Hall JM. Carcinoma arising in a dentinogenic ghost cell tumor. Oral Surg Oral Med Oral Pathol 1992;74:371–8.

92. Praetorius F, Hjorting-Hansen E, Gorlin RJ, Vickers RA. Calcifying odontogenic cyst. Range, variations and neoplastic potential. Acta Odontol Scand 1981;39:227–40.

93. Raubenheimer EJ, van Heerden WF, Sitzmann F, Heymer B. Peripheral dentinogenic ghost cell tumor. J Oral Pathol Med 1992;21:93–5.

94. Scott J, Wood GD. Aggressive calcifying odontogenic cyst—a possible variant of ameloblastoma. Br J Oral Maxillofac Surg 1989;27:53–9.

95. Tajima Y, Ohno J, Utsumi N. The dentinogenic ghost cell tumor. J Oral Pathol 1986;15:359–62.

Odontogenic Myxoma/Sinonasal Myxoma

96. Barros RE, Dominquez FV, Cabrini RL. Myxoma of the jaws. Oral Surg Oral Med Oral Pathol 1969;27:225–36.

97. Ghosh BC, Huvos AG, Gerold FP, Miller TR. Myxoma of the jaw bones. Cancer 1973;31:237–40.

98. Heffner DK. Sinonasal myxomas and fibromyxomas in children. Ear Nose Throat J 1993;72:365–8.

99. Hendler BH, Abaza NA, Quinn P. Odontogenic myxoma. Surgical management and an ultrastructural study. Oral Surg Oral Med Oral Pathol 1979;47:203–17.

100. Kangur TT, Dahlin DC, Turlington EG. Myxomatous tumors of the jaws. J Oral Surg 1975;33:523–8.

101. Katz JO, Underhill TE. Multilocular radiolucencies. Dental Clin N Am 1994;38:63–81.

102. Keszler A, Dominguez FV, Giannunzio G. Myxoma in childhood: an analysis of 10 cases. J Oral Maxillofac Surg 1995;53:518–21.

103. Kim J, Ellis GL. Dental follicular tissue: misinterpretation as odontogenic tumors. J Oral Maxillofac Surg 1993;51:762–7.

104. Lombardi T, Kuffer R, Bernard JP, Fiore-Donno G, Samson J. Immunohistochemical staining for vimentin filaments and S-100 protein in myxoma of the jaws. J Oral Pathol 1988;17:175–7.

105. McClure DK, Dahlin DC. Myxoma of bone. Report of three cases. Mayo Clin Proc 1977;52:249–53.

106. Moshiri S, Oda D, Worthington P, Myall R. Odontogenic myxoma: histochemical and ultrastructural study. J Oral Pathol Med 1992;21:401–3.

107. Nitzan DW, Gazit D, Azaz B. Childhood odontogenic myxoma. Report of two cases. Ped Dent 1985;7:140–4.

108. Peltola J, Magnusson B, Happonen RP, Borrman H. Odontogenic myxoma—a radiographic study of 21 tumours. Br J Oral Maxillofac Surg 1994;32:298–302.

109. Regezi JA, Kerr DA, Courtney RM. Odontogenic tumors: analysis of 706 cases. J Oral Surg 1978;36:771–8.

110. Slootweg PJ, van den Bos T, Straks W. Glycosaminoglycans in myxoma of the jaw: a biochemical study. J Oral Pathol 1985;14:299–306.

111. Slootweg PJ, Wittkampf AR. Myxoma of the jaws. An analysis of 15 cases. J Maxillofac Surg 1986;14:46–52.
112. Takahashi H, Fujita S, Okabe H. Immunohistochemical investigation in odontogenic myxoma. J Oral Pathol Med 1991;20:114–9.
113. Ward TO, Rooney GE. Asymptomatic expansion of the mandible. J Am Dent Assoc 1989;119:169–70.
114. White DK, Chen SY, Mohnac EM, Miller AS. Odontogenic myxoma. A clinical and ultrastructural study. Oral Surg Oral Med Oral Pathol 1975;39:901–17.
114a. Zimmerman DC, Dahlin DC. Myxomatous tumors of the jaws. Oral Surg Oral Med Oral Pathol 1958;11:1069–80.

Odontogenic Fibroma

115. Allen CM, Hammond HL, Stimson PG. Central odontogenic fibroma, WHO type. A report of 3 cases with an unusual giant cell reaction. Oral Surg Oral Med Oral Pathol 1992;73:62–6.
116. Buchner A. Peripheral odontogenic fibroma. J Craniomaxillfac Surg 1989;17:134–8.
117. Buchner A, Ficarra G, Hansen LS. Peripheral odontogenic fibroma. Oral Surg Oral Med Oral Pathol 1987;64:432–8.
118. Buchner A, Hansen LS. The histomorphic spectrum of peripheral ossifying fibroma. Oral Surg Oral Med Oral Pathol 1987;63:452–61.
119. Dahl EC, Wolfson SH, Haugen JC. Central odontogenic fibroma: review of literature and report of cases. J Oral Surg 1981;39:120–4.
120. deVillers-Slabbert H, Altini M. Peripheral odontogenic fibroma: a clinicopathologic study. Oral Surg Oral Med Oral Pathol 1991;72:86–90.
121. Gardner DG. Central odontogenic fibroma, current concepts. J Oral Pathol Med 1996;15:556–61.
122. Gunhan O, Erseven G, Ruacan S, Selasun B, Aydintug Y, Ergun E, Demiriz M. Odontogenic tumors. A series of 409 cases. Austral Dent J 1990;35:518–22.
123. Handlers JP, Abrams AM, Melrose RJ, Danforth R. Central odontogenic fibroma: clinicopathologic features of 19 cases and review of the literature. J Oral Maxillofac Surg 1991;49:46–54.
124. Inwards CY, Unni KK, Beabout JW, Shives TC. Solitary congenital fibromatosis (infantile myofibromatosis) of bone. Am J Surg Pathol 1991;15:935–41.
125. Kaffe I, Buchner A. Radiologic features of central odontogenic fibroma. Oral Surg Oral Med Oral Pathol 1994;78:811–8.
126. Kenney JN, Kaugars GE, Abbey LM. Comparison between the peripheral ossifying fibroma and the peripheral odontogenic fibroma. J Oral Maxillofac Surg 1989;97:378–82.
127. Kim J, Ellis GL. Dental follicular tissue: misinterpretation as odontogenic tumors. J Oral Maxillofac Surg 1993;51:762–7.
128. Kramer IR, Pindborg JJ, Shear M. Histologic typing of odontogenic tumors. WHO International Classification of Tumors. Hamburg: Springer, 1992.
129. Martinez V, Sissons HA. Aneurysmal bone cyst. A review of 123 cases including primary lesions and those secondary to other bone pathology. Cancer 1988;61:2291–304.
130. Odell EW, Lombardi T, Barrett AW, Morgan PR, Speight PM. Hybrid central giant cell granuloma and central odontogenic fibroma-like lesions of the jaws. Histopathology 1997;30:165–71.
131. Slootweg PJ, Muller H. Central fibroma of the jaw, odontogenic or desmoplastic. Oral Surg Oral Med Oral Pathol 1983;56:61–70.
132. Vincent SD, Hammond HL, Ellis GL, Juhlin JP. Central granular cell odontogenic fibroma. Oral Surg Oral Med Oral Pathol 1987;6:715–21.
133. Wesley RK, Wysocki GP, Mintz SM. The central odontogenic fibroma. Clinical and morphologic studies. Oral Surg Oral Med Oral Pathol 1985;40:235–45.
134. White DK, Chen SY, Hartman KS, Miller AS, Gomez LF. Central granular cell tumor of the jaws (the so-called granular cell ameloblastic fibroma). Oral Surg Oral Med Oral Pathol 1978;45:396–405.

Cementoblastoma

135. Ackermann GL, Altini M. The cementomas—a clinicopathological reappraisal. J Dent Assoc S Afr 1992;47:187–94.
136. Biggs JT, Benenati FW. Surgically treating a benign cementoblastoma while retaining the involved tooth. J Am Dent Assoc 1995;126:1288–90.
137. Cannell H. Cementoblastoma of a deciduous tooth. Oral Surg Oral Med Oral Pathol 1991;71:648.
138. Corio RL, Crawford BE, Schaberg SJ. Benign cementoblastoma. Oral Surg 1974;37:54–63.
139. Fujita S, Takahashi H, Okabe H, Watanabe C, Sonobe H. A case of benign cementoblastoma. Oral Surg Oral Med Oral Pathol 1989;68:64–8.
140. Garlick AC, Newhouse RF, Boyd DB. Benign cementoblastoma: report of a case. Mil Med 1990;155:567–70.
141. Slootweg PJ. Cementoblastoma and osteoblastoma: a comparison of histologic features. J Oral Pathol Med 1992;21:385–9.
142. Slootweg PJ. Maxillofacial fibro-osseous lesions: classification and differential diagnosis. Semin Diagn Pathol 1996;13:104–12.
143. Ulmansky M, Hjorting-Hansen E, Praetorius F, Haque MF. Benign cementoblastoma. A review and five new cases. Oral Surg Oral Med Oral Pathol 1994;77:48–55.
144. van der Waal I, Greebe RB, Elias EA. Benign osteoblastoma or osteoid osteoma of the maxilla. Report of a case. Int J Oral Surg 1983;12:355–8.
145. Zachariades N, Skordalaki A, Papanicolaou S, Ardroulakakis E, Bournias M. Cementoblastoma: review of the literature and report of a case in a seven-year-old girl. Br J Oral Maxillofac Surg 1985;23:453–61.

Ameloblastic Fibroma/Fibro-odontoma

146. Cahn LR, Blum T. Ameloblastic odontoma: case report critically analyzed. J Oral Surg 1952;10:169–70.
147. Eversole LR, Tomich CE, Cherrick HM. Histogenesis of odontogenic tumors. Oral Surg 1971;32:569–81.
148. Gardner DG. The mixed odontogenic tumors. Oral Surg 1984;57:394–7.
149. Hansen LS, Ficarra G. Mixed odontogenic tumors: an analysis of 23 new cases. Head Neck Surg 1988;10:330–43.
150. Hooker SP. Ameloblastic odontoma. An analysis of twenty-six cases. Oral Surg 1967;24:375–6.
151. Pindborg JJ, Clausen F. Classification of odontogenic tumors. A suggestion. Acta Odontol Scand 1958;16:293–301.
152. Regezi JA, Kerr DA, Courtney RM. Odontogenic tumors: analysis of 706 cases. J Oral Surg 1978;36:771–8.
153. Ruhl GH, Akuamoa-Boateng E. Granular cells in odontogenic and non-odontogenic tumors. Virchows Arch [A] 1989;415:403–9.
154. Shafer WG, Hine MK, Levy BM. A textbook of oral pathology, 4th ed. Philadelphia: WB Saunders, 1983:304–17.
155. Slootweg PJ. An analysis of the interrelationship of the mixed odontogenic tumors—ameloblastic fibroma, ameloblastic fibro-odontoma, and the odontoma. Oral Surg 1981;51:266–76.
156. Trodahl JN. Ameloblastic fibroma. A survey of cases from the Armed Forces Institute of Pathology. Oral Surg 1972;33:547–58.
157. van Wyck CW, van der Vyver PC. Ameloblastic fibroma with dentinoid formation/immature dentinoma. A microscopic and ultrastructural study of the epithelial-connective tissue interface. J Oral Pathol 1983;12:37–46.
158. Vincent SD, Hammond HL, Ellis GO, Juhlin JP. Central granular cell odontogenic fibroma. Oral Surg Oral Med Oral Pathol 1987;63:715–21.

Odontoma

159. Bellucci RJ, Zizmor J, Goodwin RE. Odontoma of the middle ear. A case presentation. Arch Otolaryngol 1975;101:571–3.
160. Budnick SD. Compound and complex odontomas. Oral Surg 1976;42:501–6.
161. Giunta JL, Kaplan MA. Peripheral, soft tissue odontomas. Two case reports. Oral Surg Oral Med Oral Pathol 1990;69:406–11.
162. Gunhan O, Erseven G, Ruacan S, et al. Odontogenic tumors. A series of 409 cases. Austral Dent J 1990;35:518–22.
163. Hirshberg A, Kaplan I, Buchner A. Calcifying odontogenic cyst associated with odontoma: a possible separate entity (odontocalcifying odontogenic cyst). J Oral Maxillofac Surg 1994;52:555–8.
164. Kaugars GE, Miller ME, Abbey LM. Odontomas. Oral Surg Oral Med Oral Pathol 1989;67:172–6.
165. Kramer IR, Pindborg JJ, Shear M. The World Health Organization histological typing of odontogenic tumors. Introducing the second edition. Oral Oncol Eur J Cancer 1993;29B:169–71.
166. Ledesma-Montes C, Perez-Bache A, Garces-Ortiz M. Gingival compound odontoma. Int J Oral Maxillofac Surg 1996;25:296–7.
167. Levy BA. Ghost cells and odontomas. Oral Surg 1973;36:851–5.
168. Lopez-Areal L, Silvestre-Donat F, Gil-Lanzo J. Compound odontoma erupting in the mouth. A four year follow-up of a clinical case. J Oral Pathol Med 1992;21:285–8.
169. McClatchey KD, Hakimi M, Batsakis JG. Retrotympanic odontoma. Am J Surg Pathol 1981;5:401–4.
170. Regezi JA, Kerr DA, Courtney RM. Odontogenic tumors: analysis of 706 cases. J Oral Surg 1978;36:771–8.

Odontoameloblastoma

171. Frissell CT, Shafer WG. Ameloblastic odontoma: report of a case. Oral Surg 1953;6:1129–33.
172. Gupta DS, Gupta MK. Odontoameloblastoma. J Oral Maxillofac Surg 1986;44:146–8.
173. Kaugars GE, Zussman HW. Ameloblastic odontoma (odonto-ameloblastoma). Oral Surg Oral Med Oral Pathol 1991;71:371–3.
174. Toretti EF, Miller AS, Peezick B. Odontomas: an analysis of 167 cases. J Pedon 1984;8:282–4.
175. Wachter R, Remagen IN, Stoll P. Is it possible to differentiate between odontoameloblastoma and fibro-odontoma? Critical position on the basis of 18 cases in DOSAK. Dtsch Zahnartzl Z 1991;46:74–7.

6
MALIGNANT ODONTOGENIC TUMORS

PRIMARY INTRAOSSEOUS CARCINOMA

Definition. Primary intraosseous carcinoma (PIOC) is a squamous cell carcinoma arising within the mandible or maxilla, presumably originating from residual odontogenic epithelial elements (1,3). In order to establish a diagnosis of PIOC, there must be no evidence of associated oral mucosal dysplasia or carcinoma in the original biopsy or main specimen and no evidence to suggest a metastatic tumor (Table 6-1) (2,9). In addition, tumors originating from salivary tissue and transformed ameloblastoma (carcinoma arising from ameloblastoma) are excluded (6).

Clinical Features. PIOC is a rare lesion with only 39 individual cases published to date (2, 4,6–10). The mean patient age is 51 years, with a range of 4 to 76 years; there is a greater than 2 to 1 male predilection. Of 32 cases in which data was available, 29 lesions arose in the mandible, with 26 of those in the posterior segments.

The most frequent presenting clinical features are swelling of the mucosa at the affected site accompanied by pain. Less common clinical findings include lymph node metastases, peripheral neuropathy, and ulceration.

Radiographically, osteolytic bony changes are noted in all cases (fig. 6-1). Margins are usually ill-defined, irregular, and diffuse. In less than one third of cases, well-defined radiographic margins have been reported. Other radiographic findings include root resorption as well as saucerization. Correlations have been drawn between rates of growth and radiographic margins, with slowly growing lesions usually presenting with well-defined, smoothly contoured borders while irregular, ragged margins are associated with more rapidly growing lesions (figs. 6-2, 6-3) (5). There are, however, no specific radiographic features which distinguish PIOC from other benign or malignant odontogenic or nonodontogenic tumors. In 39 percent of cases, metastases have been noted, however, this does not appear to influence survival time (2).

Microscopic Findings. PIOC is morphologically similar to the usual squamous cell carcinomas. No evidence of ameloblastic differentiation is noted except for a suggestion of a peripheral palisaded columnar cell population in some cases. Variable degrees of cellular pleomorphism are noted. Individual cells aggregate into cords and nests (figs. 6-4, 6-5) and may demonstrate prominent individual cell keratinization. Epithelial elements are scattered within a fibrous stroma

Table 6-1

CRITERIA FOR PRIMARY INTRAOSSEOUS CARCINOMA

1. Histology of an intraosseous squamous cell carcinoma with no evidence of associated dysplasia or carcinoma.

2. Negative chest radiograph.

3. Six month disease-free survival with no evidence of an occult primary neoplasm or an absence of primary neoplasm at autopsy.

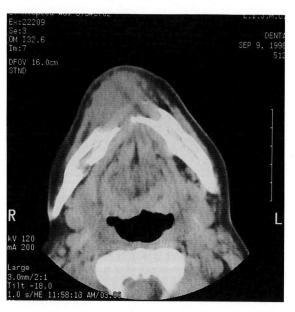

Figure 6-1

PRIMARY INTRAOSSEOUS CARCINOMA

A large, permeative, soft tissue mass extends through the labial cortical margin of the anterior mandible, producing an obvious soft tissue swelling clinically.

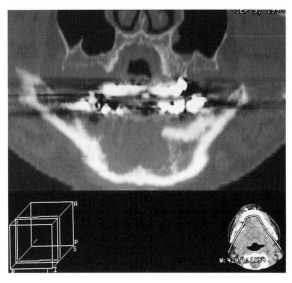

Figure 6-2
PRIMARY INTRAOSSEOUS CARCINOMA
A purely radiolucent expansile lesion produces a symmetric paramedian deformity with destruction and scalloping of the inferior mandibular margin.

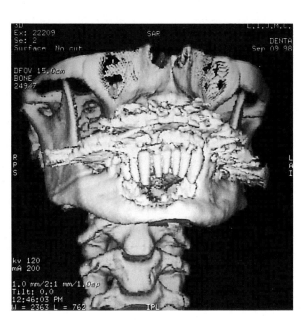

Figure 6-3
PRIMARY INTRAOSSEOUS CARCINOMA
This reconstructed three-dimensional image emphasizes the superior extension/infiltration, destroying the alveolar segment of bone and extending further toward the crestal bone apex interdentally.

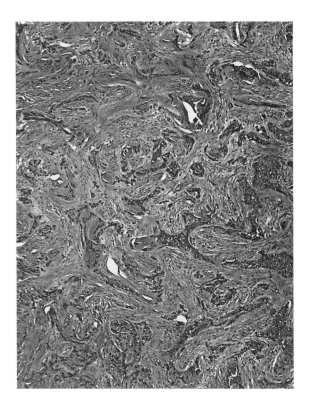

Figure 6-4
PRIMARY INTRAOSSEOUS CARCINOMA
Cords and nests of cells are scattered within a collagenous stroma in a rather haphazard pattern. Features of keratinization are seen in some islands, although this is minimal.

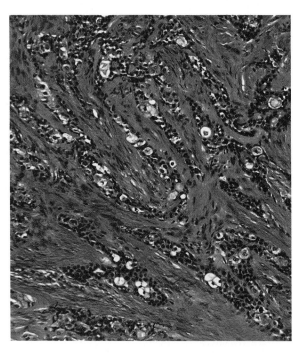

Figure 6-5
PRIMARY INTRAOSSEOUS CARCINOMA
Clear cell elements are seen within infiltrating cords of epithelial tissue, which in turn are surrounded by well-collagenized fibrous connective tissue.

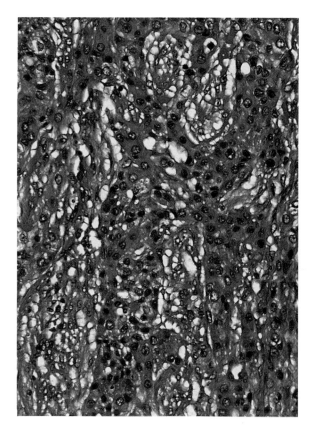

Figure 6-6
PRIMARY INTRAOSSEOUS CARCINOMA
Pleomorphic epithelial elements show prominent nuclei with coarse chromatin.

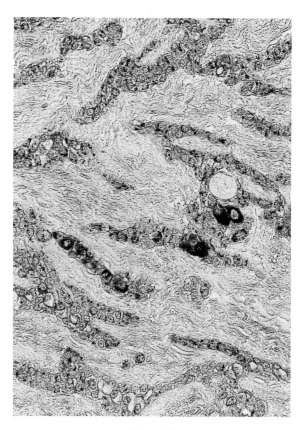

Figure 6-7
PRIMARY INTRAOSSEOUS CARCINOMA
Intense cytoplasmic staining for low molecular weight keratins is noted in all islands of tumor.

(fig. 6-6) which is generally dense with inconspicuous vascularity. The extent of keratinization varies (fig. 6-7) from slight with glassy hyalinized cytoplasm to prominent with large epithelial pearls. Permeation into the surrounding bony trabeculae as well as infiltration into the inferior alveolar nerve occurs. Occasional areas may undergo cystic breakdown, suggesting a possible relationship to a keratinizing odontogenic cyst.

Treatment and Prognosis. In cases involving the mandible, the suggested surgical management consists of a resection with elective neck dissection. Postoperative radiation therapy is an elective option. In maxillary cases, a partial to hemimaxillectomy is appropriate, depending upon the location and size of the lesion, with postoperative radiation an elective option.

The prognosis is uncertain at this time because of a paucity of reported cases with adequate follow-up. To et al. (9) have reported 12 deaths at an average period of 14.5 months; survival ranges from 6 months to 5 years. Shear (7) estimated a 30 to 40 percent survival rate. When contrasted to survival time of patients with squamous cell carcinoma developing in preexisting odontogenic cysts, those with PIOC have a less favorable prognosis (4), with two thirds demonstrating regional metastases (2).

CARCINOMA ARISING IN ODONTOGENIC CYSTS

Definition. Carcinoma may arise from a preexisting odontogenic cyst, most frequently from a dentigerous cyst (17). While squamous cell carcinoma is the predominant form of neoplastic transformation occurring within odontogenic cysts, mucoepidermoid carcinoma (15) and far less commonly, spindle cell carcinoma and verrucous

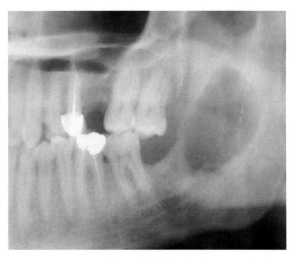

Figure 6-8
CARCINOMA ARISING IN AN ODONTOGENIC CYST
A large, radiolucent cystic lesion was initially considered to be a recurrent dentigerous cyst. Relatively well-defined margins are noted in most areas, however, the inferior and anterior borders are slightly irregular.

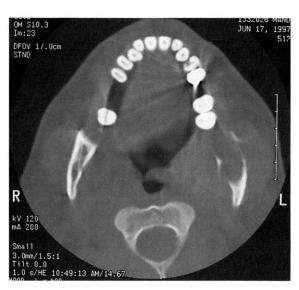

Figure 6-9
CARCINOMA ARISING IN AN ODONTOGENIC CYST
An axial CT scan shows the mid-portion of the ramus to be expanded and perforated along the buccal and lingual margins.

carcinoma may also so develop (13,14). Although other forms of salivary gland carcinoma, such as adenoid cystic malignant mixed tumor, may arise within bone (11), origin from a preexisting odontogenic cyst has not been demonstrated.

Histogenesis. Factors involved in the development of carcinoma within an odontogenic cyst are unknown. It is likely that a transition from a benign cyst lining to dysplastic epithelium occurs prior to progression to invasive carcinoma. Demonstration of this transition from an odontogenic epithelial lining to the carcinoma is essential in establishing the diagnosis (16). This sequence of transition has been demonstrated by Browne and Gough (12) with squamous metaplasia and dysplasia preceding the development of carcinoma. However, in only one fourth of cases in that series as well as in a review by Eversole et al. (15) was a metaplastic or dysplastic squamous lining seen. Demonstration of such transition remains the best evidence for excluding a noncystic source. p53-positive squamous cell carcinoma has been demonstrated within a transforming dentigerous cyst (21). Types of odontogenic cysts where such carcinomatous transformation may arise include the dentigerous cyst, odontogenic keratocyst, residual cyst, and lateral periodontal cyst.

Clinical and Radiologic Features. Pain and swelling are the most common clinical findings associated with carcinomatous transformation of an odontogenic cyst, although in most instances there is an absence of any signs or symptoms. Other features that should arouse suspicion include a rapid increase of jaw size with or without accompanying paresthesia, failure of an extraction site to heal, and cortical plate perforation. The diagnosis, however, is most often made subsequent to pathologic evaluation (22). The mean age of patients with either squamous cell or mucoepidermoid carcinoma is late in the sixth decade, with a wide age range from the third to the eighth decades (15,16). The majority of cases of squamous cell carcinoma are noted within the mandible (21) while mucoepidermoid carcinoma is almost exclusive to the mandible (95 percent) (11,15). Others found a 2 to 1 mandibular over maxillary predilection (21).

Radiographically, the affected jaw segment shows round to ovoid areas of radiolucency (fig. 6-8), often with ill-defined borders. Margins may be jagged (figs. 6-9, 6-10) as opposed to the usual well-defined and corticated margins characteristic of benign odontogenic cysts.

Microscopic Findings. The diagnosis requires documentation of microscopic transition from a

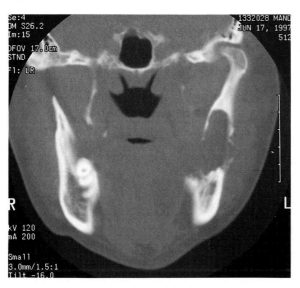

Figure 6-10
CARCINOMA ARISING IN AN ODONTOGENIC CYST
    The coronal reconstruction clearly demonstrates an uneven inferior margin which approaches the inferior alveolar canal, while medially the lingual cortex is destroyed. Along the buccal aspect a very attenuated and expanded cortex remains.

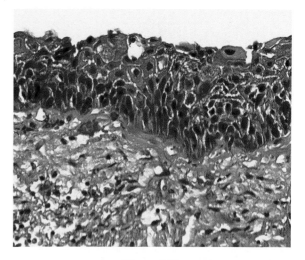

Figure 6-11
CARCINOMA ARISING IN AN ODONTOGENIC CYST
    A portion of the cyst wall shows a significant degree of epithelial dysplasia with some evidence of basal layer polarization.

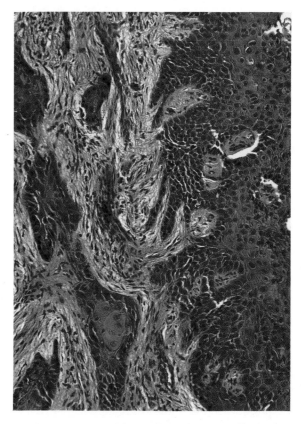

Figure 6-12
CARCINOMA ARISING IN AN ODONTOGENIC CYST
    Infiltrating islands of well-differentiated squamous cell carcinoma are noted in other areas of the cystic process.

benign cyst with its characteristic epithelial lining to an invasive carcinoma. The transition to carcinoma may be gradual or abrupt. In cases of a preexisting dentigerous cyst, dysplastic changes of the lining should be present in association with the invasive squamous cell carcinoma (fig. 6-11).

The neoplastic elements extend from the epithelial lining of the cyst deep into the connective tissue wall (figs. 6-12, 6-13). Perineural extension along the inferior alveolar nerve may be noted (20). Most carcinomas are well differentiated and are rarely papillary or spindle cell in type.

Low-grade mucoepidermoid carcinoma is the most frequent nonsquamous cell carcinoma seen associated with preexisting jaw cysts, almost always dentigerous cysts (15). Such carcinomas are usually highly differentiated and are dominated by goblet cells, with fewer epidermoid elements. Intraosseous mucoepidermoid carcinoma must be differentiated from the recently described sialo-odontogenic cyst because of their clinical, radiographic, and histologic similarities (19).

Treatment and Prognosis. Epidermoid and mucoepidermoid carcinoma are treated like any invasive carcinomas of the jaw. A mandibular resection with neck dissection is the treatment

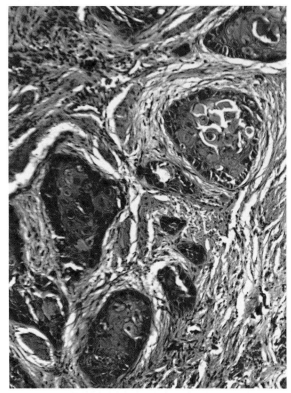

Figure 6-13
CARCINOMA ARISING IN AN ODONTOGENIC CYST
Islands of keratinizing stratified squamous epithelium retain a suggestion of a cuboidal peripheral layer.

of choice for squamous cell carcinoma. Similarly, mucoepidermoid carcinoma should be resected in a similar manner while neck dissection is elective. A risk of metastasis exists in both epidermoid and mucoepidermoid carcinomas (15, 16,18). Long-term follow-up is mandatory and the overall prognosis is good.

AMELOBLASTIC FIBROSARCOMA
(AMELOBLASTIC SARCOMA)

Definition. Ameloblastic fibrosarcoma is a mixed epithelial-mesenchymal odontogenic neoplasm in which the mesenchymal component is sarcomatous. This malignant neoplasm may arise de novo or from a preexisting cementoblastic fibroma or fibro-odontoma. The epithelial component is identical to that of the ameloblastic fibroma.

General Features. As the malignant counterpart of the ameloblastic fibroma, the ameloblastic fibrosarcoma/sarcoma is a rare odontogenic tumor

with fewer than 50 cases reported in the world literature. About half of the neoplasms arise from a preexisting ameloblastic fibroma or ameloblastic fibro-odontoma (24,27,28a,32), while the remainder arise de novo (29). Malignant transformation may follow multiple recurrences of ameloblastic fibroma or fibro-odontoma (28). The odontogenic epithelial component resembles that seen in the latter lesions.

Clinical and Radiologic Features. This clinically aggressive tumor occurs chiefly in the young, with 71 percent of cases in one study documented in patients under 21 years of age (33); a mean of 26 and 27.5 years has been documented in two other studies (24,28a). Patients are 5 to 44 years of age (24,30), with a male predilection. Nearly three fourths of cases arise in the mandible (23). In cases arising from pre-existing ameloblastic fibromas or fibro-odontomas, there is a rapid acceleration of growth. Pain and paresthesia or dysesthesia may be noted (25).

Radiographically, a destructive, generally radiolucent process is noted. Radiographic margins are irregular and ill-defined. There may be cortical expansion and perforation with associated intraoral and facial swelling (fig. 6-14).

Microscopic Findings. Bland ameloblastic epithelium, similar to but quantitatively less than that seen in the ameloblastic fibroma, is present in variable proportions from case to case and within areas of the same specimen (figs. 6-15, 6-16). A seam or band of acellular, hyaline, eosinophilic material indicative of the so-called inductive effect may be noted at the epithelial and mesenchymal interface. The fibroblastic or mesenchymal component is hypercellular, often in a patchy distribution, with less cellular intervening areas. Nuclear pleomorphism and hyperchromasia are evident and mitotic figures numerous (fig. 6-17). The cells are arranged in a storiform to herringbone pattern, with occasional tumors containing stromal eosinophilic material in a delicate branching or lacelike pattern reminiscent of that seen in osteosarcomas. Dental matrix material similar to dentin may be noted within the intercellular areas (23).

Treatment and Prognosis. Resection of the affected segment of the maxilla or mandible remains the treatment of choice. Combination or adjuvant chemotherapy has also been recommended (26).

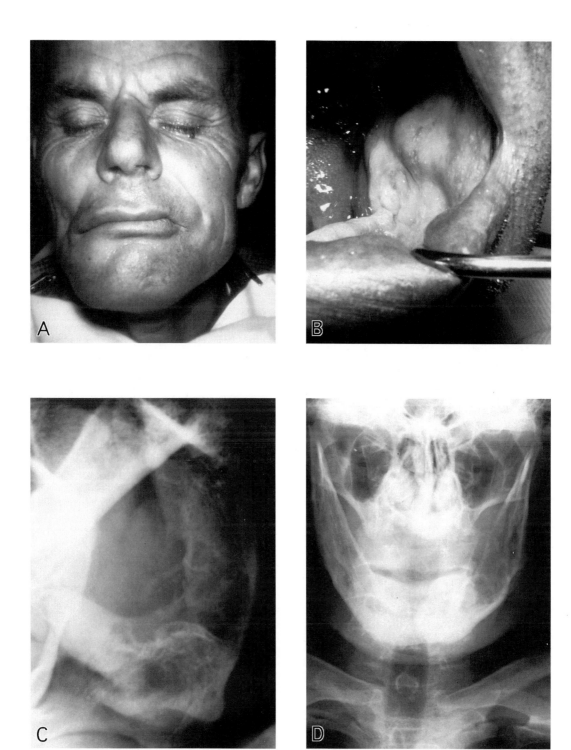

Figure 6-14
AMELOBLASTIC FIBROSARCOMA

A: Swelling and facial nerve dysesthesia is caused by a tumor in the left body and ramus of the mandible in this 43-year-old man.

B: An intraoral view of the patient in figure A shows intraoral swelling.

C: A lateral oblique radiograph shows that the tumor involves the inferior border of the body of the mandible and much of the mandibular ramus.

D: This radiogram shows a loculated lesion involving and thinning the lateral cortex of the body of the mandible. (Figs. 143–146 from Fascicle 24, 2nd Series.)

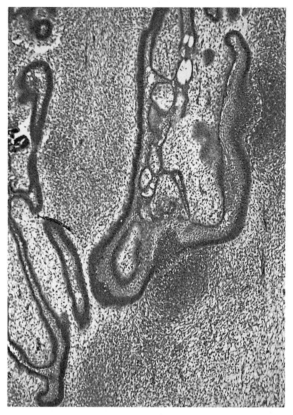

Figure 6-15
AMELOBLASTIC FIBROSARCOMA
Islands and cords of benign ameloblastic epithelial cells are seen within a hypercellular mesenchymal background.

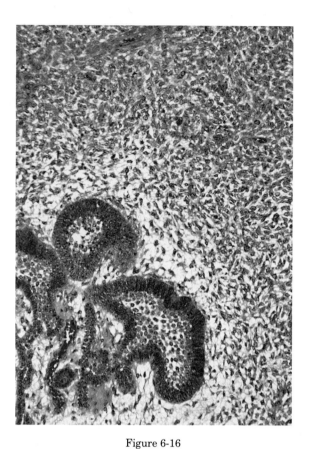

Figure 6-16
AMELOBLASTIC FIBROSARCOMA
Islands of ameloblastic epithelial cells are surrounded by a well-defined basement membrane adjacent to a hypercellular, malignant stroma.

Figure 6-17
AMELOBLASTIC
FIBROSARCOMA

A high-power view of a fibrosarcoma with hyperchromatic pleomorphic nuclei demonstrates coarse chromatin, irregular nuclear margins, and indistinct cellular borders.

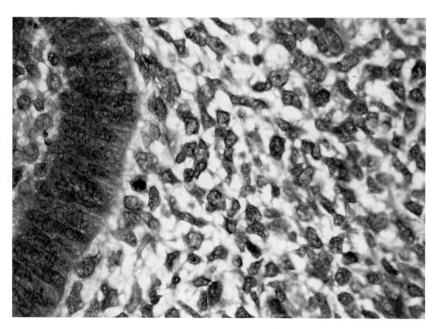

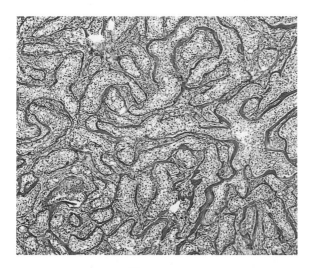

Figure 6-18
CLEAR CELL ODONTOGENIC CARCINOMA
Smoothly contoured islands of clear cells are delineated by a broad band of hyalinized stroma. The homogeneous cellular population is composed of cells with vacuolated to optically clear cytoplasm.

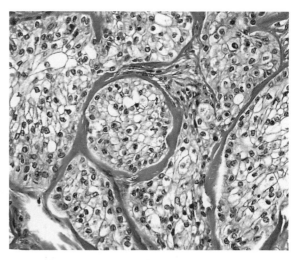

Figure 6-19
CLEAR CELL ODONTOGENIC CARCINOMA
A medium-power view shows glomeruloid structures rimmed by a thickened hyalinized basement membrane. Note the optically clear cytoplasm and centrally placed, uniformly stained nuclei.

Inadequate surgical treatment is followed by recurrence in all cases (31). While the number of cases reported is small, there appears to be a better prognosis for patients with this form of sarcoma than for those with other sarcomas of the jaw (23).

CLEAR CELL ODONTOGENIC CARCINOMA

Definition. Clear cell odontogenic carcinoma is a malignant epithelial odontogenic neoplasm in which the epithelial cell rests contain a variable proportion of glycogen-rich cells with optically clear cytoplasm. Many of these tumors contain foci of typical ameloblastoma or calcifying epithelial odontogenic tumor.

General Features. There is a wide variation in the proportion of clear cells in this tumor: some cases are composed almost exclusively of clear cells while others contain a significant number of other cellular elements. Metastases have been reported in about one third of cases (34,37,39,40). Waldron et al. (41) described a case of clear cell ameloblastoma that would currently be classified as a clear cell odontogenic carcinoma.

Clinical and Radiologic Features. On the basis of fewer than 20 reported cases, these tumors have behaved in a clinically aggressive manner with a tendency to local recurrence and metastasis in nearly two thirds of cases (35). Over 75 percent occurred in the mandible, with a distinct female predilection (76 percent) (35). Most cases are discovered between the fifth and seventh decades of life, with a peak in the fifth decade and a mean patient age of 53 years. Symptoms include mild pain and local discomfort; other patients may present with asymptomatic bony swellings and loosening of teeth. Radiologically, the lesions are radiolucent and permeative with irregular outlines, often with cortical destruction.

Microscopic Findings. The most common pattern is that of small islands or nests of epithelial cells with clear or finely granular cytoplasm surrounded by a fibrous connective tissue stroma (figs. 6-18, 6-19). The basal epithelial cell population may show some evidence of palisading, while their cytoplasm is faintly granular compared to the optically clear, more centrally placed cells within the islands (fig. 6-20). The clear cells are periodic acid–Schiff (PAS) positive and diastase labile and do not stain with Alcian blue (36). The tumor is unencapsulated and infiltrates medullary bone.

Many of these tumors are biphasic or multiphasic in that there may be islands of typical ameloblastoma and, less frequently, calcifying epithelial odontogenic tumor. Clear cells and

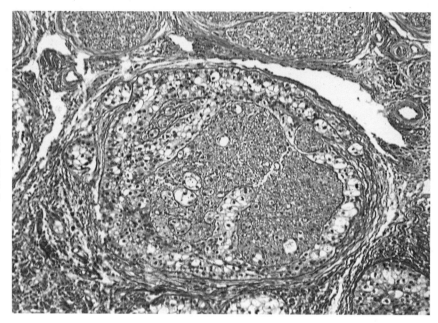

Figure 6-20
CLEAR CELL
ODONTOGENIC CARCINOMA
The centrally located population of cells within the clear cell odontogenic carcinoma has a granular cytoplasm with central nuclei. A glomeruloid architecture is also noted within the granular cell component.

more hyperchromatic polygonal cells may cluster in "glomeruloid" structures surrounded by a mature hyalinized stroma. The nuclei are oval and vary from vesicular to hyperchromatic.

Differential Diagnosis. Prior to establishing the diagnosis of a clear cell odontogenic carcinoma, metastatic renal cell carcinoma, intraosseous mucoepidermoid carcinoma, and clear cell variants of calcifying epithelial odontogenic tumor must be excluded (38).

Treatment and Prognosis. Given the high rate of pulmonary and lymphatic metastases, aggressive surgery with an adequate resection margin of normal surrounding tissue is indicated. The role of elective neck dissection has yet to be determined, given the paucity of reported cases.

REFERENCES

Primary Intraosseous Carcinoma

1. Anand VK, Arrowood JP, Krolls SO. Malignant potential of the odontogenic keratocyst. Otolaryngol Head Neck Surg 1994;111:124–9.
2. Elzay RP. Primary intraosseous carcinoma of the jaws. Review and update of odontogenic carcinomas. Oral Surg Oral Med Oral Pathol 1982;54:299–303.
3. Eversole LR, Sabes WR, Rovin S. Aggressive growth and neoplastic potential of odontogenic cysts, with special reference to central epidermoid and mucoepidermoid carcinomas. Cancer 1975;35:270–82.
4. Muller S, Waldron CA. Primary intraosseous squamous carcinoma. Report of two cases. Int J Oral Maxillofac Surg 1991;20:362–5.
5. Nolan R, Wood NK. Central squamous cell carcinoma of the mandible: report of a case. J Oral Surg 1976;34:260–4.
6. Ruskin JD, Cohen DM, Davis LF. Primary intraosseous carcinoma: report of two cases. J Oral Maxillofac Surg 1988;46:425–32.
7. Shear M. Primary intra-alveolar epidermoid carcinoma of the jaw. J Pathol 1969;97:645–51.
8. Suei Y, Tanimoto K, Taguchi A, Wada T. Primary intraosseous carcinoma: review of the literature and diagnostic criteria. J Oral Maxillofac Surg 1994;52:580–3.
9. To EH, Brown JS, Avery BS, Ward-Booth RP. Primary intraosseous carcinoma of the jaws. Three new cases and a review of the literature. Br J Oral Maxillofac Surg 1991;29:19–25.
10. Waldron CA, Mustoe TA. Primary intraosseous carcinoma of the mandible with probable origin in an odontogenic cyst. Oral Surg Oral Med Oral Pathol 1989;67:716–24.

Carcinoma Arising in Odontogenic Cysts

11. Brookstone MS, Huvos AG. Central salivary gland tumors of the maxilla and mandible. A clinicopathologic study of 11 cases with an analysis of the literature. J Oral Maxillofac Surg 1992;50:229–36.
12. Browne RM, Gough NG. Malignant change in the epithelium lining odontogenic cysts. Report of a case. Cancer 1972;29:1199–207.
13. el Mofty SK, Shannon MT, Mustoe TA. Lymph node metastasis in spindle cell carcinoma arising in an odontogenic cyst. Report of a case. Oral Surg Oral Med Oral Pathol 1991;71:209–13.
14. Enriquez RE, Ciola B, Bahn SL. Verrucous carcinoma arising in an odontogenic cyst. Oral Surg Oral Med Oral Pathol 1980;49:151–6.
15. Eversole LR, Sabes WR, Rovin S. Aggressive growth and neoplastic potential of odontogenic cysts with special reference to central epidermoid and mucoepidermoid carcinomas. Cancer 1975;35:270–82.
16. Gardner AF. The odontogenic cyst as a potential carcinoma: a clinicopathologic appraisal. J Am Dent Assoc 1969;78:746–55.
17. Johnson LM, Sapp JP, McIntire DN. Squamous cell carcinoma arising in a dentigerous cyst. J Oral Maxillofac Surg 1994;52:987–90.
18. Manganaro AM, Cross SE, Startzell JM. Carcinoma arising in a dentigerous cyst with neck metastasis. Head Neck 1997;19:436–9.
19. Manojlovic S, Grgurevic J, Knezevic G, Kruslin B. Glandular odontogenic cyst: a case report and clinicopathologic analysis of the relationship to central mucoepidermoid carcinoma. Head Neck 1997;19:227–31.
20. Maxymiw WG, Wood RE. Carcinoma arising in a dentigerous cyst: a case report and review of the literature. J Oral Maxillofac Surg 1991;49:639–43.
21. McDonald AR, Pogrel MA, Carson J, Regezi J. p53 positive squamous cell carcinoma originating from an odontogenic cyst. J Oral Maxillofac Surg 1996;54:216–8.
22. Waldron CA, Mustoe T. Primary intraosseous carcinoma of the mandible with probable origin in an odontogenic cyst. Oral Surg Oral Med Oral Pathol 1989;67:716–24.

Ameloblastic Fibrosarcoma

23. Altini M, Thompson SH, Lownie JF, Berezowski BB. Ameloblastic sarcoma of the mandible. J Oral Maxillofac Surg 1985;43:789–94.
24. Dallera P, Bertoni F, Marchetti C, Bacchini P, Campobassi A. Ameloblastic fibrosarcoma of the jaw: report of five cases. J Craniomaxfac Surg 1994;22:349–54.
25. Daramola JO, Ajagbe HA, Olawasanmi JO, Akinyemi OO, Samuel I. Ameloblastic sarcoma of the mandible. Report of a case. J Oral Surg 1979;37:432–5.
26. Goldstein G, Parker FP, Hugh GS. Ameloblastic sarcoma: pathogenesis and treatment with chemotherapy. Cancer 1976;37:1673–8.
27. Howell RM, Burkes J, Hill C. Malignant transformation of ameloblastic fibro-odontoma to ameloblastic fibrosarcoma. Oral Surg 1977;43:391–401.
28. Leider AS, Nelson JF, Trodahl JN. Ameloblastic fibrosarcoma of the jaws. Oral Surg 1972;33:559–69.
28a. Muller S, Parker DC, Kapadia SB, Budnick SD, Barnes EL. Ameloblastic fibrosarcoma of the jaws. A clinicopathologic and DNA analysis of five cases and review of the literature with discussion of its relationship to ameloblastic fibroma. Oral Surg Oral Med Oral Pathol 1995;79:468–77.
29. Pindborg JJ. Ameloblastic sarcoma in the maxilla. Cancer 1960;13:917–20.
30. Sozeri B, Ataman M, Ruacan S, Gedikoglu G. Ameloblastic fibrosarcoma. Int J Ped Otorhinolaryngol 1993;25:255–9.
31. Takeda Y, Kaneko R, Suzuki A. Ameloblastic fibrosarcoma in the maxilla, malignant transformation of an ameloblastic fibroma. Virchows Arch [A] 1984;404:253–63.
32. Tanaka T, Ohkubo T, Fujitsuka H, et al. Malignant mixed tumor (malignant ameloblastoma and fibrosarcoma) of the maxilla. Arch Pathol Lab Med 1991;115:84–7.
33. Trodahl JN. Ameloblastic fibroma. A survey of cases from the Armed Forces Institute of Pathology. Oral Surg 1972;33:547–58.

Clear Cell Odontogenic Carcinoma

34. Bang G, Koppang HS, Hansen LS, Gilhus-Moe O, Aksdal E, Persson PG. Clear cell odontogenic carcinoma: report of 3 cases with pulmonary and lymph node metastases. J Oral Pathol Med 1989;18:113–8.
35. Eversole LR, Belton CM, Hansen LS. Clear cell odontogenic tumor: histochemical and ultrastructural features. J Oral Pathol 1985;14:603–14.
36. Eversole LR, Duffey DC, Powell NB. Clear cell odontogenic carcinoma. Arch Otolaryngol Head Neck Surg 1995; 121:685–9.
37. Fan J, Kubota E, Immamura H, et al. Clear cell odontogenic carcinoma. A case report with massive invasion of neighboring organs and lymph node metastasis. Oral Surg Oral Med Oral Pathol 1992;74:768–75.
38. Hansen LS, Eversole LR, Green TL, Powell NG. Clear cell odontogenic tumor—a new histologic variant with aggressive potential. Head Neck Surg 1985;8:115–23.
39. Milles M, Doyle JL, Mesa M, Raz S. Clear cell odontogenic carcinoma with lymph node metastasis. Oral Surg Oral Med Oral Pathol 1993;76:82–9.
40. Piatelli A, Sesenna E, Trisi P. Clear cell odontogenic carcinoma. Report of a case with lymph node and pulmonary metastases. Eur J Cancer B Oral Oncol 1995;30B:278–80.
41. Waldron CA, Small IA, Silverman H. Clear cell ameloblastoma—an odontogenic carcinoma. J Oral Maxillofac Surg 1985;43:707–17.

7

FIBRO-OSSEOUS LESIONS

The noncommittal or generic terminology, "fibro-osseous lesion of bone," is widely used to connote a skeletal lesion in which the normal lamellar bone is replaced by vascularized fibrous tissue and seams of osteoid or bone, predominantly or exclusively of woven type. This definition encompasses several more specific entities, namely, fibrous dysplasia, ossifying fibroma, and juvenile or aggressive ossifying fibroma.

The dental literature is replete with articles purporting to show that fibrous dysplasia and ossifying fibroma are distinct entities, each with its own distinctive clinical, radiologic, and histologic features (1). The authors of these articles contend that fibrous dysplasia represents a developmental defect of bone in which woven bone fails to mature to lamellar bone, whereas ossifying fibroma is a true benign neoplastic process. In the majority of gnathic fibro-osseous lesions, a thorough correlation of clinical, radiographic, intraoperative, and histologic features allows a clear distinction between fibrous dysplasia and ossifying fibroma. There may be cases, however, in which it is difficult to categorize the fibro-osseous lesion as falling into one of these entities. In a recent study of 56 gnathic and extragnathic lesions from the MD Anderson Hospital, Voytek et al. (2) were able to classify 24 as fibrous dysplasia and 10 as ossifying fibroma but the remaining 22 showed overlapping histologic features. They also found that there was considerable radiologic overlap between the two entities. They proposed that fibrous dysplasia and ossifying fibroma may represent a single entity with a continuum of clinical, radiologic, and histologic features. In the jaw bones we believe that the two entities can be distinguished by careful clinicopathologic evaluation and that the term "fibro-osseous, not otherwise specified" be reserved for the few cases in which such differentiation cannot be made.

FIBROUS DYSPLASIA

Historical Features. Examples of polyostotic fibrous dysplasia were probably first included in cases described by von Recklinghausen as deforming osteitis fibrosa in 1891 (4a). In 1937, Albright et al. (3) and McCune and Burch (10) independently documented the occurrence of skin pigmentation and precocious sexual development in females in association with disseminated bone lesions. The term "polyostotic fibrous dysplasia" was coined by Lichtenstein in 1938 (8) and in 1942 Lichtenstein and Jaffe (9) categorized fibrous dysplasia into monostotic and polyostotic forms.

Clinical Features. Fibrous dysplasia may involve only a single bone (monostotic), multiple bones (polyostotic), multiple bones confined to one side of the body, or multiple bones and an association with melanin pigmentation of the skin and precocious sexual development in females (McCune-Albright syndrome).

About 70 percent of cases of fibrous dysplasia are of monostotic type, with the jaw and facial bones comprising about 10 percent of the total. The maxilla is involved more frequently than the mandible. The remaining 30 percent of cases are of polyostotic type while about 3 percent manifest as McCune-Albright syndrome. Polyostotic fibrous dysplasia involves the craniofacial region in 50 to 100 percent of cases; the neural cranium and the facial cranium are almost equally affected (7). Polyostotic lesions may be limited to the craniofacial bones. The disease is usually diagnosed during childhood, with a peak incidence in the second and third decades. Progression of disease occurs during the period of bone growth and tends to stabilize with cessation of bone growth. However, lesional growth and activity may persist into adulthood. Females are more often affected than males and there is no particular racial predilection.

The lesion expands the involved bone without eroding the overlying cortex. This bony expansion may cause significant cosmetic deformity during the period of active bone growth. The deformity may result in malocclusion of teeth (7); lesions in the maxilla and cranial bones may produce orbital deformity and rarely diplopia with proptosis as well as deformity of the paranasal sinuses and nasal passages resulting in nasal obstruction.

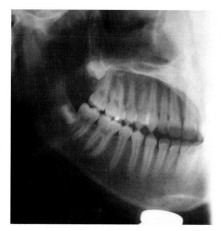
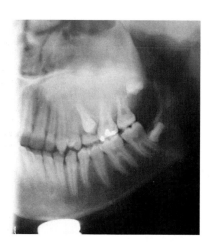

Figure 7-1
FIBROUS DYSPLASIA
OF MAXILLA

Typical radiologic features of fibrous dysplasia in a 14-year-old girl: poorly delimited radiodense lesion with a "ground glass" appearance involving the right maxilla including antrum. The lesion envelopes but does not displace or resorb involved teeth. (Figures 7-1, 7-3, and 7-4 are from the same patient.)

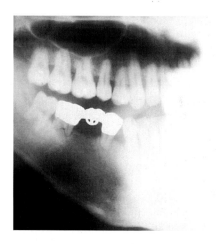
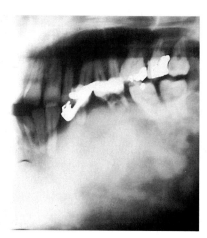

Figure 7-2
FIBROUS DYSPLASIA
OF MANDIBLE

The right side of the body of the mandible shows features similar to those seen in figure 7-1.

Radiologic Findings. During the early active phase of the lesion, the presence of vascularized fibrous tissue and poorly mineralized woven bone produces an osteolytic lesion. As the myriad of woven bone plates within the lesion become more densely mineralized, they produce the characteristic "ground-glass" or "orange peel" radiologic appearance (figs. 7-1, 7-2). The margins of the lesion are usually ill-defined. The lesional tissue wraps around teeth rather displacing them; however, segmental alveolar displacement may occur with corresponding tooth malposition and occlusal table alterations. The lesion expands the involved bone but does not transgress the cortical plates. Occasionally, the margins are more sharply defined and internal trabeculation may produce a unilocular or multilocular cystic appearance. During the late healing or maturational phase, the lesion may acquire a more densely sclerotic appearance.

Superior displacement of the mandibular canal is a rare radiologic finding (5).

Pathologic Findings. Fibrous dysplasia is composed of variably shaped spicules of woven bone set in a vascularized fibrous stroma. The woven bone spicules are fairly evenly distributed throughout the lesion and in their variety of shapes, have been compared to letters in the Chinese alphabet (figs. 7-3, 7-4). Individual trabeculae have a curvilinear shape. The stromal cellularity is variable from case to case and in an individual lesion. Conversely, the amount of collagen varies and is usually inversely proportional to the degree of cellularity. The nuclei of the stromal fibroblasts may be plump and ovoid or slender. However, they never exhibit atypism and are devoid of mitoses. Of particular importance is the fact that the stromal fibroblasts produce the bony matrix without morphologic evidence of transformation into polygonal

142

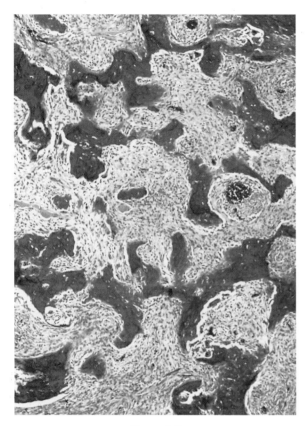

Figure 7-3
FIBROUS DYSPLASIA OF MAXILLA
The typical pattern of fibrous dysplasia is comprised of variously shaped spicules of woven bone, described as resembling characters in the Chinese alphabet, separated by moderately cellular fibrovascular stroma.

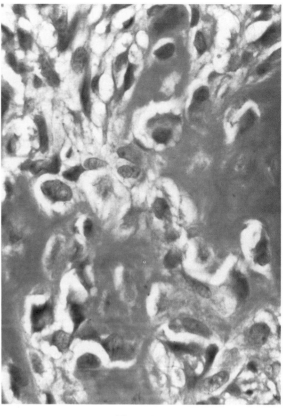

Figure 7-4
FIBROUS DYSPLASIA OF MAXILLA
High magnification of figure 7-3 shows woven bone surrounded by plump ovoid to spindle-shaped fibroblast nuclei with finely dispersed chromatin and small nucleoli. No well-defined layer of rimming osteoblasts is seen.

osteoblastic cells that align themselves at the periphery of the lamellae, as is seen in reactive callus bone and in ossifying fibroma. In the jaw bones, mineralized matrix in the form of spherical, concentrically laminated cementum or cementum-like material may be present in addition to the woven bone.

In about 10 percent of cases of fibrous dysplasia in extragnathic locations, islands of cartilage constitute part of the matrix. When the cartilagenous element is abundant, the lesion may be misinterpreted as an enchondroma or even a low-grade chondrosarcoma. Cartilage has not been described as a component of the matrix in fibrous dysplasia of jaw bones.

As the lesion has been considered by many authorities to be a developmental defect in the

maturation of woven to lamellar bone, the presence of lamellar bone should preclude a diagnosis of fibrous dysplasia. Some authors, however, have described lamellar bone in association with fibrous dysplasia (11). This may represent a maturational phenomenon that occurs during healing of the lesion. Lamellar bone may also be derived from nonlesional tissue curetted from the periphery of the lesion. We have recently had the opportunity to study material from a patient over 80 years of age who had polyostotic fibrous dysplasia since childhood. Although the stromal element was inactive and relatively acellular, the matrix was composed almost exclusively of thicker trabeculae of woven bone. The only lamellar bone detected was at the periphery of the lesion and this was associated with bone marrow elements, suggesting its derivation from non-lesional bone.

Molecular Pathology. Molecular alterations have been detected in fibrous dysplasia. These involve the intracellular guanine nucleotide–binding proteins (G proteins) associated with signal transduction via cell surface receptors. Such alterations permit abnormal cell growth and tumorigenesis without the need for receptor occupancy. The mutant gene is usually present in small amounts and requires a polymerase chain reaction–based technique for its detection. Using such a technique, Candeliere et al. (4) demonstrated a somatic mutation in all eight fibrous dysplasia cases studied in DNA obtained from both the osseous lesions and from blood leukocytes, but no such alterations in the 13 control cases. Of particular interest was the unique mutation involving the substitution of arginine for serine in a patient with panostotic fibrous dysplasia as compared to the more typical substitution of arginine for histidine or cysteine. The more typical substitutions have been demonstrated in multiple tissues of patients with McCune-Albright's syndrome (13). These molecular techniques may in the future enable us to define subsets of fibrous dysplasia with distinctive biologic characteristics.

Differential Diagnosis. Judicious correlation of clinical, radiologic, and histologic features usually ensures a correct diagnosis. However, as indicated above, the radiologic features may vary from the typical ill-defined lesion with ground-glass texture to a more circumscribed cystic-appearing lesion to a densely sclerotic lesion. The radiologic differential diagnosis is thus quite broad and includes odontogenic cysts, ameloblastoma, osteomyelitis, desmoplastic fibroma, and osteosarcoma. Histologically, the most important differential diagnoses are osteomyelitis, desmoplastic fibroma, and central low-grade osteosarcoma. The reactive bone present in chronic osteomyelitis can readily be distinguished from the woven bone matrix of fibrous dysplasia. The former resembles callus in that the woven bone spicules exhibit a more orderly, often parallel, arrangement and are typically lined by plump epithelioid-shaped osteoblasts with distinct basophilic cytoplasm. Scattered chronic inflammatory cells can be identified within the fibrovascular stroma. Desmoplastic

fibroma resembles its soft tissue counterpart, the desmoid tumor (fibromatosis), and is devoid of bone except for residual islands of lamellar bone entrapped by the process. The most important distinction is from low-grade central osteosarcoma. As discussed in the section dealing with osteosarcoma of the jaws, the low-grade central osteosarcoma bears a striking superficial histologic resemblance to fibrous dysplasia. The neoplastic woven bone spicules are more haphazardly distributed in the sarcoma, the stromal neoplastic cells usually show a mild but definite degree of atypia, and there is a tendency for the neoplastic bone to be laid down in direct apposition to fragments of residual lamellar bone surviving within the lesion.

Treatment and Prognosis. Most authorities recommend a conservative approach to the treatment of fibrous dysplasia. If the patient can be tided over until termination of skeletal growth when the lesion is likely to stabilize, definitive surgery can be effected at that time. If surgical intervention is then required only for cosmetic purposes, a limited contouring procedure is recommended. More radical and earlier intervention may be required should the lesion produce significant functional or psychologic disability. Curettage is the usual surgical modality but, rarely, resection of the lesion with subsequent reconstruction may be required (fig. 7-5). Surgical intervention during the active growth phase of the lesion is often followed by rapid and prompt recurrence. Under no circumstances should radiotherapy be utilized because of its limited effectiveness and danger of subsequent radiation-induced sarcoma. The rate of sarcomatous transformation in fibrous dysplasia is reported to be 0.4 percent. Twelve of 29 patients with malignancy complicating fibrous dysplasia had received radiotherapy at an average of 14 years prior to diagnosis of the sarcoma (6). Another review of 33 cases of fibrous dysplasia with malignant transformation included 13 with facial bone involvement; the authors estimated an incidence of malignant transformation following radiotherapy of 44 percent (12). Any lesion of fibrous dysplasia that manifests a sudden accelerated growth spurt or severe pain should be suspected of having undergone malignant change.

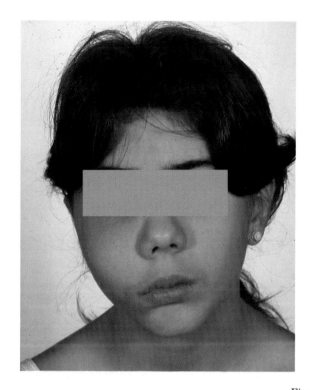
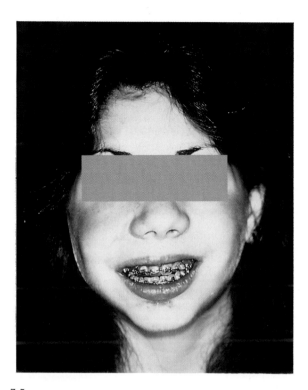

Figure 7-5
FIBROUS DYSPLASIA OF MAXILLA
Left: The 14-year-old girl whose radiographs and histology are seen in figures 7-1, 7-3, and 7-4, prior to cosmetic surgical intervention.
Right: Following surgery.

OSSIFYING FIBROMA (CEMENTO-OSSIFYING FIBROMA)

Clinical Features. Ossifying fibroma occurs most frequently in the second and third decades of life. It is more common in the mandible than in the maxillofacial region and in females. Its presentation is similar to that of fibrous dysplasia in that it causes expansion of the bone without violating the cortical plate. It may cause cosmetic deformities and malocclusion; if the maxillary region is affected, nasal, antral, or orbital deformity may result. In neglected cases, the deformity may be severe (fig. 7-6) (15).

Radiologic Findings. The involved bone is expanded by a well-delineated radiolucent or mixed radiolucent and radiopaque lesion. The margin may be slightly sclerotic. As the lesion expands, it tends to cause displacement and root resorption of teeth rather than enveloping them as in fibrous dysplasia (figs. 7-7, 7-8). It may also displace the mandibular canal.

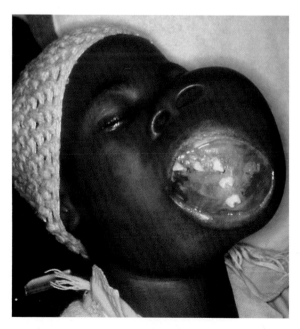

Figure 7-6
OSSIFYING FIBROMA OF MANDIBLE
A 13-year-old black girl with a huge ossifying fibroma of left maxilla. (Courtesy of Prof. Erich J. Raubenheimer, Medunsa, South Africa). (Figures 7-6 and 7-9 are from the same patient.)

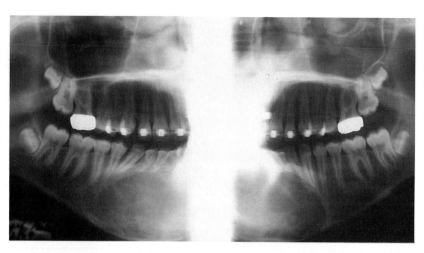

Figure 7-7
OSSIFYING
FIBROMA OF MANDIBLE
Panoramic radiograph of mandible shows a sharply circumscribed lesion in the anterior body. The lesion is displacing the roots of the overlying teeth rather than enveloping them as in fibrous dysplasia.

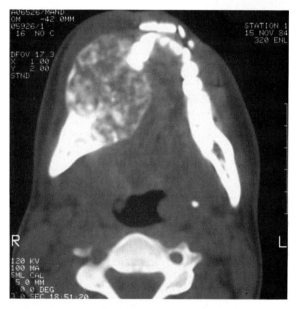

Figure 7-8
OSSIFYING FIBROMA OF MANDIBLE
This CT axial image demonstrates the well-circumscribed appearance of an expansile lesion with multiple radiopaque foci of mineralization. (Figures 7-8, 7-10, and 7-11 are from the same patient.)

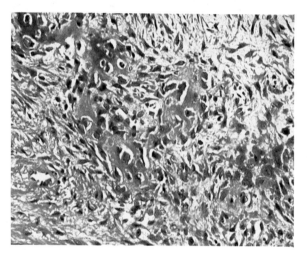

Figure 7-9
OSSIFYING FIBROMA
Typical pattern of anastomosing trabeculae of woven bone lined by active osteoblasts and separated by cellular fibrovascular stroma.

Pathologic Findings. Grossly, the lesion is extremely well circumscribed, with a smooth outer contour. For this reason, it can be readily surgically dissected from adjacent normal bone. Histologically, ossifying fibroma shows architectural features similar to those of fibrous dysplasia: spicules of osteoid or woven bone of varying shape are set in a vascularized fibrous stroma. Unlike fibrous dysplasia, in which matrix formation proceeds directly from the stromal fibrocytic type cells, the stromal cells in ossifying fibroma evolve into rimming osteoblasts which line the bony spicules (figs. 7-9, 7-10). As in fibrous dysplasia, cementicles might constitute a minor or major portion of the mineralized matrix. The term *juvenile ossifying fibroma* has been applied to lesions with a highly cellular stroma and cell-rich osteoblastic cords (14a). Patients with this variant are usually diagnosed at an earlier age.

Differential Diagnosis. Radiologically, the circumscribed cystic appearance of the lesion resembles odontogenic cyst and ameloblastoma. Histologically, it is usually not confused with other lesions except fibrous dysplasia.

Treatment and Prognosis. The sharp circumscription of the lesion lends itself readily to surgical enucleation (fig. 7-11). Sciubba and Younai (14) noted only a single recurrence in 18 cases of ossifying fibroma, the majority of which were treated by conservative excision.

Juvenile Ossifying Fibroma

Definition. Juvenile ossifying fibroma (JOF) is a variant of ossifying fibroma characterized clinically by rapid evolution in a young age group and histologically by a cellular fibrous stroma containing a network of osteoid seams rimmed by plump, active osteoblasts. Synonyms include *aggressive ossifying fibroma, young ossifying fibroma, juvenile active ossifying fibroma, trabecular desmo-osteoblastoma, active fibrous dysplasia, psammo-osteoid fibroma, psammomatoid desmo-osteoblastoma,* and *psammomatoid ossifying fibroma.*

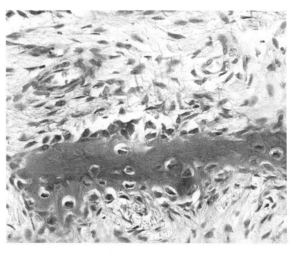

Figure 7-10
OSSIFYING FIBROMA OF MANDIBLE
The histologic appearance differs from fibrous dysplasia in that the fibrocytic cells show differentiation into plump polygonal osteoblasts which rim the newly formed trabeculae of woven bone.

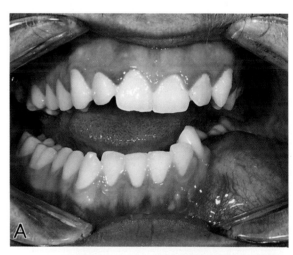

Figure 7-11
OSSIFYING FIBROMA OF MANDIBLE
Presurgical appearance of lesion causing prominent swelling of the right mandibular body and severe dental malocclusion (A). Postsurgical restoration of dental occlusion following simple enucleation of lesion (B,C).

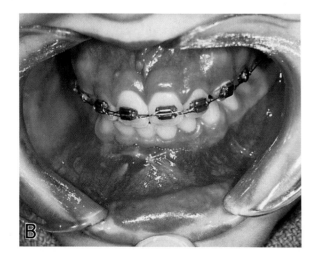

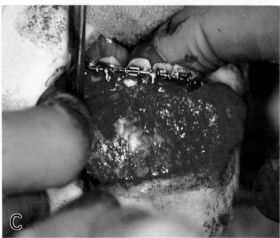

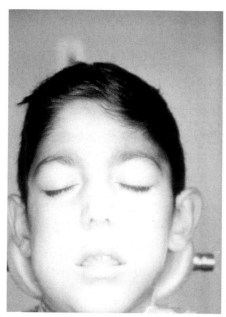
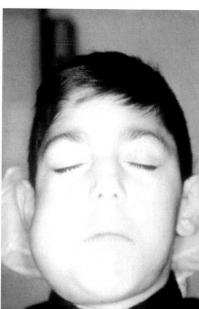

Figure 7-12
JUVENILE
OSSIFYING FIBROMA
Rapid clinical progression of this lesion in the body of the right mandible is evident in these two photographs taken 5 months apart. (Figures 7-12, 7-13, and 7-15 from the same patient.)

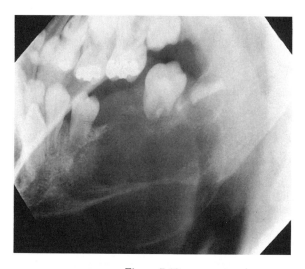

Figure 7-13
JUVENILE OSSIFYING FIBROMA
A radiolucent expansile lesion of the mandibular body has a well-defined sclerotic margin.

Clinical and Radiologic Features. JOF usually manifests between the ages of 5 and 15 years and exhibits rapid growth over a period of several weeks rather than the typical slow growth pattern over months and years of the nonjuvenile form (fig. 7-12) (17–19). It involves the maxilla and paranasal sinuses more frequently than the mandible (21). As with its nonaggressive counterpart, it is radiologically a well-delineated ra-

diolucent lesion but may show foci of mineralization (fig. 7-13) (16). However, as a consequence of its rapid growth it may cause erosion and even disappearance of adjacent bone (fig. 7-14).

Pathologic Findings. The histologic features are very similar to those described for ossifying fibroma. The stromal cellularity is of a higher order, with less collagen formation and a few mitotic figures (figs. 7-15–7-23). The network of woven bone seams is rimmed by plump, active, polygonal osteoblasts as in ossifying fibroma (figs. 7-18, 7-19) (18). Cementum-like or psammomatous structures might constitute a minor, major, or even exclusive component of the mineralized matrix. In an analysis of 33 cases of JOF, Slootweg et al. (20) found that 23 showed a predominant psammomatous pattern of matrix mineralization and that this subset occurred in an older age group. They recommended that this group be designated "cemento-ossifying fibroma" rather than juvenile ossifying fibroma. However, as psammomatous mineralization is not infrequently seen as a component of fibro-osseous lesions in odontogenic locations and even in extragnathic fibro-osseous lesions, we question the validity of separating this subset simply on the basis of this histologic feature. JOF may also show foci with osteoclastic type giant cells, often associated with intralesional hemorrhage and cystic degeneration (20). We believe this may

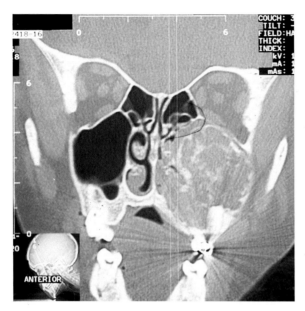

Figure 7-14
JUVENILE OSSIFYING FIBROMA

CT scan from an 11-year-old boy with swelling of left
maxillary region. The lesion has caused expansion of the
maxillary antrum and has extended into the nasal cavity.
Most of the lesion is still delimited by an attenuated bony
shell. (Figures 7-14, 7-16–7-23 are from the same patient.)

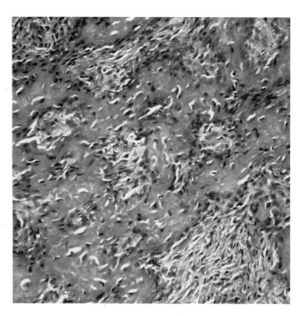

Figure 7-15
JUVENILE OSSIFYING FIBROMA

A network of osteoid seams is rimmed by a layer of active
osteoblasts and separated by a moderately cellular fibrous
stroma.

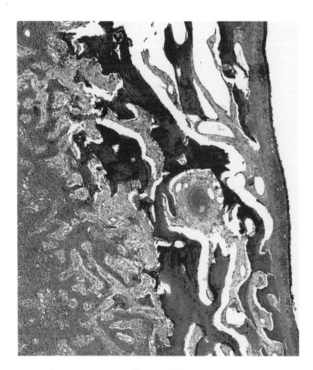

Figure 7-16
JUVENILE OSSIFYING FIBROMA

A shell of residual lamellar bone separates lesional tissue
from overlying antral mucosa.

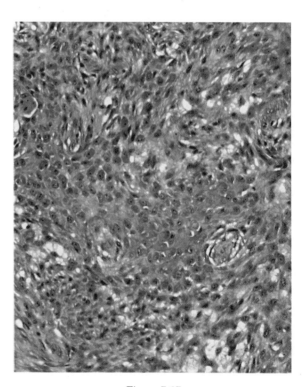

Figure 7-17
JUVENILE OSSIFYING FIBROMA

The cellular stroma is composed of spindle- to ovoid-
shaped fibrocytic cells. An incipient focus of osteoid matrix
formation is in the center of the photomicrograph.

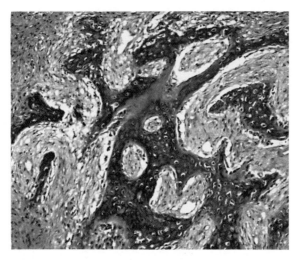

Figure 7-18
JUVENILE OSSIFYING FIBROMA
A network of osteoid seams is rimmed by a layer of osteoblasts and separated by moderately cellular fibrovascular stroma.

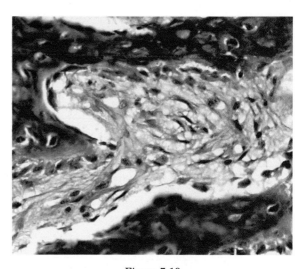

Figure 7-19
JUVENILE OSSIFYING FIBROMA
High-power view of figure 7-18 shows the lining osteoblasts and stromal fibroblasts in detail.

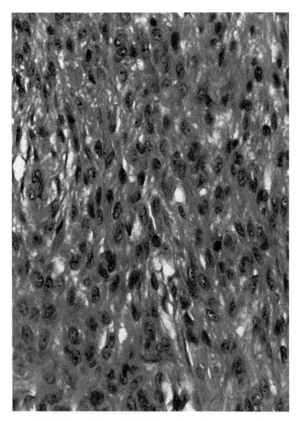

Figure 7-20
JUVENILE OSSIFYING FIBROMA
Areas of tumor lack osteoid formation. Mitotic figures are not infrequent. A biopsy from this area could raise concern about a diagnosis of low-grade fibrosarcoma or desmoplastic fibroma.

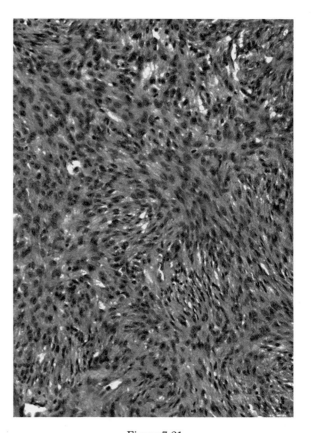

Figure 7-21
JUVENILE OSSIFYING FIBROMA
An area of tumor that lacks osteoid formation and has a storiform growth pattern.

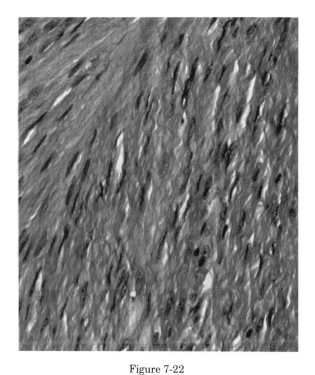

Figure 7-22
JUVENILE OSSIFYING FIBROMA
This area of tumor lacks osteoid formation and is comprised of elongated fibrocytic nuclei with abundant collagen resembling desmoplastic fibroma.

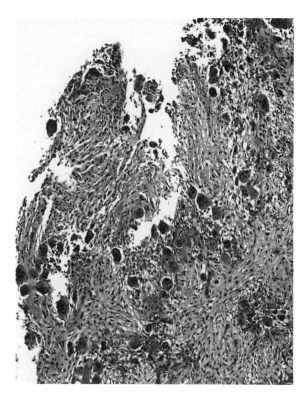

Figure 7-23
JUVENILE OSSIFYING FIBROMA
A cystic focus with numerous osteoclast giant cells in the adjacent tissue is indicative of secondary aneurysmal bone cyst formation.

represent foci of secondary aneurysmal bone cyst formation (fig. 7-23).

Treatment and Prognosis. The recurrence rate for JOF is 30 to 58 percent, which is greater than that for the nonjuvenile form (21). For this reason, a more radical surgical approach has been advocated by some although many surgeons still prefer conservative curettage or resection (fig. 7-24). Radiotherapy is contraindicated. There has been no report of evolution into a sarcoma.

PERIAPICAL CEMENTAL DYSPLASIA

Definition. Periapical cemental dysplasia is the most common member of the group of "cemento-osseous dysplasias" with postulated origin from the periodontal membrane (22). While related to florid cemento-osseous dysplasia and focal cemento-osseous dysplasia, this entity is nearly always a self-limited condition occurring at the apex of mandibular incisor teeth. Synonyms include *periapical cemento-osseous dysplasia* and *periapical cementoma*.

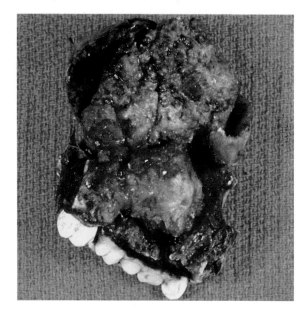

Figure 7-24
JUVENILE OSSIFYING FIBROMA
A more radical resection was performed in this patient.

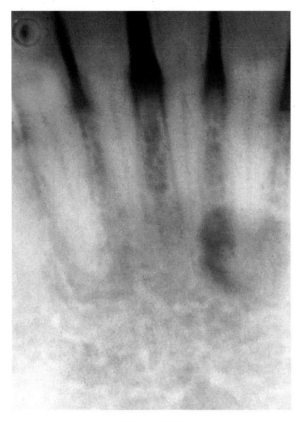

Figure 7-25
PERIAPICAL CEMENTAL DYSPLASIA
A periapical radiograph demonstrates early to intermediate signs of apical alteration characterized by a well-defined periapical radiolucency within which are signs of early mineralization at the tooth apex.

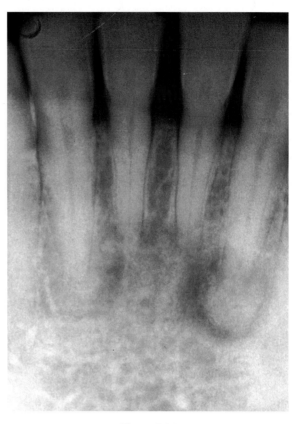

Figure 7-26
PERIAPICAL CEMENTAL DYSPLASIA
This periapical film of the same patient nearly 3 years later shows increased radiodensity at the apices of the mandibular lateral incisor teeth. The peripheral lucent halo is less dominant, while the centrally located opacification has increased significantly in size.

Clinical and Radiologic Features. Periapical cemental dysplasia is an asymptomatic condition involving the apical region of the mandibular anterior teeth. It occurs in the fourth and fifth decades. It may be focal and involve only a single or a few adjacent teeth; less frequently, lesions may occur synchronously in the mandible and maxilla (23). Involvement of the premolar and molar regions has been reported in Japan (23).

In the early stages of development the lesion is radiolucent, periapical in location, and ranges from a few millimeters to less than a centimeter in diameter. Rarely, it may reach a diameter of greater than 1 cm. The lucent phase of development is characterized by a well-defined periphery which is not corticated (fig. 7-25). The periapical lamina dura is usually lost; however, on occasion the lesion may develop at a slight distance from the apex with preservation of the lamina dura. Persistence of the lamina dura indicates a vital tooth pulp.

When the lesion has been present for a decade or longer, increasing radiodensity is noted, culminating in near complete opacification (fig. 7-26). Maturation usually occurs in a centrifugal pattern. A thin, circumferential, lucent line may be noted along the outer margin of the opacity and this lucency is contiguous with the periodontal membrane space along the tooth root. The radiographic differential diagnosis includes the common periapical granuloma or radicular cyst and focal cemento-osseous dysplasia.

Histologic Findings. The earliest osteodestructive phase consists of a fibrovascular proliferation: individual fibroblasts are plump and bipolar and the vessels thin walled (fig. 7-27). An

152

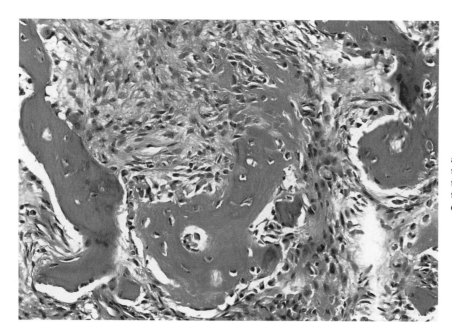

Figure 7-27
PERIAPICAL
CEMENTAL DYSPLASIA
A fibroblastic cellular stroma is associated with immature dysplastic bony tissue representing the intermediate phase of development of this periapical cemento-osseous dysplastic process.

Figure 7-28
PERIAPICAL
CEMENTAL DYSPLASIA
Droplet type of cemental mineralization demonstrates annular incremental rings. Adjacent droplets fuse to form larger irregular masses of cementum and bony conglomerates.

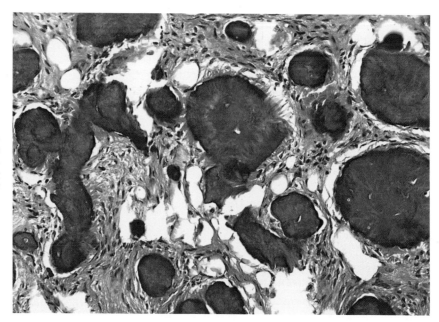

intermediate phase may be noted with cementoblastic cell proliferation and deposition of matrix in irregular droplet form. Maturation is characterized by fusion and coalescence of cementum (fig. 7-28). Masses or sheets of cementum with a gently contoured or molded periphery ultimately form. Collagen fibers extend from the cementum into the stroma perpendicular to the cemental surface. A diminishing volume of stroma characterizes the later phases of maturation.

Treatment and Prognosis. Management should not extend beyond establishing the diagnosis. This may include a pulp vitality test after radiographic documentation is obtained. To be avoided is overzealous surgical intervention or endodontic pulpal extirpation.

FLORID CEMENTO-OSSEOUS DYSPLASIA

Definition. Florid osseous dysplasia is a non-neoplastic condition of bone and cementum which is unique to the jaws. Confusion concerning terminology over the years has resulted in a plethora of synonymous terms for this process which have included *gigantiform cementoma, familial multiple cementomas, sclerotic cemental masses, multiple periapical fibro-osteomas, florid osseous dysplasia,* and *florid cemental dysplasia.*

General Features. Sclerosing osteitis and chronic sclerosing osteomyelitis are unrelated to this entity, however, secondarily infected florid cemento-osseous dysplasia may resemble osteomyelitis clinically and pathologically. Young et al. (31) categorized an extremely rare familial form of florid cemento-osseous dysplasia as familial gigantiform cementoma. They reported a large kindred of over five generations with a deforming, multiquadrant presentation; the anterior mandible was the most severely affected site (figs. 7-29, 7-30). Familial relationship, early age of onset, extensive jaw expansion, relatively rapid growth, and absence of ɔimple type bone cysts are necessary criteria of familial gigantiform cementoma. Finally, an entity termed *multiple familial ossifying fibroma* has been described in relation to two affected generations (30).

Clinical and Radiologic Features. Florid cemento-osseous dysplasia is usually asymptomatic and has a predilection for black females; the peak incidence is between the fourth and fifth decades of life. On occasion, a dull aching sensation may be noted, while pain, swelling, and low-grade fever may be present when infection supervenes (26). Posterior segments of the mandible are preferentially involved and unifocal lesions outnumber multifocal ones by a 2 to 1 ratio (29). Controversy exists regarding the role of genetic factors, with some authors advocating an autosomal dominant mode of inheritance and separation of familial from sporadic ethnically related cases (29,31).

There may be hard buccal and lingual expansion (fig. 7-31) associated with radiographic evidence of diffusely distributed lobular, irregular, dense radiopacities within the alveolar segment of the jaw (figs. 7-32–7-34). A ground-glass appearance is associated with these opacities,

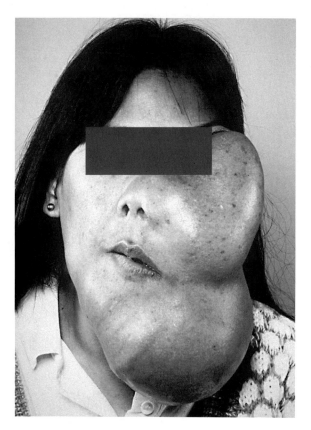

Figure 7-29
FAMILIAL GIGANTIFORM CEMENTOMA

This lesion had been present for 11 years in a 26-year-old female. It started as a small lump on the patient's chin. The disease was familial, involving several members of the patient's family. (Courtesy of Dr. Lester E. Wold, Rochester, MN.)

while on anteroposterior and panoramic radiographic projections, a pagetoid appearance can be seen (fig. 7-35) (26). Root apex involvement is common, and usually associated with dissolution or obfuscation of the lamina dura. A radiolucent periphery commonly surrounds the opaque masses while, less frequently, more obvious cystic changes may be seen in tooth-bearing areas (24). Such cystic spaces are radiographically consistent with traumatic cysts and are seen more frequently in black females over 30 years of age. Over time, a gradual waxing and waning of the radiopaque and radiolucent components of the lesion may be observed (25). Similar radiographic changes may be noted in the more limited form of this condition, *focal cemento-osseous dysplasia.* This focal lesion of periodontal membrane origin may occasionally progress to multifocal or "florid" involvement (27).

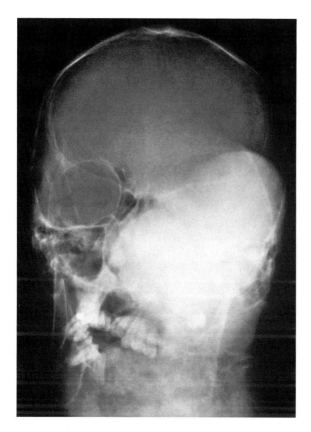 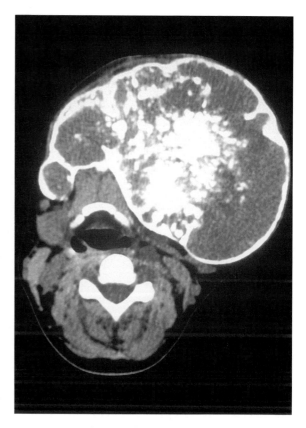

Figure 7-30
FAMILIAL GIGANTIFORM CEMENTOMA

Left: Massive involvement of left maxilla and much of the mandible. Note the "ground glass" appearance and relative sharp circumscription of the maxillary lesion.

Right: CT scan showing good circumscription of the lesion despite its massive proportions. (Courtesy of Dr. Lester E. Wold, Rochester, MN.)

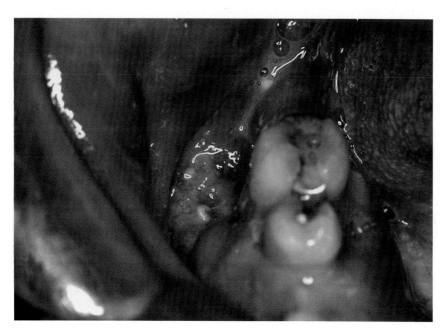

Figure 7-31
FLORID OSSEOUS DYSPLASIA

Alveolar expansion is noted in the mandibular molar area of a middle-aged female. Exposure of the underlying cemental mass is appreciated along the buccal aspect.

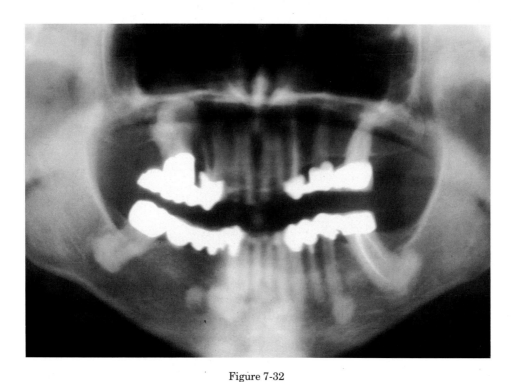

Figure 7-32
FLORID OSSEOUS DYSPLASIA
A panoramic radiograph shows multiple, scattered cemental masses at the periapical level within the mandible and maxilla.

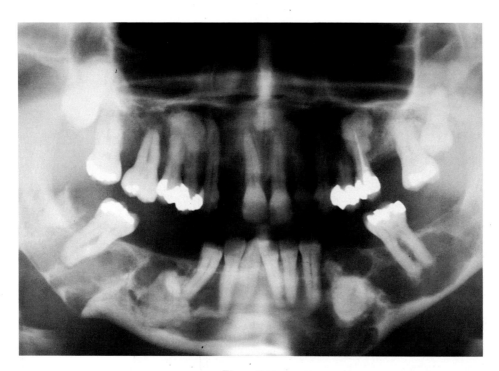

Figure 7-33
FLORID OSSEOUS DYSPLASIA
Multiquadrant alteration of the maxillary and mandibular bone is characterized by large cystic radiolucencies around the roots of the posterior dentition. Many such lucencies also contain lobulated opacities at the root apex level.

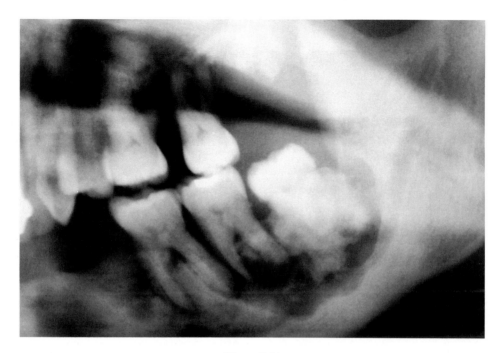

Figure 7-34
FLORID OSSEOUS DYSPLASIA
The posterior portion of the mandible shows a mixed radiolucency and opacity with undulating peripheral margins, broad areas of lucency, and a cotton wool type of alteration seen adjacent to the terminal molar tooth.

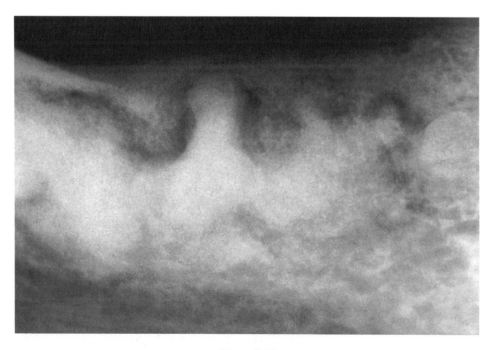

Figure 7-35
FLORID OSSEOUS DYSPLASIA
The posterior portion of the mandible shows multinodular confluent masses of pagetoid type mineralization characteristic of the postextraction state of florid osseous dysplasia.

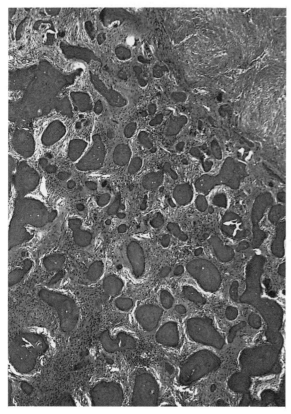

Figure 7-36
FLORID OSSEOUS DYSPLASIA
Numerous cementum type droplets of various size are scattered within a fibroblastic stroma.

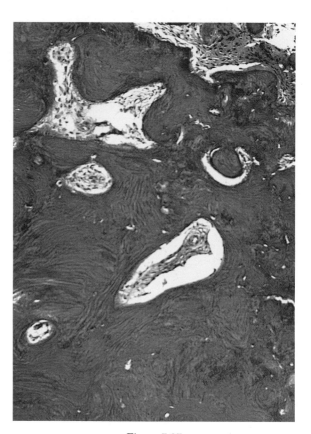

Figure 7-37
FLORID OSSEOUS DYSPLASIA
Sheets of mature cemento-osseous tissue within a cellular fibroblastic stroma characterize the radiopaque nodular masses.

Histologic Findings. Accumulating masses of bone and cementum within a fibrovascular background characterize both florid and focal cemento-osseous dysplasia (28). The latter entity occupies a position along a spectrum from periapical cemental dysplasia to florid cemento-osseous dysplasia (27). A cellular fibrovascular stroma contains irregularly scattered foci of mineralized tissue in the form of droplets or irregular trabeculae of cementum (fig. 7-36). Cementum droplets fuse into rounded forms with a purple periphery, creating large bosselated structures with a "pagetoid" appearance (fig. 7-37). Preexisting lamellar bone may be incorporated within the deposits of cementum. Some bone trabeculae may be lined by plump osteoblasts, while foci of osteoclasts may be noted within resorptive lacunae.

When present, simple bone cysts are lined by a narrow band of vascularized fibrous connective tissue (fig. 7-38). Occasionally, osteoid seams

with variable degrees of mineralization may be present within the lining of these cysts.

Differential Diagnosis. Fibrous dysplasia, ossifying fibroma, chronic sclerosing osteomyelitis, and Paget's disease must be considered in both the radiographic and histologic differential diagnoses. In fibrous dysplasia, early age of onset, diffuse radiographic margins, and unilateral location are distinguishing features; ossifying fibroma is unifocal, exhibits centrifugal growth, and is radiographically well delineated; Paget's disease has a late age of onset and serum alkaline phosphatase elevation. There may be difficulty in separating infected florid cemento-osseous dysplasia from diffuse sclerosing osteomyelitis. Multiple quadrant presentation, clear radiographic demarcation, and tooth root/alveolar proximity favor florid cemento-osseous dysplasia.

Treatment and Prognosis. If the patient is asymptomatic and has the typical radiologic

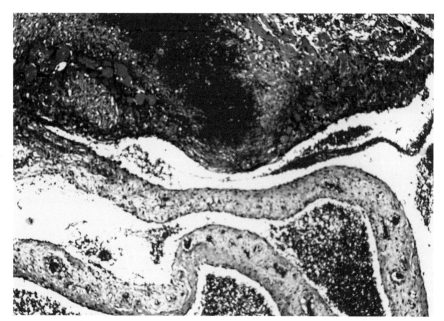

Figure 7-38
FLORID OSSEOUS
DYSPLASIA

A simple bone cyst is noted on occasion in direct association with florid osseous dysplasia. The bone cyst is characterized by compressed granulation tissue at the periphery and an absence of an epithelial lining, as noted in this photomicrograph.

features of this self-limiting condition, periodic examination for dental caries and periodontal prophylaxis is all that is required. Inopportune surgical exposure of the highly mineralized, poorly vascularized masses often results in long-term superimposed chronic osteomyelitis which is difficult to manage. The infected areas may require saucerization and sequestrectomy in conjunction with antibiotic therapy if conservative antibiotic therapy alone fails.

The prognosis of untreated patients is excellent, but as mentioned above, surgical intervention or the development of a dental or periodontal inflammatory process may have long-term adverse consequences.

REFERENCES

Fibro-Osseous Lesions

1. Eversole LR, Sabes WR, Rovin S. Fibrous dysplasia: a nosologic problem in the diagnosis of fibro-osseous lesions of the jaws. J Oral Pathol 1972;1:189–220.

2. Voytek TM, Ro JY, Edeiken J, Ayala AG. Fibrous dysplasia and cemento-ossifying fibroma. A histological spectrum. Am J Surg Pathol 1995;19:775–81.

Fibrous Dysplasia

3. Albright F, Butler AM, Hampton AO, Smith P. Syndrome characterized by osteitis fibrosa disseminata, areas of pigmentation and endocrine dysfunction, with precocious puberty in females: report of five cases. N Engl J Med 1937;216:727–46.

4. Candeliere GA, Roughley PJ, Glorieux FH. Polymerase chain reaction-based technique for the selective enrichment and analysis of mosaic arg 201 mutations in G alpha s from patients with fibrous dysplasia of bone. Bone 1997;21:201–6.

4a. Eversole LR, Sabes WR, Rovin S. Fibrous dysplasia: a nosologic problem in the diagnosis of fibro-osseous lesions of the jaws. J Oral Pathol 1972;1:189–220.

5. Goldberg MH, Sperling A. Gross displacement of the mandibular canal: a radiographic sign of benign fibro-osseous bone disease. Oral Surg Oral Med Oral Pathol 1981;51:225–8.

6. Kinnman JE, Hong CE, Lee EB, Shin HS. Fibrous dysplasia of the face and skull. Pract Otorhinolaryngol 1969;31:11–21.

7. Kreutziger KL. Giant fibrous dysplasia of the mandible: surgical management. Laryngoscope 1989;99:618–31.
8. Lichtenstein L. Polyostotic fibrous dysplasia. Arch Surg 1938;36:874–98.
9. Lichtenstein L, Jaffe HL. Fibrous dysplasia of bone. Arch Pathol 1942;33:777–816.
10. McCune DJ, Burch H. Osteodystrophia fibrosa. Am J Dis Child 1937;54:806–46.

11. Slootweg PJ, Muller H. Differential diagnosis of fibro-osseous jaw lesions. A histologic investigation of 30 cases. J Craniomaxillofac Surg 1990;18:210–4.
12. Slow IN, Stern D, Friedman EW. Osteogenic sarcoma arising in a pre-existing fibrous dysplasia: report of a case. J Oral Surg 1971;29:126–9.
13. Spiegel AM. The molecular basis of disorders caused by defects in G proteins. Horm Res 1997;47:89–96.

Ossifying Fibroma

14. Sciubba JJ, Younai F. Ossifying fibroma of the mandible and maxilla: review of 18 cases. J Oral Pathol Med 1989;18:315–21.
14a. Slootweg PJ, Muller H. Differential diagnosis of fibro-osseous lesions. A histologic investigation of 30 cases. J Craniomaxillofac Surg 1990;18:210–4.

15. van Heerden WF, Raubenheimer EJ, Weir RG, Kreidler J. Giant ossifying fibroma: a clinicopathologic study of 8 tumors. J Oral Pathol Med 1989;18:506–9.

Juvenile Ossifying Fibroma

16. Bendet E, Bakon M, Tadmor R, Talmi Y, Kronenberg J. Juvenile cemento–ossifying fibroma of the maxilla. Ann Otol Rhinol Laryngol 1997;106:75–8.
17. Koury ME, Regezi JA, Perrott DH, Kaban LB. "Atypical" fibro-osseous lesions: diagnostic challenges and treatment concepts. Int J Oral Maxillofac Surg 1995;24:162–9.
18. Makek MS. So called "fibro-osseous lesions" of tumorous origin. Biology confronts terminology. J Cranio Max Fac Surg 1987;15:154–68.

19. Schofield ID. An aggressive fibrous dysplasia. Oral Surg Oral Med Oral Pathol 1974;38:29–35.
20. Slootweg PJ, Panders AK, Koopmans R, Nikkels PG. Juvenile ossifying fibroma. An analysis of 33 cases with emphasis on histopathologic aspects. J Oral Med Pathol 1994;23:385–8.
21. Wiedenfeld KR, Neville BW, Hutchins AR, Bell RA, Brock TR. Juvenile ossifying fibroma of the maxilla in a 6-year-old male: case report. Ped Dentistry 1995;17:365–7.

Periapical Cemental Dysplasia

22. Neville BW, Albenesius RJ. The prevalence of benign fibro-osseous lesions of periodontal ligament origin in black women: a radiographic survey. Oral Surg Oral Med Oral Pathol 1986;62:340–4.

23. Tanaka H, Yoshimoto A, Toyama Y, Iwase T, Hayasaka N, Moro I. Periapical cemental dysplasia with multiple lesions. Int J Oral Maxillofac Surg 1987;16:757–63.

Florid Cemento-Osseous Dysplasia

24. Ariji Y, Ariji E, Higuchi Y, Kubo S, Nakayama E, Kauda S. Florid cemento-osseous dysplasia. Radiographic study with special emphasis on computed tomography. Oral Surg Oral Med Oral Pathol 1994;78:391–6.
25. Kaugars GE, Cale AE. Traumatic bone cyst. Oral Surg Oral Med Oral Pathol 1987;63:318–24.
26. Melrose RJ, Abrams AM, Mills BG. Florid osseous dysplasia. Oral Surg Oral Med Oral Pathol 1976;41:62–82.
27. Slootweg PJ. Maxillofacial fibro-osseous lesions: classification and differential diagnosis. Semin Diagn Pathol 1996;13:104–12.

28. Summerlin DJ, Tomich CE. Focal cemento-osseous dysplasia: a clinicopathologic study of 221 cases. Oral Surg Oral Med Oral Pathol 1994;78:611–20.
29. Thompson SH, Altini M. Gigantiform cementoma of the jaws. Head Neck 1989;11:538–44.
30. Yi WY, Pederson GT, Bartley MH. Multiple familial ossifying fibromas: relationship to other osseous lesions of the jaws. Oral Surg Oral Med Oral Pathol 1989;68:754–8.
31. Young SK, Markowitz NR, Sullivan S, Seale TW, Hirschi R. Familial gigantiform cementoma: classification and presentation of a large pedigree. Oral Surg Oral Med Oral Pathol 1989;68:740–7.

❖❖❖

8

NONODONTOGENIC LESIONS

GIANT CELL LESIONS

Giant Cell Granuloma

Definition. Giant cell granuloma is a localized osteolytic lesion of variably aggressive nature that affects the jaw bones. It encompasses both asymptomatic, incidentally discovered small lesions cured by simple curettage as well as symptomatic, large, locally destructive lesions that frequently recur and require more aggressive surgical therapy. Several aspects of this lesion remain controversial: its terminology, whether it represents a reactive or a neoplastic process, whether the nonaggressive and aggressive variants represent a continuum of a single disease process or perhaps two distinct entities, and the relationship of the lesion, especially the aggressive variant, to extragnathic giant cell tumor (osteoclastoma). Synonyms include *giant cell tumor* and *central giant cell lesion.*

Terminology. The name "giant cell reparative granuloma" was coined by Jaffe in 1953 (10) since he considered the lesion to be reparative in nature; the term "giant cell" drew attention to the prominence of multinucleate giant cells in the lesion and the term "granuloma" alluded to the heterogenous population of fibrocytic, giant cell, and even osteoblastic components. There is currently unanimity among authors in the field that this terminology is not well chosen although it has become hallowed by frequent use. The lesion does not appear to be a repair process to any known destructive event and it does not fulfill the usual histologic criteria required for diagnosis of a granulomatous process. This has led to a proposal in recent years that the entity be re-named "central giant cell lesion" in view of its uncertain nature or even "giant cell tumor" by those who believe the lesion to be a neoplasm closely related to extragnathic giant cell tumor (4).

Clinical Features. There is a fairly wide patient age spectrum, with a mean of about 20 years; most lesions manifest before patients are 30 years of age. Females outnumber males by a ratio of about 3 to 2. Mandibular involvement is twice as frequent as involvement of the maxilla and the lesions tend to be more often anteriorly located (18,20). However, a recent radiologic evaluation of 80 cases by Kaffe et al. (11) demonstrated that the lesions occurred with almost equal frequency in the anterior and posterior regions of the jaws.

There is a fairly distinctive bimodal pattern of presentation. In the majority of cases, the lesion is nonaggressive, asymptomatic, usually small, and detected coincidentally at the time of radiologic dental evaluation. In the remainder of the cases the lesion has an aggressive clinical appearance manifested by pain, paresthesia, jaw swelling resulting from its large size, and radiologic evidence of erosion of cortical plates, dental root resorption, and displacement of teeth. The aggressive lesions are more commonly located in the maxilla. There have been several reports of multiple giant cell granulomas within the jaws in the absence of hyperparathyroidism (13).

Radiologic Findings. The incidentally discovered, nonaggressive variant is a radiolucent, fairly well-circumscribed lesion that is not particularly related to the teeth (figs. 8-1, 8-2). It does not usually expand the involved bone or cause cortical erosion.

The aggressive variant is usually a large lytic lesion at the time of diagnosis and is more frequently multilocular than unilocular (ratio of about 3 to 2) (figs. 8-3, 8-4). Its appearance may closely resemble that of an ameloblastoma. Root resorption was seen in 40 percent of cases and displacement of teeth in 35 percent in the large series of 142 cases reported by Whitaker and Waldron (20). As the lesion expands, it erodes the cortical plates. In a study of 31 cases, Minic and Stajcic (13) noted cortical perforation and soft tissue extension in 7 cases. All except 1 of these 31 cases were treated by curettage and recurrences were seen in 5 patients. These 5 patients all showed microscopically confirmed cortical perforation at the time of first occurrence. There was no correlation between the finding of cortical perforation and histologic pattern. These authors concluded that radiologic or histologic evidence of cortical perforation constitutes the most

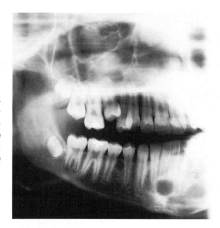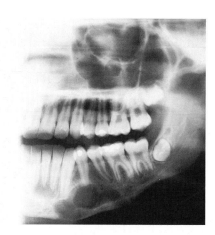

Figure 8-1
CENTRAL GIANT
CELL GRANULOMA
This panoramic radiograph shows a well-circumscribed, multi-locular, radiolucent lesion involving the anterior segment of the body of the mandible. (Figures 8-1 and 8-2 are from the same patient.)

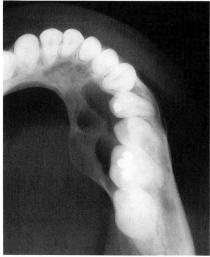

Figure 8-2
CENTRAL GIANT CELL GRANULOMA
The occlusal radiograph shows a well-circumscribed, multilocular, radiolucent lesion that is mildly expanding the inner cortical plate.

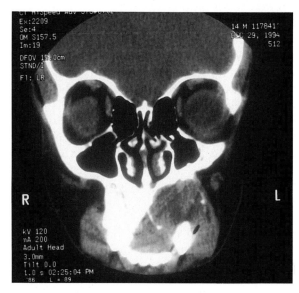

Figure 8-3
CENTRAL GIANT CELL GRANULOMA
Coronal CT scan shows an expansile, destructive, radiolucent lesion of the anterior portion of the left maxilla. A thin shell of cortical bone is preserved around much of the lesion. (Figures 8-3–8-7, 8-10, and 8-12 are from the same patient.)

useful prognostic indicator with regard to likelihood of recurrence.

Pathologic Findings. While there are histologic features that are unique to both the nonaggressive lesions and the large aggressive variant, this distinction is by no means absolute and overlapping histologic features are observed, even within a single lesion. Nevertheless, for didactic purposes we have chosen to describe the usual histologic features associated with each variant.

The nonaggressive variant indeed resembles tissue seen in a reactive or reparative lesion as suggested by Jaffe (10). Within a background of proliferating fibroblasts set in a stroma of collagenous tissue and myxoid ground substance, there are irregularly distributed clusters of osteoclast type cells (figs. 8-5–8-9). The giant cells tend to be smaller and have fewer nuclei than cells of a typical giant cell tumor of bone (1). Endothelial-lined vascular channels in association with proliferating fibroblasts within the lesion closely resemble reparative granulation tissue (fig. 8-10). Mitoses may be frequent; they numbered

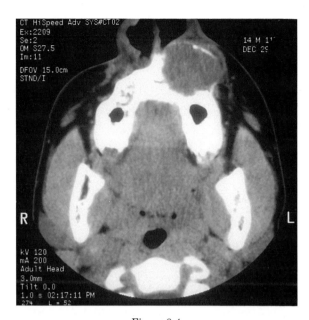

Figure 8-4
CENTRAL GIANT CELL GRANULOMA
An axial CT scan shows an expansile, destructive, radiolucent lesion in the anterior portion of the left maxilla. The thin shell of cortical bone is well shown.

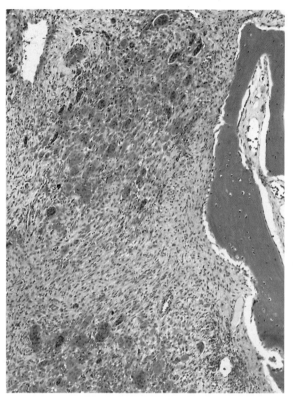

Figure 8-5
CENTRAL GIANT CELL GRANULOMA
Nests of osteoclast type giant cells alternate with fibrovascular stroma. The lamellar bone on the right side corresponds to the thin shell of surviving cortical bone shown in figures 8-3 and 8-4.

between 2 and 19 (mean, 6.3) per 50 high-power fields in the 31 cases reported by Minic and Stajcic (13). Focal deposition of hemosiderin within the lesion is indicative of prior intralesional hemorrhage. A final constituent of the lesion is the presence of some spicules of woven bone which resemble reactive callus type bone (figs. 8-6, 8-9). Foci of residual lamellar bone may also be entrapped within the lesion or be seen as a surviving shell at its periphery (figs. 8-5, 8-6).

The aggressive form of the lesion histologically resembles giant cell tumor of bone. The stromal cells have more uniformly ovoid nuclei and the giant cells are more evenly distributed, are larger, and have more nuclei than the non-aggressive variant (figs. 8-11, 8-12). Mitotic figures are more numerous in the stromal mononuclear cells but are not abnormal (fig. 8-12). Indeed, the features may be identical to those of giant cell tumor of the extragnathic skeleton so that without knowledge of the location of the lesion, the proffered histologic diagnosis would be giant cell tumor of bone.

There have been attempts to correlate clinical behavior with the histologic features enumerated above. Chuong et al. (4) and Ficcara et al.

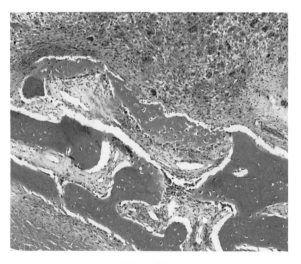

Figure 8-6
CENTRAL GIANT CELL GRANULOMA
The lesional tissue is surrounded by a layer of reactive woven bone which in turn is surrounded by a shell of cortical lamellar bone.

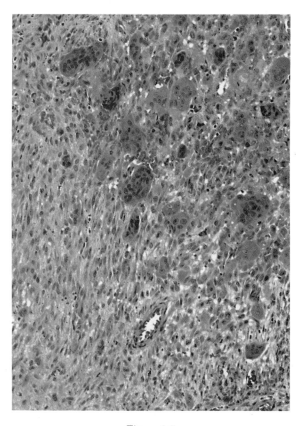

Figure 8-7
CENTRAL GIANT CELL GRANULOMA
Nests of osteoclast type giant cells in the upper right alternates with fibrovascular stroma in the lower left of the photomicrograph.

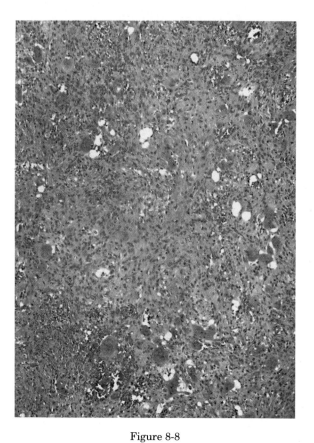

Figure 8-8
CENTRAL GIANT CELL GRANULOMA
Osteoclast type giant cells are irregularly distributed in a fibroblast-rich stroma. (Figures 8-8 and 8-9 are from the same patient.)

Figure 8-9
CENTRAL GIANT
CELL GRANULOMA

High-power photomicrograph shows clustering of osteoclast type giant cells, fibrovascular stroma, and scattered trabeculae of reactive bone.

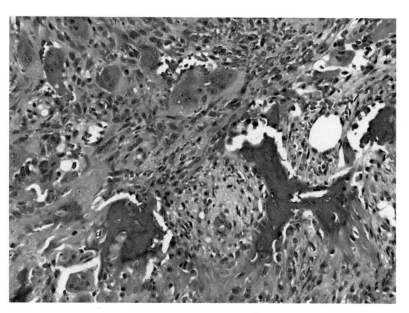

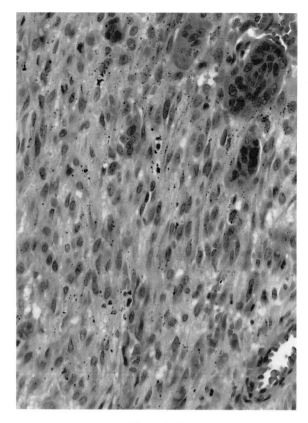

Figure 8-10
CENTRAL GIANT CELL GRANULOMA
The fibrovascular stroma is composed of uniform, plump fibrocytic cells. Scattered hemosiderin deposits are also present.

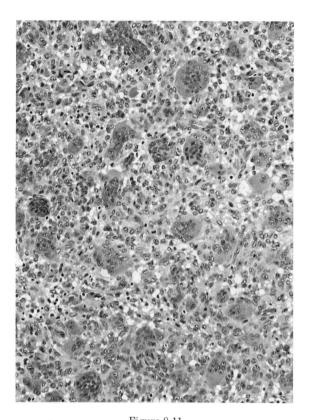

Figure 8-11
CENTRAL GIANT CELL GRANULOMA
This area of lesion is composed of uniformly distributed and abundant osteoclast type giant cells separated by ovoid to polygonal mononuclear stromal cells. This pattern resembles giant cell tumor (osteoclastoma) of bone.

(6) have indeed shown significant correlation between aggressive clinical behavior, including recurrent disease, and larger sized giant cells and uniform distribution of such giant cells within the lesion. However, Auclair et al. (2), in a study using computer-aided image analysis, were unable to confirm these findings. A study of AgNOR counts has shown a higher count in recurrent as compared to nonrecurrent and non-aggressive lesions (19).

Pathogenesis. The pathogenesis of giant cell granuloma remains enigmatic. For those who believe that this is a reactive ("reparative") lesion, there remains the difficulty in explaining the aggressive clinical behavior of the larger lesions which histologically resemble giant cell tumor. Conversely, those who believe the lesion to be neoplastic and perhaps related to giant cell tumor would have difficulty in including the nonaggressive small lesions in that category. In

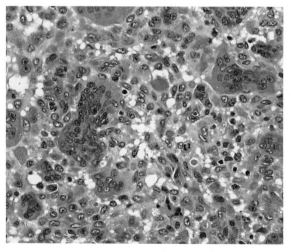

Figure 8-12
CENTRAL GIANT CELL GRANULOMA
High-power view of figure 8-11 illustrates the ovoid to polygonal shape of mononuclear cells between uniformly distributed osteoclasts. Mitotic figure can be seen in the center.

fact, such lesions in the extragnathic skeleton have been termed *extragnathic giant cell reparative granuloma* and are separate from giant cell tumor of bone. Stolovitzky et al. (17) believe that the disease may be closely related to giant cell tumor of bone and propose a continuum of clinical behavior and histologic features from the nonaggressive to the aggressive end of a spectrum.

A further consideration is whether the aggressive variant represents a separate entity, namely, a gnathic manifestation of giant cell tumor. There are, however, several differences between aggressive giant cell granuloma and giant cell tumor. Giant cell granuloma occurs in a younger mean age group (20 versus 30 years); has a lower recurrence rate (13 to 35 percent versus 60 percent); and exhibits a virtual absence of reports of malignant transformation and metastatic disease (as compared to a 6 to 10 percent rate of development of sarcoma and a 2 percent rate of metastasis in giant cell tumors). Furthermore, giant cell tumor of bone develops only in bones preformed from cartilage and not from membrane bone. Whitaker and Waldron (20) have countered these arguments by suggesting that the discrepancies in age distribution and recurrence rate may be related to earlier diagnosis of the more visible jaw lesions and more effective treatment at an earlier stage in the biologic evolution of the disease. In addition, Quick et al. (16) in an article dealing with maxillary giant cell tumors in children illustrated the presence of cartilage within the membrane bone of the facial bones of a 15 week human fetus. To date, there have been only anecdotal case reports of giant cell lesions within the jaw bones that have developed metastatic disease (12,14).

The giant cells in giant cell granuloma have been shown by in vitro tissue culture studies and immunohistochemistry to be osteoclasts (7). In tissue culture, the cells have digested bone substrate; this activity is inhibited by calcitonin. By immunohistochemistry, the cells are decorated by monoclonal antibody against osteoclast cells. O'Malley et al. (15), in an immunohistochemical study of 28 giant cell granulomas, demonstrated that only the mononuclear cells were in cell cycle and that the majority of these cells stained only for the fibroblast-associated antigen, prolyl 4-hydroxylase. They concluded that the lesion is primarily a fibroblastic/myofibroblastic tumor in which the macrophages and osteoclasts play a secondary role. They observed no phenotypic differences between aggressive and nonaggressive lesions.

Bhambhani et al. (3) described the development of a recurrent giant cell tumor of the mandible, in addition to a giant cell tumor of the L3 vertebral body, in a patient with Paget's disease who was born in Avellino, Italy. Several other patients from Avellino have developed giant cell tumors within pagetic bone (9). By electron microscopy, these authors demonstrated the presence of paramyxovirus-like inclusions in the giant cells. El-Labban (5) described similar inclusions in a recurrent "giant cell tumor" of the maxilla in a patient with Paget's disease. Mills (12) also demonstrated paramyxovirus type inclusions in the giant cells of a malignant "giant cell tumor" of the mandible unassociated with Paget's disease.

Differential Diagnosis. The nonaggressive variant of giant cell granuloma is histologically identical to the "brown tumor" of hyperparathyroidism and the lesional tissue of cherubism (4). The distinction from hyperparathyroidism requires a careful search for the clinical and radiologic stigmata of that disease. Even in the absence of such findings, it is almost axiomatic that a serum calcium or parathormone assay should be performed to exclude that diagnosis. The differentiation from cherubism is usually not difficult because of the distinctive clinical presentation of that disease and the more posterior location of the lesion. The noncystic elements of an aneurysmal bone cyst may be indistinguishable from giant cell granuloma. Indeed, in the extragnathic skeleton, the terms solid variant of aneurysmal bone cyst and giant cell granuloma have been used interchangeably. An unusual association of multiple fibro-osseous lesions devoid of giant cells has been described with hereditary hyperparathyroidism (8). Unlike the brown tumor, these jaw lesions tend to progress even after surgical correction of the cause of hypercalcemia. However, such jaw lesions more closely resemble fibrous dysplasia or ossifying fibroma than giant cell granuloma.

Treatment and Prognosis. Despite the controversy concerning several aspects of the disease, there is consensus that small nonaggressive lesions require no more than simple curettage while larger aggressive lesions should be more thoroughly curetted or more completely resected because of a significant incidence of recurrence.

Cherubism

Definition. Cherubism is a lesion of probable developmental origin usually affecting all four quadrants of the jaw in a symmetric fashion and resulting in a characteristic clinical facies. The histologic features are identical to those of giant cell granuloma.

Historical Features. The lesion was first described by Jones in 1933 (26). He coined the descriptive term "cherubism" in 1938 (26a). To date, over 150 cases have been documented in the literature (29).

Clinical Features. The disease is familial, with a mendelian dominant mode of inheritance of variable penetrance, 100 percent in males and 50 to 70 percent in females (27). This accounts for the 2 to 1 male to female ratio. The lesion first manifests in early childhood between the ages of 1 and 4 years, and is progressive until about the age of puberty, after which regression occurs with clinical improvement of the facial disfigurement (25). The lesion usually involves all jaw bones symmetrically although unilateral involvement may occasionally occur. Unilateral involvement may be the initial presentation; in such cases, distinction from giant cell granuloma is usually not possible and confirmation of the diagnosis requires the appearance of a contralateral lesion during the course of follow-up. Arnott (21) documented a 2-year hiatus between initial unilateral presentation in a 9-year-old boy and the subsequent radiologic development of contralateral disease. Peters (28) reported a single case of unilateral disease in a study of 20 cases from a single family.

In the mandible, the lesion initially involves the angle and subsequently extends into the ramus and body. The coronoid process may be involved but the condylar process is uniformly spared. The posterior aspect of the maxilla is first involved, with later extension of the lesion into anterior portions of the maxilla and orbital region. The symmetric enlargement of jaw bones associated with retraction of the lower eyelids, exposing the sclera inferiorly, produces what has been described as the "raised-to-heaven" look and the resemblance to the cherubs so ubiquitous in Re-

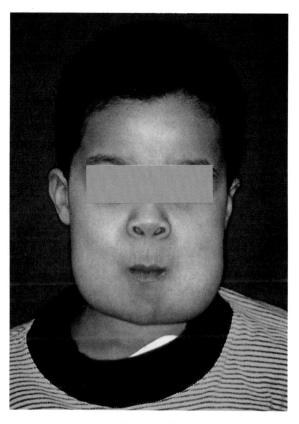

Figure 8-13
CHERUBISM
Both sides of the mandible are involved in this child with cherubism. (Courtesy of Dr Howard D. Dorfman, Bronx, NY.) (Figures 8-13–8-20 are from the same patient.)

naissance art (fig. 8-13). Of functional significance is the displacement and even loss of teeth (fig. 8-14). There may be destruction of tooth buds, a feature not seen in giant cell granuloma. Cervical lymphadenopathy, resulting from hyperplasia and fibrosis, may also occur (27).

Radiologic Findings. The involved jaw bones are expanded by a well-defined radiolucent lesion; trabeculation produces a "soap bubble" appearance (figs. 8-15–8-17). The cortical margins are usually intact but may become perforated. Teeth are displaced, absent, or may be observed "floating" within the lytic lesion. During the later healing phase of the lesion, bone replaces the lesional tissue, with progressive sclerosis of the lytic areas (25).

Pathologic Findings. The basic nature of the lesion is still uncertain but is generally thought to result from maldevelopment of the bone-forming

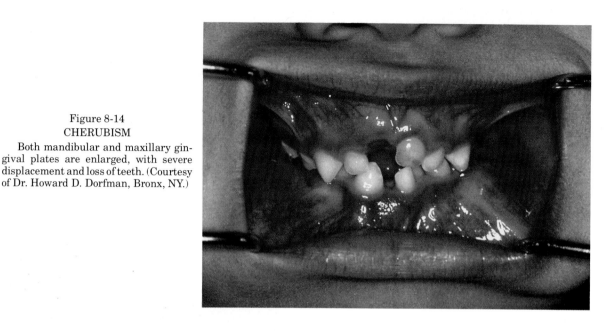

Figure 8-14
CHERUBISM
Both mandibular and maxillary gingival plates are enlarged, with severe displacement and loss of teeth. (Courtesy of Dr. Howard D. Dorfman, Bronx, NY.)

Figure 8-15
CHERUBISM
The well-defined, radiolucent, expansile lesion involves the angle, body, and lower half of the ramus of mandible. Note the sparing of the mandibular condyles. Trabeculation produces a "soap bubble" appearance. Displaced teeth appear to be "floating" within the lytic lesion. (Courtesy of Dr. Howard D. Dorfman, Bronx, NY.)

mesenchyme of the jaw during the period of active bone growth. Histologically, the lesion is indistinguishable from giant cell granuloma, the solid variant of aneurysmal bone cyst (an entity probably synonymous with the aforementioned lesion), and the "brown tumor" of hyperparathyroidism. All of these lesions are comprised of a reactive-looking fibrovascular stroma within which are areas of denser fibrous tissue, giant cells of osteoclast type irregularly dispersed within the lesion and often focally aggregated, deposition of hemosiderin, and occasional seams of osteoid or woven bone (figs. 8-18–8-20). Any one or more of the above elements may predom-inate in a particular lesion, in different areas of the same lesion, and, even in different areas of the same histologic section. This heterogeneity is quite typical of these lesions and the overall histologic impression is that of a "reactive" process. A histologic feature said to be unique to cherubism, as opposed to the other histologic look-alikes, is the deposition of pericapillary eosinophilic material thought to be collagen (23). However, this is difficult to demonstrate and of little diagnostic value. Although the histologic features of the various diseases mentioned above are identical, cherubism can readily be distinguished because of its characteristic clinical and radiologic features. The

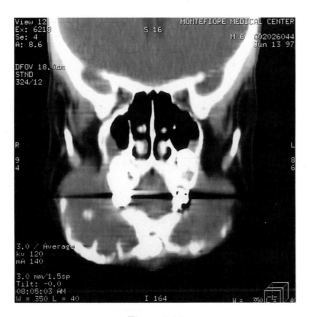

Figure 8-16
CHERUBISM
The CT scan shows lesional tissue expanding the body and ramus of the mandible bilaterally but sparing the condyles. (Courtesy of Dr. Howard D. Dorfman, Bronx, NY.)

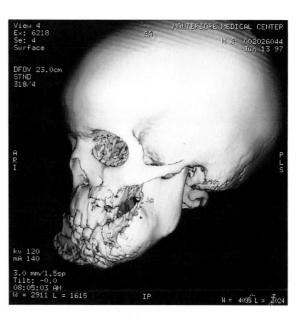

Figure 8-17
CHERUBISM
The expansion and distortion of the mandible can be readily appreciated in this three-dimensional radiologic reconstruction. (Courtesy of Dr. Howard D. Dorfman, Bronx, NY.)

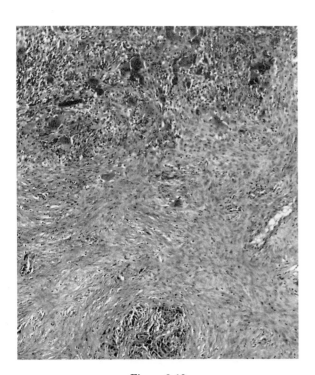

Figure 8-18
CHERUBISM
Fibrous stroma surrounds a nest of osteoclast type giant cells in the upper half and an aggregate of hemosiderin-laden macrophages in the lower half of the photomicrograph. (Courtesy of Dr. Howard D. Dorfman, Bronx, NY.)

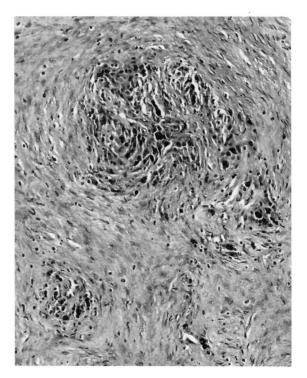

Figure 8-19
CHERUBISM
Fascicles of uniform, plump fibroblasts surround aggregates of hemosiderin-laden macrophages. (Courtesy of Dr. Howard D. Dorfman, Bronx, NY.)

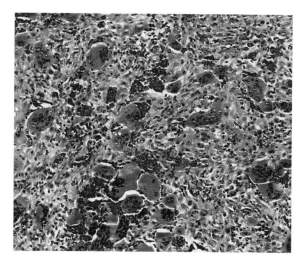

Figure 8-20
CHERUBISM
There is an admixture of uniform, plump fibrocytic cells and osteoclast type giant cells. (Courtesy of Dr. Howard D. Dorfman, Bronx, NY.)

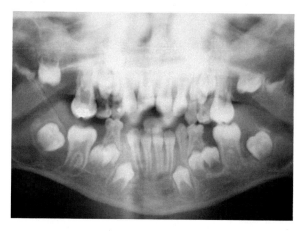

Figure 8-21
NOONAN-LIKE MULTIPLE GIANT CELL
GRANULOMA SYNDROME
The osteolytic expansile lesions involve both angles and rami of the mandible of a child.

"brown tumor" is accompanied by biochemical features of hyperparathyroidism.

Treatment and Prognosis. Therapy should be withheld until cessation of bone growth since the lesion regresses in time. Residual deformity at that time can be corrected by cosmetic contouring. Functional impairment may necessitate corrective surgery at an earlier date. Radiotherapy is contraindicated: there is a report of a patient with cherubism who developed a maxillary sarcoma following treatment with radiotherapy (28).

Noonan Syndrome/Cherubism. There have been several reported cases of an association of multiple giant cell granulomas of the jaws with a phenotype resembling Noonan's syndrome, namely, the bodily habitus of Turner's syndrome, hypertelorism, downward slanting palpebral fissures, ptosis, low set ears, cryptorchidism, increased anteroposterior thoracic dimension, pulmonary valve stenosis and other cardiac defects, and mental retardation (fig. 8-21) (22,24). Oral features include micrognathia, high arched palate, dental malocclusion, delayed tooth eruption, bifid uvula, and rarely, cleft palate. Giant cell granulomas have also occurred in the extragnathic skeleton and a pigmented villonodular synovitis-like lesion has been described in the joints. The relationship of this Noonan-like/multiple giant cell granulomatous lesion to Noonan's syndrome and cherubism is uncertain at the present time.

Aneurysmal Bone Cyst

Definition. Aneurysmal bone cyst is a blood-filled, unilocular or multilocular pseudocyst occurring within bone either as a primary lesion or a secondary complication engrafted upon some other bone lesion. Its etiology and pathogenesis have not been elucidated but it has been postulated to result from abnormal capillary-venous communications within bone.

Clinical Features. Aneurysmal bone cyst affects young individuals in the first three decades. By 1993, 51 cases had been documented within jaw bones: 31 in the mandible and 20 in the maxilla with no particular locus of predilection (31). In 1997 Bataineh (30) reviewed 31 cases involving the maxilla. The lesion may evolve rapidly and cause an alarming expansion of the involved bone (fig. 8-22).

Radiologic Findings. The lesion produces a fairly well-circumscribed, unilocular or multilocular cystic expansion of the involved bone. This expansion may be so impressive as to justify the frequently used term, "blow-out" lesion (fig. 8-23). The overlying cortical bone is attenuated and may eventually be completely eroded, allowing the lesion to expand into adjacent soft tissues. Teeth may be displaced but their viability is maintained (33). The bony expansion is usually well demonstrated on computed tomography (CT) scans. A distinctive radiologic feature is the

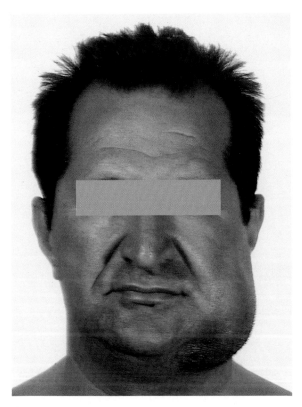

Figure 8-22
ANEURYSMAL BONE CYST OF MANDIBLE
The rapidly evolving expansile nature of the lesion has produced this large swelling of the jaw. (Figures 8-22–8-27 are from the same patient.)

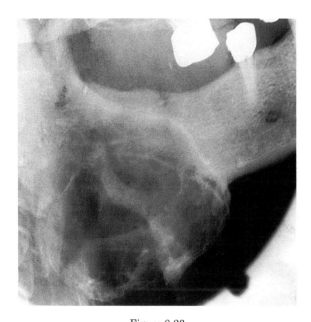

Figure 8-23
ANEURYSMAL BONE CYST
A large, expansile, lytic lesion in the region of the mandibular ramus. The lesion is multilocular. A thin delimiting cortical shell is present at the periphery.

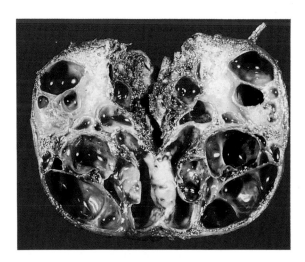

Figure 8-24
ANEURYSMAL BONE CYST
Transected gross specimen shows exquisite delimitation of the lesion, multilocularity, and the presence of blood within the locules.

presence of fluid-filled levels within the loculated spaces resulting from sedimentation of solid constituents of the blood (32). The cell-poor serum and cell-rich sediment produce bright and low intensity signals, respectively, on the T2-weighted images, with a fairly sharp interface.

Pathologic Findings. In the primary form of aneurysmal bone cyst, no other bony lesion can be identified, whereas in the secondary form there is an associated bone lesion, usually chondroblastoma, osteoblastoma, or a fibro-osseous lesion. Grossly, the lesion is hemorrhagic, well circumscribed, and multilocular (fig. 8-24). Histologically, nonendothelial-lined spaces of varying size are separated by fibrovascular septa (fig. 8-25). The septa vary in thickness and not infrequently form more solid nodules or sheets of lesional tissue (figs. 8-26, 8-27). The cellular and stromal constituents of the septa are identical to those seen in giant cell reparative

granuloma, namely, fibroblasts, scattered osteoclast type giant cells, macrophages, spicules of newly formed woven bone rimmed by osteoblasts, and focal hemosiderin deposits (fig. 8-27). A notable feature in most lesions is the tendency

171

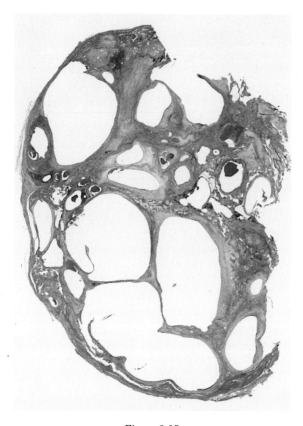

Figure 8-25
ANEURYSMAL BONE CYST
A whole mount preparation of a multilocular cystic lesion. Some of the locules still contain blood.

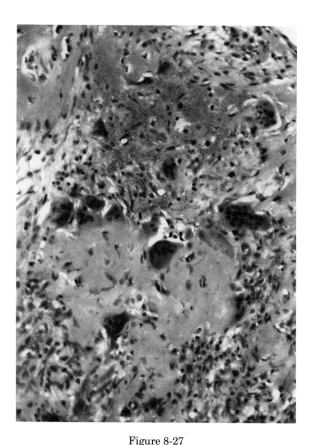

Figure 8-27
ANEURYSMAL BONE CYST
Within this thickened fibrovascular septum, osteoclast type giant cells and woven bone spicules can be seen.

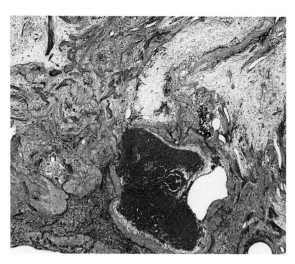

Figure 8-26
ANEURYSMAL BONE CYST
The septal lining is composed of fibrovascular tissue and reactive bone trabeculae. Blood is present within the lumen of some of the locules.

for the giant cells to protrude into the blood lakes. In some lesions focal deposits of amorphous granular material may be seen.

Differential Diagnosis. The most significant differential diagnosis is that of telangiectatic osteosarcoma. At low magnification, the two lesions are remarkably similar. However, careful evaluation of the cytologic features at higher magnification usually allows for distinction between these lesions. The stromal cells in telangiectatic osteosarcoma are malignant and show the usual histologic evidence of sarcoma cells. The matrix may be sparse but when present takes the forms of irregular lace-like formations and the associated osteoblasts are distinctly pleomorphic. Mitoses may be frequent and even include abnormal forms.

When the aneurysmal bone cyst has a more solid configuration it may be difficult to differentiate from giant cell granuloma (31); indeed, it is

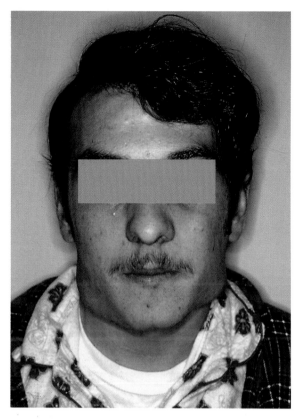

Figure 8-28
OSTEOMAS OF MANDIBLE
IN GARDNER'S SYNDROME
Deformity of both sides of the mandible is produced by
multiple mandibular osteomas. (Figures 8-28–8-30 are from
the same patient.)

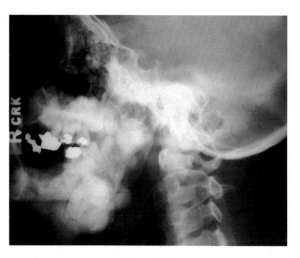

Figure 8-29
OSTEOMAS OF MANDIBLE
IN GARDNER'S SYNDROME
Dense, sclerotic, circumscribed masses are present
within the body of the mandible.

likely that the solid variant of aneurysmal bone cyst and giant cell granuloma are closely related if not identical. The solid component may represent a later stage of the lesion.

Treatment and Prognosis. The standard therapy is curettage or enucleation. This may be supplemented by cryosurgery because of the high incidence (26 percent) of local recurrence (31,33).

OSSEOUS LESIONS

Osteoma

Definition. This is a benign, bone-forming neoplasm composed of mature, lamellar type bone. The lesion may be either centrally or peripherally located. Peripheral lesions may be sessile or pedunculated. Nearly all osteomas occur in the craniofacial region.

Clinical Features. Solitary osteomas of the jaw bones are rare (40). Most occur on the lingular aspect of the angle of the mandible. Craniofacial osteomas occur most commonly in the frontal and ethmoid sinuses but involvement of the maxillary sinus has been reported (36,38). Other unusual sites of jaw involvement include the coronoid process, the condylar notch, and the genial tubercle (34,37,39). The lesion has been reported to occur at the site of a previous jaw fracture (35).

Multiple jaw osteomas are an intrinsic component of the *familial adenomatous polyposis (Gardner) syndrome,* a mendelian dominant disorder, characterized by the presence of multiple colonic adenomatous polyps developing early in life and invariably complicated by the development of colonic adenocarcinoma by the age of 35 to 40 years (figs. 8-28–8-30). These patients also develop epidermoid inclusion cysts and about 10 percent develop fibromatosis. The fibromatous lesions are located within the mesentery in about 75 percent of cases. Multiple osteomas occur in 70 to 90 percent of patients with Gardner's syndrome. They are located with greatest frequency in the region of the angle of the mandible (42). In addition to jaw osteomas, patients develop dental abnormalities including misplaced and supernumerary teeth and odontomas (41). Both the dental anomalies and jawbone osteomas

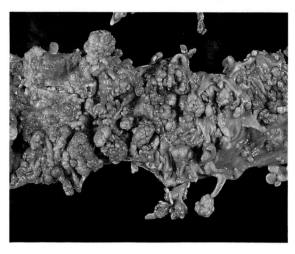

Figure 8-30
MULTIPLE ADENOMATOUS
POLYPS IN GARDNER'S SYNDROME
The mucosa is studded with adenomatous polyps of varying size.

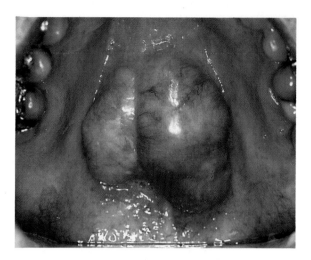

Figure 8-32
PALATAL TORI
Dome-shaped, smooth, exophytic masses arise from the midline of the hard palate. The overlying mucosa is intact.

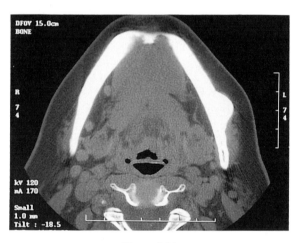

Figure 8-31
OSTEOMA OF MANDIBLE
Sagittal CT scan shows a dome-shaped exophytic and densely sclerotic lesion of body of mandible.

constitute useful clinical markers for the syndrome as they may be detected at an earlier age than the colonic polyps.

Radiologic Findings. Osteomas usually manifest radiologically as dense, osteosclerotic, well-circumscribed lesions occurring in either a central or exophytic location (figs. 8-29, 8-31). The central lesions are often difficult to differentiate from other densely sclerotic, well-delimited lesions such as ossifying fibroma or fibrous dys-

plasia, osteoblastoma, and bone islands (enostosis) (38). Some of the pedunculated peripheral lesions may represent end-stage osteochondromas in which the cartilage cap has undergone complete endochondral ossification (37).

Differential Diagnosis. Osteomas should be differentiated from the more frequently occurring tori and exostoses. Tori are dome-shaped, single or multiple bony excrescences covered by oral mucosa and arise from the palatal midline or lingual aspect of the mandible, where they are usually bilateral (figs. 8-32, 8-33). There appears to be a hereditary predisposition more frequently observed in Native Americans, blacks, Asians, and Eskimos. Exostoses are also single or multiple, dome-shaped bony excrescences covered by oral mucosa but arise on the buccal aspect of the alveolar bone, most frequently in the posterior portions of the maxilla and mandible (fig. 8-34). Exostoses may be irritational in origin, secondary to occlusional dental stress. Histologically, tori and exostoses resemble compact osteomas but are readily identified by their typical clinical features. They usually require no therapy unless necessitated by dental prosthetic surgery.

Pathologic Findings. Histologically, osteoma is composed of lamellar bone. There are two histologic variants. In the *compact variant (osteoma eburnum),* only small and scant fibrovascular spaces are present within the compact mass of

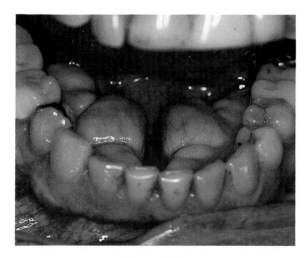

Figure 8-33
MANDIBULAR TORI
Bilateral, dome-shaped, smooth, exophytic masses arise from the lingular aspect of the mandible and are covered by intact mucosa.

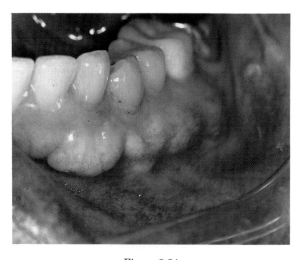

Figure 8-34
MANDIBULAR EXOSTOSES
Multiple, coalescing, dome-shaped bony excrescences arise on the buccal aspect of the alveolar bone posteriorly.

lamellar bone (figs. 8-35, 8-36), whereas in the *cancellous variant (osteoma spongiosa),* plates or sheets of lamellar bone are separated by more abundant marrow spaces containing fatty or even hematopoietic elements (figs. 8-37, 8-38) (40).

Treatment and Prognosis. Many of these lesions are discovered incidentally during radiologic examination and usually require no therapy unless they produce cosmetic or functional problems, in which case they should be locally resected.

Osteoblastoma/Osteoid Osteoma

Definition. Osteoblastoma is a benign bone-forming neoplasm most commonly occurring in the vertebrae, long bones, and small bones of the hands and feet.

Clinical Features. There have been over 30 documented cases of involvement of jaw bones by osteoblastoma; the jaw is said to constitute 15 percent of all sites involved by this neoplasm. It occurs most frequently in patients in the second decade of life and involves the mandible more often than the maxilla (46,53). Within the mandible, most cases involve the body but isolated reports describe cases in the ramus, coronoid process, and condyle (54). As with many other jaw neoplasms, pain, tenderness, and swelling constitute the usual triad of symptoms.

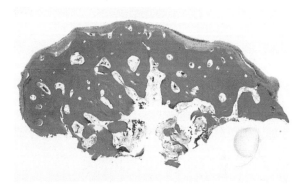

Figure 8-35
OSTEOMA OF MAXILLA
A polypoid exophytic bony mass is covered on one surface by respiratory mucosa of sinus. (Figures 8-35 and 8-36 are from the same patient.)

Radiologic Findings. The neoplasm is usually sharply circumscribed and may expand the involved bone. It may be purely osteolytic or have a mixed lytic and sclerotic pattern, reflecting the degree of mineralization of the matrix within the lesion (fig. 8-39). Radiologically, the lesion most closely resembles an ossifying fibroma.

Pathologic Findings. The histologic features are identical to those of lesions in extragnathic locations. Anastomosing spicules of woven bone are rimmed by a single layer of plump, uniform osteoblastic cells and separated

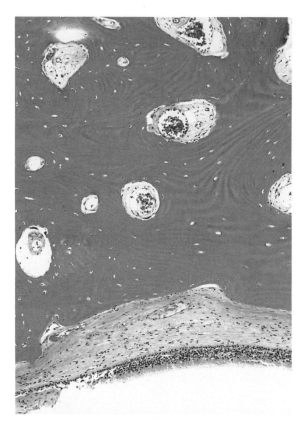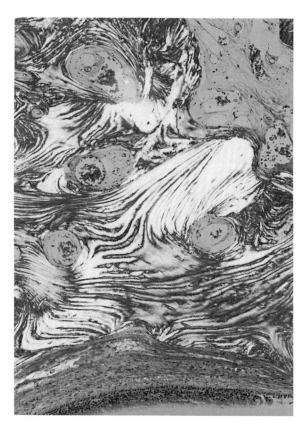

Figure 8-36
OSTEOMA OF MAXILLA

Left: The osteoma is composed of dense lamellar type bone with scanty intervening fibrovascular stroma and surface lining of respiratory mucosa.

Right: The lamellar configuration of the bone is best demonstrated using polarized light.

Figure 8-37
OSTEOMA OF MAXILLA

This osteoma is composed of a peripheral rim of dense, sclerotic lamellar bone and a central component of trabeculae of lamellar bone separated by vascularized adipose tissue. (Figures 8-37 and 8-38 are from the same patient.)

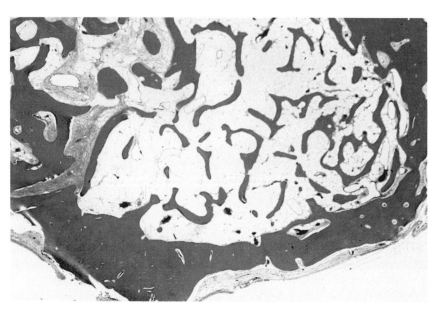

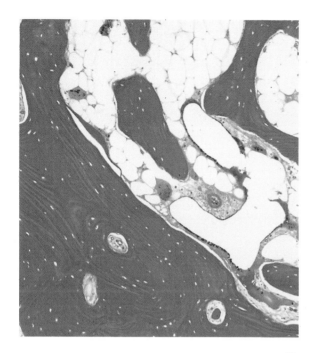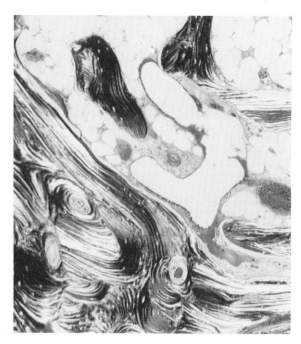

Figure 8-38
OSTEOMA OF MAXILLA
Left: Compact and trabecular lamellar bone is seen at high magnification.
Right: A corresponding section as viewed with polarized light.

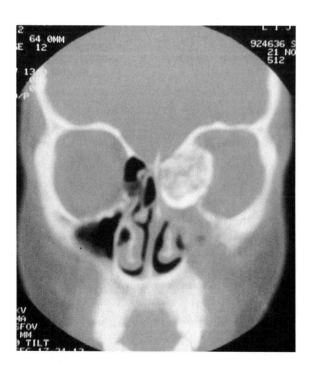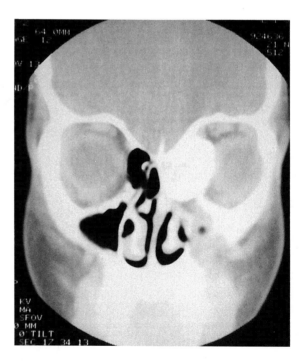

Figure 8-39
OSTEOBLASTOMA OF MAXILLA
Left: CT scan of the skull of an 11-year-old boy with proptosis. A well-circumscribed osteoblastic lesion involves the left maxillary sinus and orbit. This cut shows the densely sclerotic margin, with irregular sclerotic foci more centrally.
Right: Another level in which the entire lesion appears densely sclerotic. (Figs. 8-39 to 8-44 are from the same patient.)

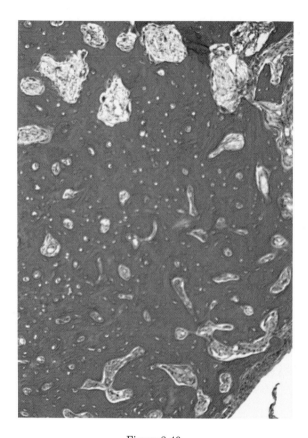

Figure 8-40
OSTEOBLASTOMA OF MAXILLA
A peripheral component of the lesion is composed of
compact lamellar bone resembling an osteoma.

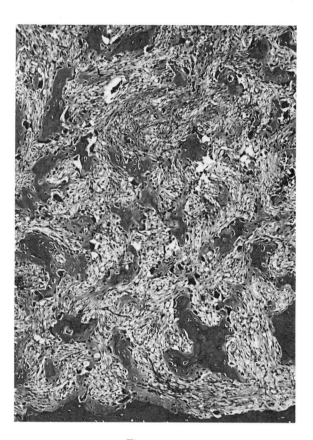

Figure 8-41
OSTEOBLASTOMA OF MAXILLA
A central component of the lesion is comprised of trabeculae of woven bone of uniform width separated by fibrovascular stroma.

by a loose fibrovascular stroma, resembling granulation tissue (figs. 8-40–8-42). The osteoid and
bone spicules and intervening stroma are of similar width, imparting to the neoplasm an overall
organized architectural configuration when
viewed at low power. Another conspicuous component is the presence of fairly numerous osteoclast
type giant cells within the stroma. The margins of
the lesion are sharply circumscribed, with no evidence of infiltration or entrapment of surrounding
uninvolved bone or soft tissue. Osteoblastoma in
the jaw bones may be complicated by the development of an aneurysmal bone cyst (51).

A variant of osteoblastoma has been categorized as "aggressive" by Dorfman and Weiss (44)
and as "malignant" by Schajowicz and Lemos (49).
This variant constituted 15 of 102 osteoblastomas
reviewed by Dorfman and Weiss and exhibited a
50 percent recurrence rate as compared to 13
percent for usual osteoblastomas; no metastases

developed, however. Histologically, the aggressive variant is characterized by large but uniform, polygonal rimming osteoblasts with prominent eosinophilic nucleoli described as having
epithelioid features (figs. 8-43, 8-44). In addition,
the osteoid or bony matrix may have a sheet-like
or lace-like architectural pattern rather than the
more uniform architectural pattern described
above. Mitoses may be present. However, the
osteoblasts show no pleomorphic features and
mitoses are never atypical. The aggressive variant has been described in the maxilla (48).

In addition to the aggressive variant, we have
observed several examples of a benign osteoblastic
neoplasm within the paranasal sinuses which en-
compass the histologic features of both a sinus
osteoma and osteoblastoma. Radiologically, these
circumscribed lesions are more densely sclerotic
than the usual osteoblastoma but contain focal

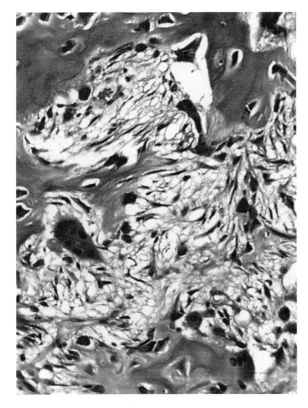

Figure 8-42
OSTEOBLASTOMA OF MAXILLA
Higher magnification of figure 8-41 illustrates the woven bone trabeculae with rimming osteoblasts and multinucleate osteoclasts.

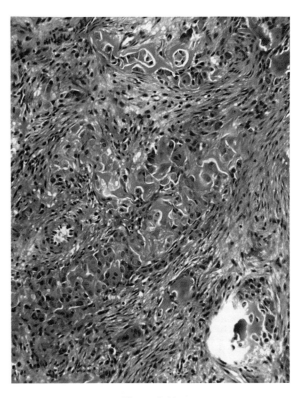

Figure 8-43
OSTEOBLASTOMA OF MAXILLA
The osteoid trabeculae have a more delicate, ribbon-like quality and the osteoblasts are large with epithelioid characteristics. These areas fulfill the histologic criteria for "aggressive osteoblastoma."

lucent areas (fig. 8-39, left). Histologically, the more lucent areas show lesional tissue resembling osteoblastoma while the densely sclerotic component corresponds to dense bone as seen in a sinus osteoma (figs. 8-40, 8-41). This lesion has been referred to as *multifocal sclerosing osteoblastoma*. It raises the possibility of a histogenetic relationship of sinus osteoblastoma to sinus osteoma.

The vexing question of whether an osteoblastoma can undergo malignant transformation cannot be answered at this time. The few reported cases of such an event usually include a caveat that the lesion may have been a low-grade osteosarcoma from its inception (52).

Differential Diagnosis. The most important entity in the differential diagnosis of osteoblastoma, particularly the aggressive variant, is low-grade osteosarcoma or osteoblastoma-like osteosarcoma. The distinction is aided by careful

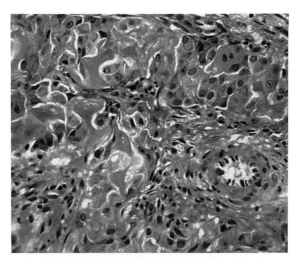

Figure 8-44
OSTEOBLASTOMA OF MAXILLA
Higher magnification of figure 8-43 demonstrates the presence of large epithelioid type osteoblasts with prominent eosinophilic nucleoli surrounding delicate spicules of woven bone. This lesion recurred twice following local resection.

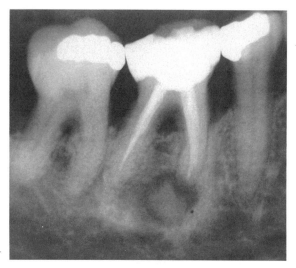

Figure 8-45
OSTEOID OSTEOMA OF MANDIBLE
A panoramic radiograph shows the lesion adjacent to premolar teeth. A radiodense nidus is surrounded by a narrow radiolucent zone. Note the small size of the lesion. (Figures 8-45, 8-46 are from the same patient.)

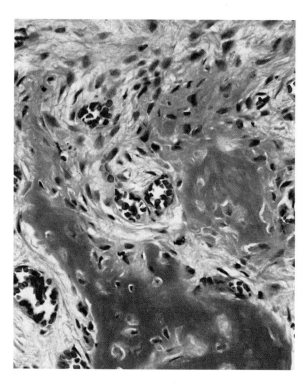

Figure 8-47
OSTEOID OSTEOMA OF MANDIBLE
High-power view of trabeculae of woven bone surrounded by fibrovascular stroma.

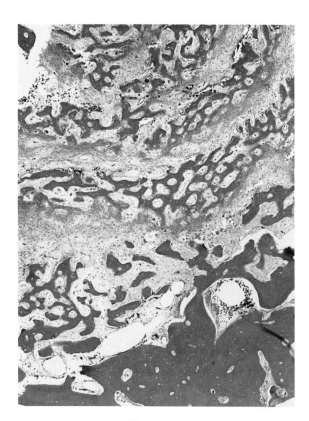

Figure 8-46
OSTEOID OSTEOMA OF MANDIBLE
Nidus composed of anastomosing trabeculae of bone is surrounded by a rim of more densely sclerotic bone.

radiologic-pathologic correlation. Osteosarcomas are seldom well circumscribed radiologically, and careful histologic evaluation usually reveals significant atypism of the osteoblasts, more haphazard matrix formation, and an infiltrative destructive growth pattern. Of the benign fibro-osseous lesions, osteoblastoma most closely resembles ossifying fibroma. Both exhibit similar radiologic features, and, histologically, both contain lamellae of woven bone fairly uniformly distributed and rimmed by plump osteoblasts. However, ossifying fibroma has a more fibrous and less vascularized stroma, with fewer osteoclast type giant cells. Cementoblastoma also bears a close radiologic and histologic resemblance to osteoblastoma. However, this lesion always develops in direct apposition to teeth (50). Histologically, the nidus of an osteoid osteoma is identical to the lesional tissue of an osteoblastoma but can be distinguished by its smaller size (less than 2 cm) and surrounding rim of reactive sclerotic bone. Only a few such lesions have been well documented in the jaw (figs. 8-45–8-47) (55).

Treatment and Prognosis. The recurrence rate for osteoblastoma at all sites is about 10 percent but only sporadic recurrences have been noted in the jaw bones (43). There have also been two reports of osteoblastoma within the jaw bones having undergone regression following only biopsy or incomplete removal (45,47). For the above reasons, the treatment of choice for such tumors in the jaw is curettage or local excision.

Osteosarcoma

Definition. This is a sarcoma in which the neoplastic mesenchymal cells show evidence of production of osteoid or bone. Osteosarcomas of the jaw bones originate in the mandible, the maxilla, and adjacent palatal bones.

Incidence. Osteosarcomas of the jaw bones account for about 6.5 percent of all osteosarcomas (65,67). Over 400 cases have been reported (75). The largest series of 131 cases from the Armed Forces Institute of Pathology was analyzed in the second series Fascicle of the Atlas of Tumor Pathology dealing with intraosseous and parosteal tumors of the jaws (80). Another large series of 66 cases was derived from a total of 998 osteosarcomas from all sites from the Mayo Clinic (67). By 1986, 84 of 1,274 osteosarcomas seen at the Mayo Clinic involved jaw bones (69). Osteosarcomas affect about 1 in 100,000 individuals and those of the jaw about 0.07 in 100,000 (65,67,75). There have been several reports of osteosarcomas of the jaw in patients from Nigeria where they constitute a larger percentage of all reported osteosarcomas (about 19 percent) and where the patients present with advanced lesions (56,57). The peak incidence of osteosarcoma of the jaw, namely in the third decade, is a decade later than that for extragnathic osteosarcomas. The mean age in several large series has been 32, 34, and 39 years, respectively (61,65,67,89). However, the age range is wide, with reports of patients from ages 4 to 82 years. Most series report a 2 to 1 male to female ratio for tumors in the maxilla and an equal sex incidence for those in the mandible, although a slight female predominance has been noted in Mexico and Japan (70,74,95). The mandible has generally been involved more frequently than the maxilla, with one literature review revealing a 1.7 to 1 ratio (61). The series from the Mayo Clinic showed an equal sex incidence (67). Mandibular osteosarcoma has been described as a component of the mendelian dominant familial cancer syndrome, the *Li-Fraumeni syndrome* (77).

Etiologic Factors. Fibrous dysplasia has been observed in association with about 0.5 percent of cases of osteosarcoma (74). In a review of 89 cases of fibrous dysplasia associated with malignancy, 60 percent were osteosarcomas; 36 of the 89 cases involved craniofacial bones. Of the 89 cases, 39 were monostotic, 39 polyostotic, and the remaining 11 exhibited features of Albright's syndrome (72). Irradiation may be an important factor in the induction of malignant change in some of these cases; radiation treatment was given in 28 percent of the 83 cases of fibrous dysplasia associated with malignancy reported by Yabut et al. (99).

Irradiation plays a significant role in the development of osteosarcomas of the jaw. Of the 66 cases from the Mayo Clinic, 9 were considered to be irradiation induced (67). Irradiation to the head and neck region has been used to treat both non-neoplastic and malignant diseases such as fibrous dysplasia, retinoblastoma, and oral and nasopharyngeal cancers (71). The latent period between application of the radiotherapy and the development of the sarcoma ranges from 7 to 23 years and the dose of radiotherapy from 4,500 to 23,000 rads (58).

Paget's disease is a well-known predisposing factor for the development of sarcoma, including osteosarcoma, within bone. Tillman (96) reported 3 osteosarcomas developing within a series of 24 cases of Paget's disease of the jaw bones. Sarcoma has been reported to involve from 1 to 15 percent of patients with Paget's disease, with the higher incidence in those with polyostotic disease (10 percent) (59,98); 16 percent of osteosarcomas arising in polyostotic Paget's disease are multifocal (98). Patients who develop osteosarcoma complicating Paget's disease are usually in an older age group than those whose sarcoma develops ab initio. The sarcoma should be suspected in the presence of a lytic focus within the lesion of Paget's disease and in patients with a marked increase in the level of serum alkaline phosphatase (59). Smith et al. (93) demonstrated that there is an intense and uniform uptake of the radionucleotide Tc-99 in pagetoid bone but a marked decrease in uptake at the site of the Paget sarcoma (figs. 8-48, 8-49). By contrast,

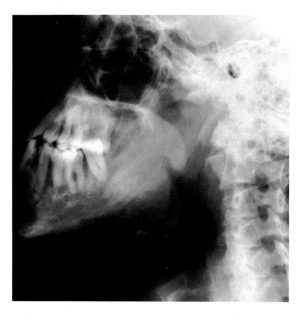
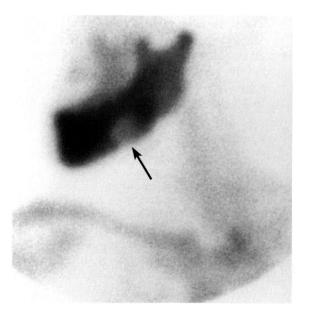

Figure 8-48

OSTEOSARCOMA ARISING IN PAGET'S DISEASE

Left: Radiograph of a mandibular lesion in a 71-year-old man known to have Paget's disease of the mandible, ilium, and femur. The patient developed painful swelling of right mandible of 3 months' duration. Note the coarse trabeculation indicative of involvement by Paget's disease.

Right: Tc-99m isotope scan shows intense uptake with sharp borders by pagetoid bone and decrease in uptake at site of the Paget sarcoma (arrow). (Courtesy of Dr. Howard D. Dorfman, Bronx, NY.) (Figures 8-48 and 8-49 are from the same patient.)

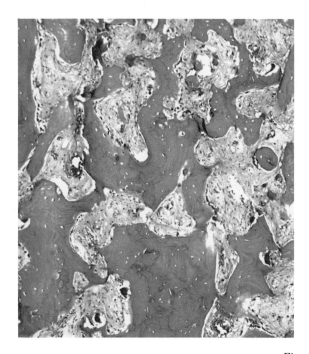
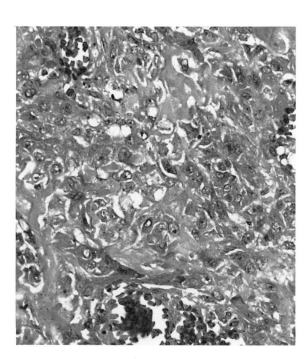

Figure 8-49

OSTEOSARCOMA ARISING IN PAGET'S DISEASE

Left: Typical pattern of Paget's disease showing appositional cement lines, fibrovascular stroma, and tunneling resorption of bone.

Right: This area of osteosarcoma is composed of sheets of large atypical osteoblasts with formation of lace-like osteoid lamellae. (Courtesy of Dr. Howard D. Dorfman, Bronx, NY.)

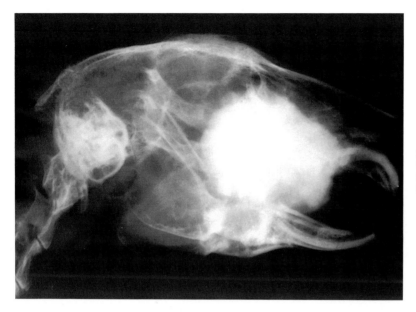

Figure 8-50
OSTEOSARCOMA
OF JAW IN RABBIT
A radiograph of a dense osteosclerotic mass, with marginal "sun-ray" spiculation, in the maxilla of a rabbit. (Courtesy of Dr. S.K. Liu, New York, NY.) (Figures 8-50 and 8-51 are from the same animal.)

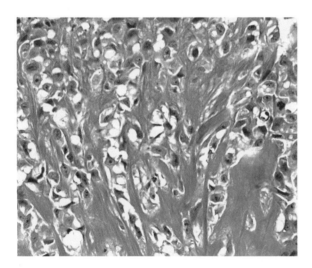 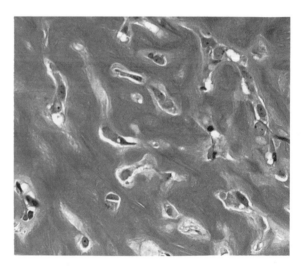

Figure 8-51
OSTEOSARCOMA OF JAW IN RABBIT
Left: There are irregular ribbons of neoplastic osteoid with intervening atypical osteoblasts with prominent nucleoli.
Right: A dense sclerotic region of the sarcoma shows osteoblasts sandwiched between anastomosing trabeculae of bone. (Courtesy of Dr. S.K. Liu, New York, NY.)

gallium is only minimally increased in pagetoid bone, but markedly increased in the sarcoma.

In the jaw, Paget's disease affects the maxilla more frequently than the mandible. Smith et al. (93) documented only one case of sarcoma involving the mandible and two affecting the maxilla out of a total of 85 patients from Memorial Sloan Kettering Cancer Institute with bone sarcoma complicating Paget's disease.

Jaw osteosarcoma also occurs in other vertebrate species (figs. 8-50, 8-51). Osteosarcomas have been reported to be associated with stainless steel implants in dogs: 17 such cases were documented by 1990, including 6 from the Animal Medical Center in New York City (86). Osteosarcoma accounts for between 46 and 85 percent of all canine bone tumors and 8 percent of these involve skull bones (86).

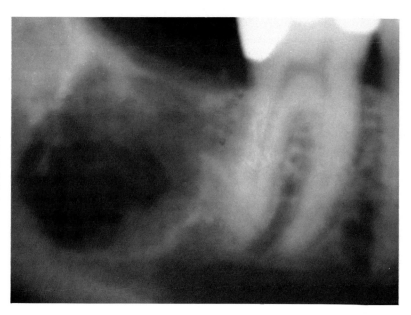

Figure 8-52
HIGH-GRADE
OSTEOBLASTIC
OSTEOSARCOMA
This 35-year-old female was initially diagnosed as suffering from a dental problem, which resulted in removal of a loose lower second molar tooth. Note the fairly well-delimited lucent lesion at the site of the extracted tooth. (Figures 8-52–8-54 are from the same patient.)

Some osteosarcomas, as well as certain other malignancies and retinoblastoma, share a deletion in chromosome 13 which results in inactivation of an antioncogene, the retinoblastoma gene. This explains the increased incidence of osteosarcoma in children with familial bilateral retinoblastoma. Such patients inherit one inactive retinoblastoma gene and require only a single "hit" to inactivate the second gene (73).

Clinical Features. Osteosarcoma of the jaw most frequently presents as a mass or swelling with pain (65,67,74). There is frequently a long delay in diagnosis because the disease may masquerade as an odontogenic infection and extraction of affected, frequently loose teeth, precedes the definitive diagnosis. There are several warning signs that should alert the clinician to the possibility of an underlying osteosarcoma. These include a periapical lucency associated with a vital tooth, tooth mobility without periodontal disease, root resorption, an irregular peridental lucent outline, regional nerve anesthesia, and failure to respond clinically and radiologically to adequate endodontic therapy (figs. 8-52, 8-53) (81). Distalization of the last molar tooth may occur (Cernea's sign). Paresthesia related to tumor infiltration of the inferior alveolar nerve (Vincent's sign) or the supraorbital and infraorbital nerves is a less frequent symptom. Trismus may result from tumor infiltration of the pterygoid muscles. In addition, osteosarcomas of the maxilla may cause signs and symptoms secondary to extension into the orbit (exophthalmos, diplopia), nasal cavity (obstruction), and paranasal sinuses. The serum alkaline phosphatase is elevated in only a few cases (65). The duration of symptoms prior to the establishment of a diagnosis is usually between 3 and 6 months (67,70,75).

Radiologic Findings. The early radiologic features may be subtle and nonspecific, and may be related to the odontogenic apparatus. These features include irregular resorption of the roots of the teeth, displacement of teeth, "floating teeth" in which the affected teeth are unsupported by surrounding bone, absence or attenuation of the lamina dura, and a widened periodontal ligament space (fig. 8-55) (60). The latter results from invasion of sarcoma into the ligament with resorption of interdental alveolar bone. This finding is an important early radiologic manifestation of the disease. A similar appearance may be seen in scleroderma, in which case the phenomenon is generalized as compared to its localization in osteosarcoma (76,78).

In more advanced stages of the disease, the bone exhibits an ill-defined, "moth-eaten" lytic appearance, with or without foci of sclerosis. However, this radiologic feature can be mimicked by other disorders such as osteomyelitis, Ewing's sarcoma, and lymphoma. Destruction of the cortical margins with extension of a mass lesion into the soft tissue, especially in association

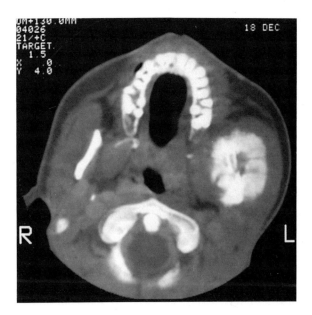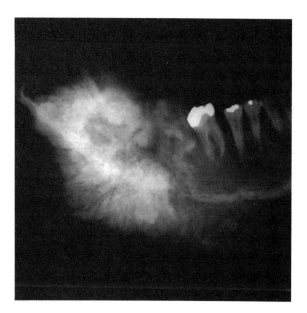

Figure 8-53
HIGH-GRADE OSTEOBLASTIC OSTEOSARCOMA
Left: CT scan taken about 12 months later shows the development of an expansile osteoblastic neoplasm with excessive new bone formation.
Right: Specimen radiograph of the resected mandible illustrates the characteristic peripheral "sun-ray" spiculation of this osteoblastic osteosarcoma.

with evidence of mineralization in the soft tissue component, is a more diagnostic feature (fig. 8-56). The typical "sun burst" appearance in which reactive or tumor bone is laid down in the soft tissue perpendicular to the long axis of the underlying cortex has been observed in only about 25 percent of cases (figs. 8-50, 8-53) (78). Within the mandible, a particularly helpful radiologic feature results from neoplastic invasion of the mandibular canal. The canal may be widened, with loss of clear definition of its cortical margins (85). Within the maxilla, growth of the neoplasm may produce clouding of the antrum and destruction of its walls. In addition to routine imaging studies, CT is an excellent modality for the demonstration of tumor mineralization, cortical involvement, and soft tissue and intramedullary involvement (figs. 8-53, left, 8-57A). Magnetic resonance imaging (MRI) demonstrates the extent of the lesion, including soft tissue and intramedullary involvement, and delineates the soft tissue and bony elements of the neoplasm (figs. 8-57, 8-58) (84).

Gross Findings. By the time of surgical resection, the neoplasm is frequently of large size and it may be difficult to determine its exact site of origin. Within the mandible, the body is the most frequent site of origin, followed in descending order of frequency by the symphysis, angle, and ramus (67). Sites of predilection in the maxilla are the alveolar ridge followed by antrum (fig. 8-58D) (67). Resected specimens from maxillectomy, hemimandibulectomy, or partial mandibulectomy should be properly oriented, if necessary with the assistance of a maxillofacial surgeon. All resection margins should be inked prior to dissection and carefully evaluated to assess the adequacy of resection.

Microscopic Findings. The initial histologic diagnosis is often dependent on examination of small fragments of biopsy material. These are frequently superficial and show intensely inflamed, exuberant granulation tissue which may mask the presence of a sarcoma or fail to be representative of a deeper seated lesion. In such an event, the clinical and radiologic features

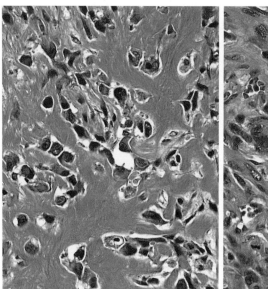
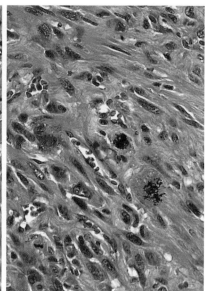

Figure 8-54
HIGH-GRADE
OSTEOBLASTIC
OSTEOSARCOMA

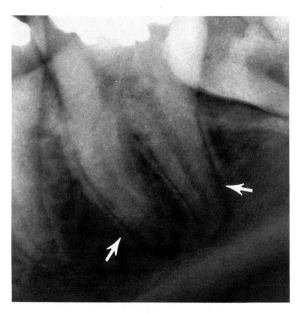

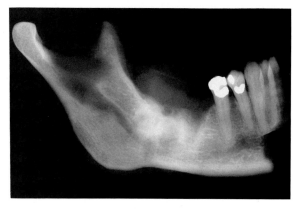

Figure 8-56
OSTEOSARCOMA OF MANDIBLE
Specimen radiograph demonstrate a mixed lytic-sclerotic pattern and extension of the neoplasm beyond the cortical margin.

Figure 8-55
OSTEOSARCOMA
Radiograph of a relatively early osteosarcoma involving the posterior mandible. Bone destruction is evident, as is the widening of the periodontal ligament space (arrows). (Fig. 165 from Fascicle 24, 2nd Series.)

discussed previously may alert the surgeon and pathologist to the need for repeat and more adequate biopsy of the lesion.

Histologically, osteosarcoma of the jaw bones is similar to that seen in extragnathic locations. The establishment of the diagnosis requires the dem-onstration of a sarcomatous stroma with osteoid matrix production by the neoplastic cells. In high-grade lesions, this is usually easily accomplished (figs. 8-54, 8-59) but in low-grade lesions, the distinction from reactive and non-neoplastic lesions such as callus and fibrous dysplasia may be difficult. Occasionally, there is abundant acid mucopolysaccharide–rich ground substance, producing a myxoid histologic pattern that resembles odontogenic myxoma (figs. 8-60, 8-61). Such lesions require detailed clinicopathologic and radiologic correlation and thorough evaluation of histologic and cytologic features.

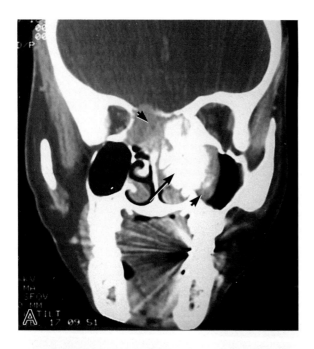
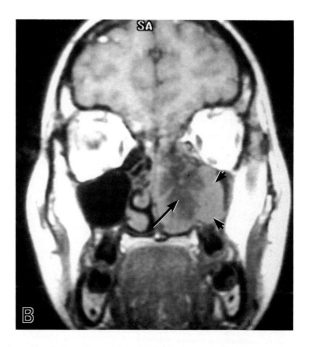
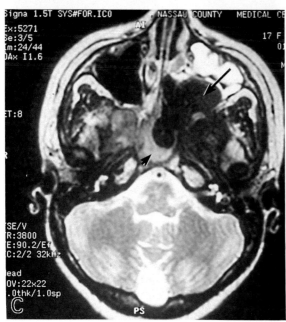
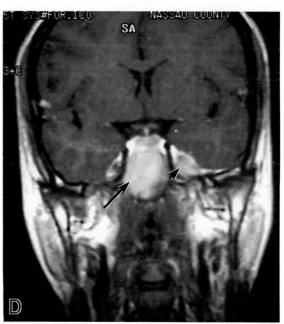

Figure 8-57

OSTEOSARCOMA OF MAXILLARY SINUS

A: CT scan from a 19-year-old female with osteosarcoma of the left paranasal sinuses. This extensive lesion has a central, homogeneous, hyperdense component (long arrow) and a more peripheral soft tissue density (short arrows). The scan clearly delineates involvement of left maxillary sinus, left nasal cavity, bilateral ethmoid and sphenoid sinuses, and floor of anterior cranial fossa.

B: T1-weighted MRI shows a central hypointense component corresponding to the osteoblastic element of the lesion (long arrow) and a peripheral component isointense with soft tissue (tongue) (short arrows) corresponding to the fibrosarcomatous element.

C: T2-weighted MRI shows a central hypointense osteoblastic component (long arrow) and soft tissue component of intermediate signal intensity involving the sphenoid sinuses (short arrow). Note the anterior hyperintense component in left maxillary sinus which represents retention of mucus.

D: T1-weighted MRI with contrast shows involvement of sphenoid sinus (long arrow) and extension of lesion through the floor of the middle cranial fossa (short arrow). (Figures 8-57 and 8-58 are from the same patient.)

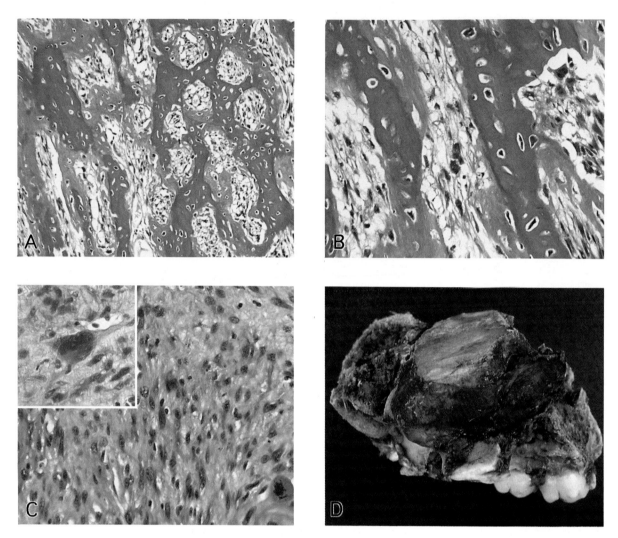

Figure 8-58
OSTEOSARCOMA OF MAXILLARY SINUS

A,B: The central bony component of the neoplasm shows features of well-differentiated osteoblastic osteosarcoma. Note the moderate atypism of some of the nuclei.

C: A peripheral nonosseous component shows a pattern of moderately differentiated fibrosarcoma. Note the atypical mitosis in right lower corner and multinucleate tumor giant cells in inset.

D: Maxillectomy specimen shows tumor involving maxillary and ethmoid sinuses.

Osteosarcoma may be predominantly osteoblastic, in which case the tumor osteoid and woven bone are haphazardly deposited in a lacelike pattern or in a more diffuse, irregular, sheetlike pattern. The sarcoma cells usually show readily identifiable pleomorphism, hyperchromasia, and brisk mitotic activity including abnormal forms (figs. 8-50, 8-51, 8-59). Destruction of preexisting lamellar bone with deposition of neoplastic bone on remnants of normal bone may be seen. The sarcoma may extend into surrounding soft tissue and entrap and destroy normal structures such as skeletal muscle and myelinated nerve bundles; it may also extend into vascular and lymphatic channels.

In chondroblastic osteosarcoma, abundant neoplastic cartilage predominates but the lesion requires the demonstration of some tumor bone to exclude a diagnosis of chondrosarcoma. In most series of gnathic osteosarcoma, osteoblastic lesions outnumber chondroblastic lesions, except in the Mayo Clinic and Mexican reports (67,70). Dahlin

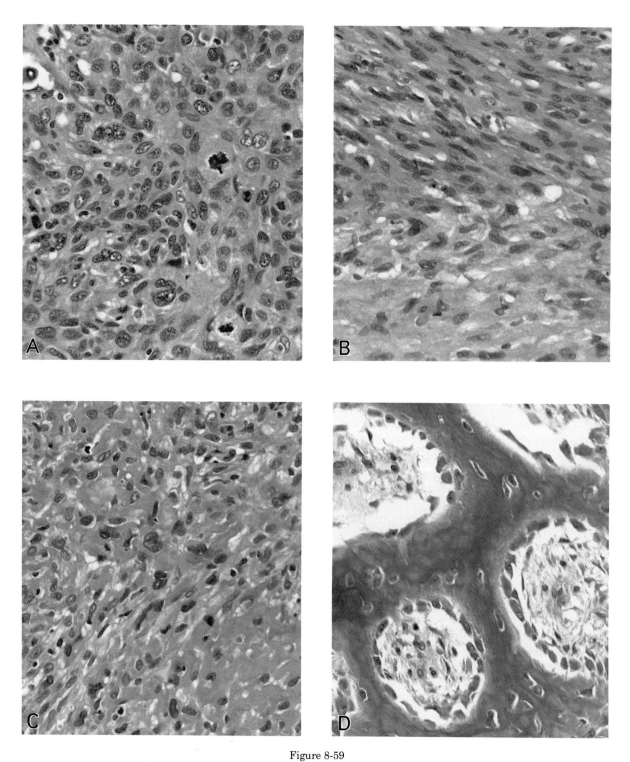

Figure 8-59
HIGH-GRADE OSTEOSARCOMA WITH HETEROGENEOUS PATTERNS

A: The pleomorphic component resembles malignant fibrous histiocytoma. (Figures A–D are from the mandible of a 64-year-old female.)

B: Fibrocytic component resembles fibrosarcoma.

C: Osteoblastic component with abundant lace-like osteoid production.

D: Reactive callus with a symmetric pattern of osteoid production and a surface layer of reactive osteoblasts from a pathologic fracture that complicated this lesion.

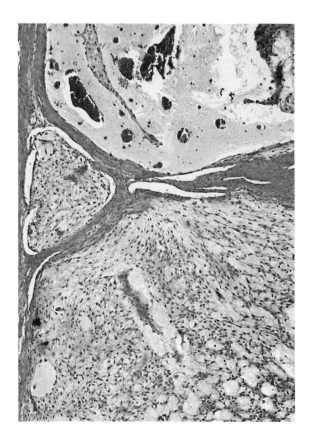 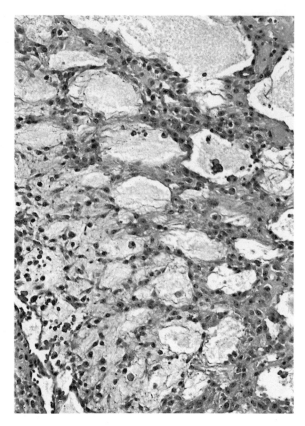

Figure 8-60

OSTEOSARCOMA WITH PROMINENT MYXOID FEATURES

Left: A prominent, lobulated, myxoid component of osteosarcoma from the mandible of 18-year-old male. A mucinous lake is seen in the upper third of the photomicrograph.

Right: Accumulation of stromal mucin has resulted in a cribriform pattern. (Figures 8-60 and 8-61 are from the same patient.)

and Unni (69) attribute the higher incidence of the chondroblastic type in their study to the fact that such cases are probably classified as chondrosarcomas in other series. They point out that small peripheral or central foci of tumor osteoid can usually be identified in these cases. In any event, they believe the distinction is only of academic interest since the behavior of chondroblastic osteosarcoma and chondrosarcoma of the jaw is identical.

A third histologic pattern is one in which a fibrosarcomatous pattern predominates, the fibroblastic type (fig. 8-62). A low-grade osteosarcoma of fibroblastic type may be difficult to distinguish from desmoplastic fibroma of bone (figs. 8-63–8-65) (82). Both may present with the similar radiologic features of a lytic lesion, with variably defined borders (figs. 8-63). Histologically, both

may be comprised of uniform ovoid to spindle-shaped cells with a variable quantity of intercellular collagenous matrix (fig. 8-64, left). Desmoplastic fibroma, like the desmoid, its soft tissue counterpart, tends to be of uniform cellularity, has a fairly conspicuous collagenous matrix, and has mitoses that are absent or extremely sparse. By contrast, low-grade fibrogenic osteosarcoma tends to show variation in cellular content from one area to another, and in the more cellular foci, it tends to contain less collagenous matrix than the desmoplastic fibroma (figs. 8-64, right, 8-65, left). Mitoses may be inconspicuous but can usually be demonstrated by thorough examination. The most helpful distinguishing feature is the production of tumor osteoid or bone in the osteosarcoma, but its presence may be focal and not demonstrable in biopsy specimens (fig. 8-65).

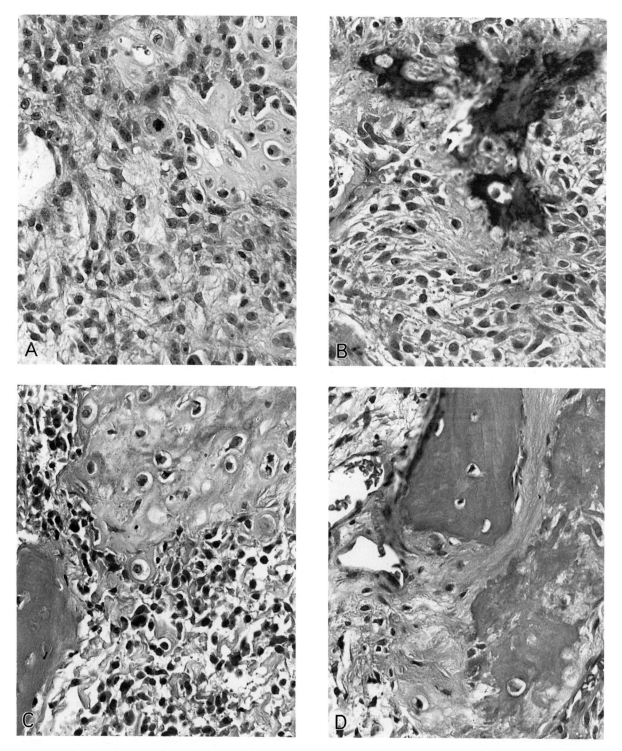

Figure 8-61
OSTEOSARCOMA WITH PROMINENT MYXOID FEATURES

A: The cellular area of the neoplasm contains cells with large round to ovoid nuclei and prominent nucleoli. Moderate mitotic activity is seen. Note the incipient osteoid formation in the right upper corner of photomicrograph.

B: An area of tumor bone is formed by spindle-shaped sarcoma cells.

C: A focus of malignant cartilage within a cellular area of the sarcoma.

D: Neoplastic woven bone is laid down in apposition to surviving fragments of preexisting lamellar bone.

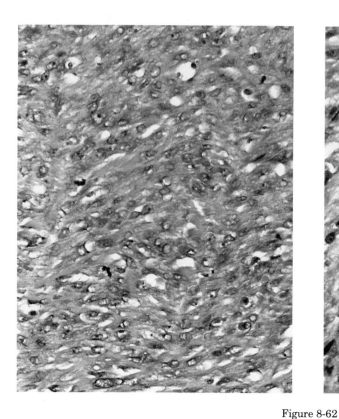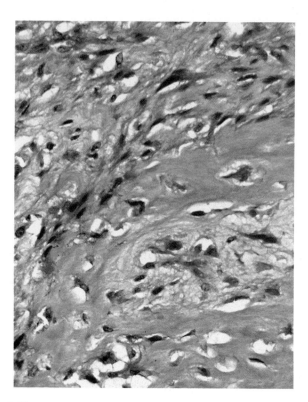

Figure 8-62
OSTEOSARCOMA: FIBROBLASTIC TYPE
Left: A predominantly fibrosarcomatous pattern is seen, with numerous mitotic figures.
Right: A focal area shows osteoid production by sarcoma cells. (Courtesy of Dr. Andrew Huvos, New York, NY.)

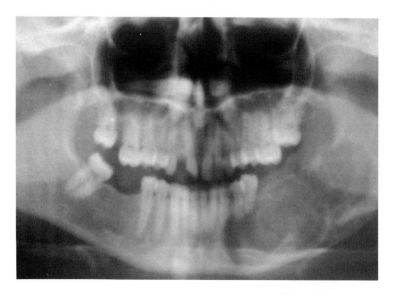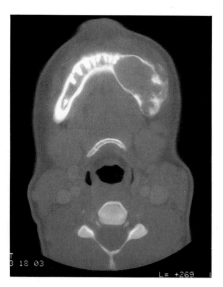

Figure 8-63
LOW-GRADE FIBROBLASTIC OSTEOSARCOMA
Left: The radiograph shows a lobulated expansile lesion with fairly well-defined borders and root resorption of premolar teeth. The patient was a 23-year-old female with an extended history of left mandibular enlargement.
Right: CT scan shows expansion of the body of left mandible with attenuated but intact cortex. These radiologic images are suggestive of a benign, slow growing lesion. (Figures 8-63–8-65 are from the same patient.)

192

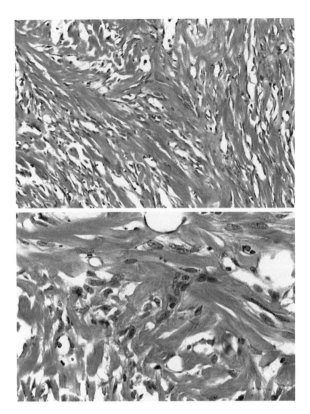
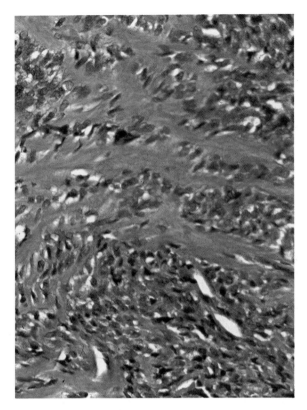

Figure 8-64
LOW-GRADE FIBROBLASTIC OSTEOSARCOMA
Left: The biopsy specimen shows a fibroblastic lesion with abundant collagen production and uniformly bland nuclei. The lesion resembles a desmoplastic fibroma.
Right: Aggregation of cells between acellular collagen bundles is inconsistent with the pattern of a desmoplastic fibroma. A diagnosis of low-grade fibroblastic osteosarcoma was rendered.

In our experience, it is not uncommon for individual osteosarcomas of the jaws to be heterogeneous with regard to the three elements described above (figs. 8-59, 8-65). The high-grade variant comprises 54 to 90 percent of osteosarcomas of the jaw (62,70).

Osteosarcoma Subtypes. Apart from the three histologic patterns described above, several well-defined subtypes of osteosarcoma have been delineated. Each of these has been documented as occurring within jaw bones although the number of cases is limited.

Telangiectatic Osteosarcoma. This variant has the architectural features of an aneurysmal bone cyst, with blood-filled lakes surrounded by septa comprised of mesenchymal cells, osteoblasts, and matrix (figs. 8-66, 8-67A). It differs from an aneurysmal bone cyst in that the mesenchymal cells are malignant and are responsi-

ble for the production of tumor osteoid and bone (fig. 8-67B,C). Failure to carefully examine the cytologic features of the mesenchymal cells may result in an erroneous diagnosis of telangiectatic osteosarcoma as aneurysmal bone cyst as evidenced by such an occurrence in a case report from Hong Kong (66). The diagnosis of an osteosarcoma of the jaw may be further complicated by the development of a secondary aneurysmal bone cyst within an osteosarcoma. This was the case in 8 of 75 (11 percent) jaw osteosarcomas reported by Struthers and Shear (94).

Small Cell Osteosarcoma. Only a single case of the small cell variant of osteosarcoma of the jaw has been reported in an 8-year-old child (79). It is essential to distinguish such a lesion from other small round cell tumors such as Burkitt's lymphoma, embryonal rhabdomyosarcoma, and metastatic neuroblastoma.

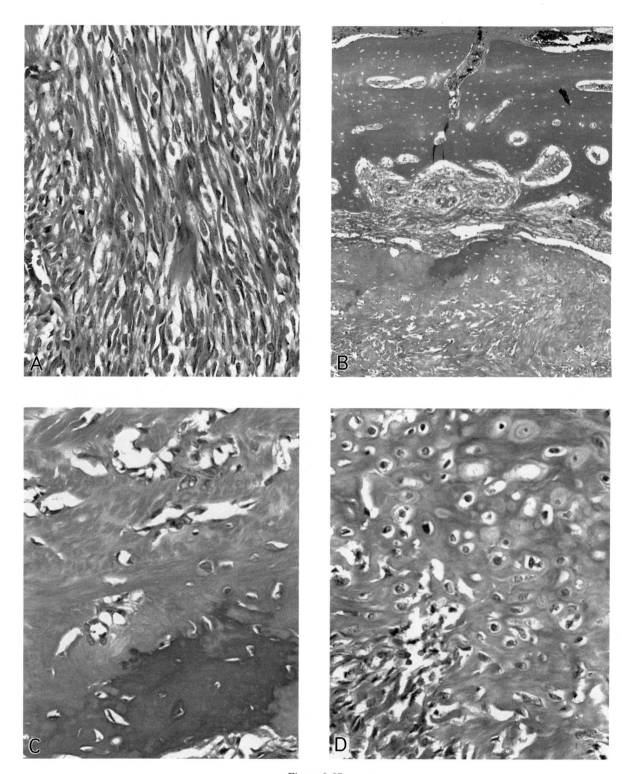

Figure 8-65
LOW-GRADE FIBROBLASTIC OSTEOSARCOMA
A: Partial mandibulectomy specimen with a hypercellular, fibroblastic, lesional component. Rare mitotic figures are evident.
B: Erosion of cortical bone (top) by broad sheets of neoplastic woven bone (bottom).
C: Higher magnification of sheet of irregular woven bone.
D: A focal area of atypical cartilage differentiating from the fibroblastic component which is seen in the left lower corner.

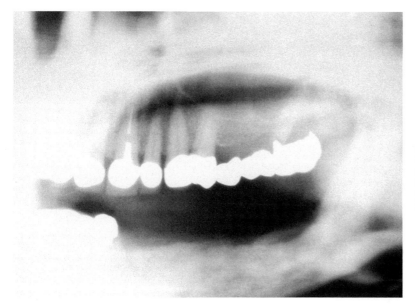

Figure 8-66
POSTIRRADIATION
TELANGIECTATIC
OSTEOSARCOMA
Radiograph of an ill-defined, lytic and sclerotic lesion in an edentulous portion of body of mandible of a 44-year-old female. Patient had received radiation therapy for carcinoma of tongue 18 years previously. (Figures 8-66 and 8-67 are from the same patient.)

Figure 8-67
POSTIRRADIATION
TELANGIECTATIC OSTEOSARCOMA
A: The lesion is composed of septa of varying width, a pattern suggestive of an aneurysmal bone cyst.
B: High magnification illustrates severe cellular anaplasia and mitotic activity of septal cells, indicative of a malignant process. Note the presence of some benign osteoclast type giant cells.
C: A focal area of osteoid production by malignant osteoblasts.

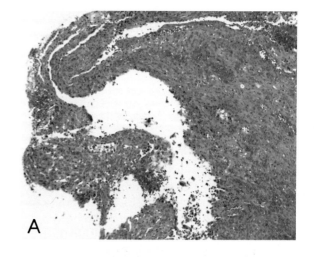

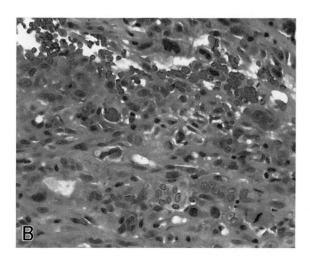

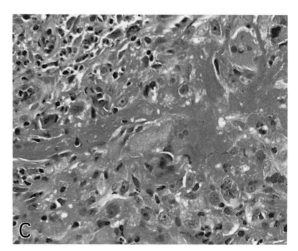

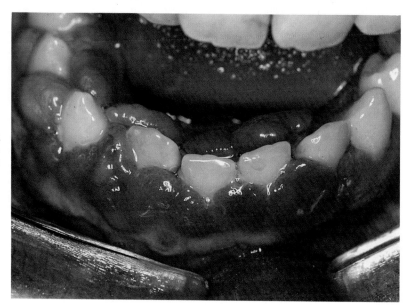

Figure 8-68
LOW-GRADE
CENTRAL OSTEOSARCOMA
Hyperplastic gingival tissue present since a pregnancy several months previously. (Figures 8-68–8-70 are from the same patient.)

Osteosarcoma–Malignant Fibrous Histiocytoma Subtype. This subtype differs from the garden variety osteosarcoma in that it resembles a soft tissue malignant fibrous histiocytoma (fig. 8-59A) but with evidence of tumor osteoid or bone production by the neoplastic cells. In a comparison of 4 examples of this subtype with 11 of the usual type within the jaw, the malignant fibrous histiocytoma subtype was found to be purely lytic, the mean age of occurrence was about 40 years, and mandible and maxilla were equally involved (68). By definition, this subtype is of high histologic grade.

Well-Differentiated Central Osteosarcoma. This subtype originates centrally within the bone and is composed of a fibrovascular stroma and spicules of neoplastic woven bone (figs. 8-68–8-70). The mesenchymal cells within the fibrovascular stroma show only mild nuclear atypism. Histologically, this pattern closely resembles that seen in fibrous dysplasia (fig. 8-70C). Radiologically, the lesion has rather ill-defined margins and irregular areas of radiolucency or radiodensity (fig. 8-69). Fibrous dysplasia has a uniform ground glass appearance, ill-defined margins but with an intact cortical margin, and a normal periodontal ligament space; teeth may or may not be displaced. Although the bone may be expanded, the lesion is always confined to the bone. By contrast, well-differentiated central osteosarcoma manifests irregular lucency and

density, its margins are ill-defined with a "moth-eaten" appearance, the cortical margin may be destroyed with extension into soft tissues, and there is widening of the periodontal ligament space; the teeth are usually not displaced (63). Histologically, the woven bone spicules in fibrous dysplasia are more evenly distributed throughout the lesion and the fibrocytic cells are not atypic. By contrast, the woven bony spicules of central low-grade osteosarcoma are haphazardly distributed and are more variable in size (fig. 8-70C). Of particular diagnostic help is the deposition of neoplastic bone in direct apposition to fragments of residual, partially resorbed lamellar bone (fig. 8-61D). Extension of the process into surrounding soft tissue with entrapment and destruction of normal tissue components firmly establishes a diagnosis of malignancy (fig. 8-70D), as does the presence of metastasis (fig. 8-70E). Although the neoplasm is well differentiated, careful histologic examination usually reveals a mild degree of nuclear pleomorphism and hyperchromasia, and occasional mitotic figures.

This variant of osteosarcoma may also be difficult to distinguish from reparative bone in chronic osteomyelitis and from reactive callus. Of particular help in this regard is the presence of a maturation or zoning phenomenon similar to that seen in myositis ossificans in reactive processes. Some areas show reparative granulation tissue

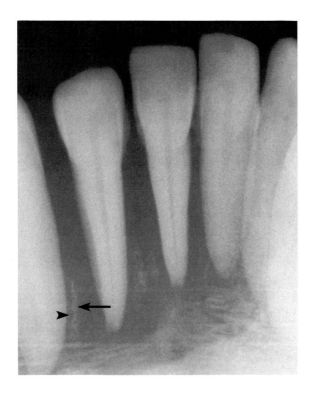

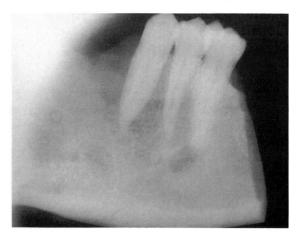

Figure 8-69
LOW-GRADE CENTRAL OSTEOSARCOMA
Left: Radiograph shows bone destruction at the apices of incisor and canine teeth. Note the persistence of portions of lamina dura (long arrow) and the suggestion of a widened periodontal ligament space (arrow head).
Above: Specimen radiograph shows an ill-defined lytic lesion involving the roots of incisor and canine teeth.

with a variable inflammatory cell infiltrate. This merges imperceptibly with foci in which early hyaline matrix, representing early osteoid formation, is deposited within the granulation tissue. This in turn merges with areas of provisional callus formation. The callus exhibits a fairly uniform lattice-like formation and the individual seams of callus are rimmed by a uniform layer of plump active osteoblasts (figs. 8-71, 8-72). Careful evaluation of these features should enable the pathologist to distinguish a reactive from a neoplastic process with a high degree of confidence.

Parosteal Osteosarcoma. This is one of three subtypes of osteosarcoma arising on the surface of the bone external to the cortex. There is some inconsistency in terminology in the literature in that the terms "parosteal" and "juxtacortical" are regarded by some authors as synonymous whereas others use the term "juxtacortical" to include the two surface osteosarcomas, parosteal and periosteal. We use the former terminology.

Radiologically, the tumor is seen attached to the surface of the bone and may partially encircle it. It may be heavily mineralized. A rather characteristic, wedge-shaped separation of tumor from bone is seen at the proximal and distal extremities of the lesion. Histologically, this lesion resembles low-grade central osteosarcoma, having a relatively bland-appearing fibrocytic component and forming variable-sized spicules or sheets of tumor osteoid or bone. In the early stages of its evolution, there is little tendency to invade underlying cortex or medulla. A review of 12 cases involving jaw bones had been reported in the literature by 1990 but this included examples of both periosteal and low-grade parosteal osteosarcomas (64,87).

Periosteal Osteosarcoma. This surface osteosarcoma is a higher grade lesion than the parosteal type described above. Radiologically, it is confined to the surface of the bone where it forms a poorly defined mass with irregular areas of mineralization. It may have a sunburst appearance. Histologically, there is a predominantly cartilaginous component but there is evidence of bone formation by tumor cells. The lesion is of an intermediate to high grade of malignancy. Periosteal osteosarcoma is an extremely rare lesion in the jaw and only a few isolated cases have been reported (88,100).

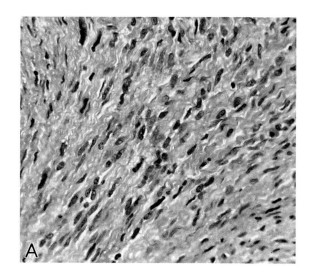

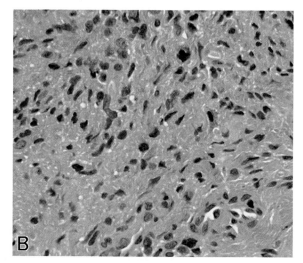

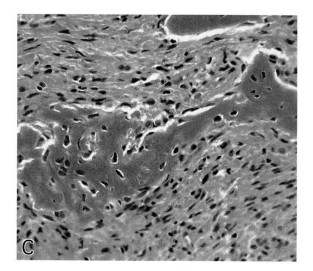

Figure 8-70
LOW-GRADE CENTRAL OSTEOSARCOMA

A: Fascicles of fairly uniform fibrocytic cells and abundant wavy collagen fibers are seen. This pattern is reminiscent of a desmoplastic fibroma.

B: Area of tumor shows mild but definite atypia of spindle cells with occasional enlarged hyperchromatic nuclei.

C: Focal irregular osteoid production by tumor cells.

D: Extension of tumor through eroded cortex into soft tissue adjacent to salivary gland.

E: Cervical lymph node shows metastatic sarcoma. A residual germinal center is in right lower corner.

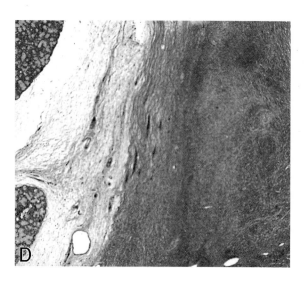

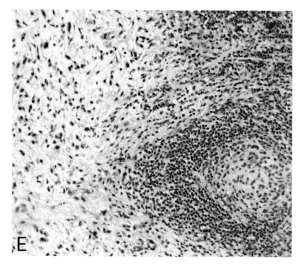

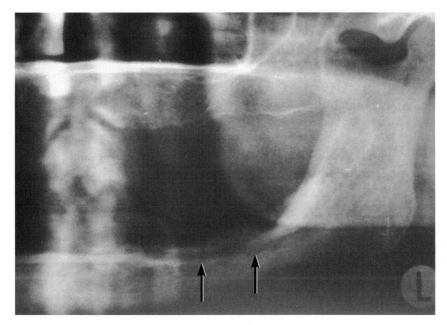

Figure 8-71
REACTIVE CALLUS
Radiograph of left mandible from 71-year-old female with a history of several episodes of pain and swelling. An ill-defined lucency is in the body of the mandible but the margins of the mandibular canal (arrows) are preserved. (Figures 8-71 and 8-72 are from the same patient.)

Immunohistochemical Findings. Immunohistochemical evaluation is occasionally helpful in distinguishing osteosarcoma from other neoplasms of nonmesenchymal type (83,90). In particular, it is occasionally difficult to differentiate a sarcoma from a spindle cell squamous carcinoma by routine hematoxylin and eosin staining. While the presence of cytokeratins within the spindle cells might suggest an epithelial derivation, aberrant cytokeratin staining is frequently observed in osteosarcoma of the jaws. Regezi et al. (90) noted cytokeratin staining in 7 of 16 jaw osteosarcomas that they evaluated. Chondroid tissue within an osteosarcoma is decorated by an antibody to S-100 protein antigen. However, focal cytokeratin staining has been reported in chondroblastic areas of an osteosarcoma as well (90).

Treatment and Prognosis. The standard form of therapy for osteosarcoma of the jaw bones is ablative radical surgery. In the mandible, this usually involves a hemimandibulectomy and in the maxilla, maxillectomy with or without orbital exenteration. The pathologist is frequently requested to assist in assessing the adequacy of the procedure by evaluating by frozen section technique multiple soft tissue biopsy specimens from the resection margin. There is insufficient data to assess the value of other therapeutic modalities such as adjuvant chemotherapy or radiotherapy.

The prognosis of patients with gnathic osteosarcoma is better than that for those with osteosarcoma at other sites. A 40 percent 5-year survival rate was reported from the Mayo Clinic but figures have ranged from 12 to 58 percent (67,92). Most series report a better prognosis for those with mandibular lesions than maxillary lesions. The M.D. Anderson Hospital found a 71 percent 5-year survival rate for patients with osteosarcoma of the mandible, compared to a 50 percent 5-year survival rate for those with maxillary osteosarcoma (91). Other series have reported a 24 to 50 percent survival rate for patients with mandibular and 19 to 30 percent rate for those with maxillary lesions (97). This trend was reversed in a series from Memorial Sloan Kettering Cancer Institute in which a 33 percent 5-year survival rate was documented for those with maxillary osteosarcoma as compared to 24 percent for mandibular osteosarcoma (65).

The behavior of osteosarcoma of the jaw differs from extragnathic osteosarcoma in that local recurrence is more common than distant metastases. The local recurrence rate in the Mayo Clinic cases was 70 percent (73 percent for the maxilla and 66 percent for the mandible); only 4 of the 66 tumors metastasized (67). The Memorial Sloan Kettering Cancer Institute cases manifested an 80 percent local recurrence rate for lesions of the maxilla and a 47 percent rate for those

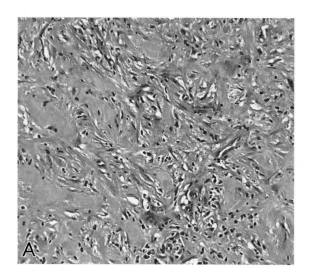

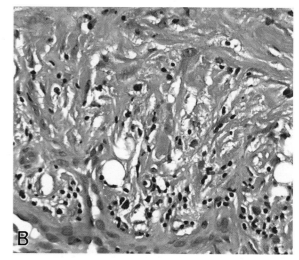

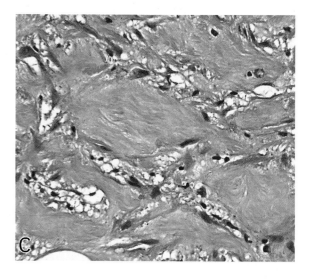

Figure 8-72
REACTIVE CALLUS

Maturation phenomenon in biopsy material from a patient with chronic inflammation and reparative bone formation. This was misinterpreted at a prestigious cancer hospital as low-grade intramedullary osteosarcoma.

A: Typical granulation tissue with myofibroblasts and neovascular endothelial-lined channels.

B: Higher magnification shows myofibroblasts, endothelial cells, and chronic inflammatory cells.

C: Deposition of fibrillar acellular material in an organized pattern represents early osteoid formation.

D: Production of trabeculae of woven bone in an orderly array. These trabeculae are rimmed by a uniform layer of osteoblastic cells.

E: Further maturation of reactive bone. Note the lining layer of uniform osteoblastic cells differentiating from underlying bland fibrocytic cells.

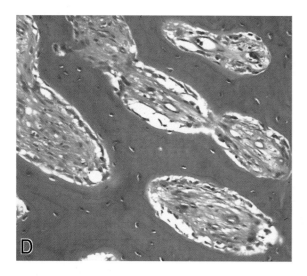

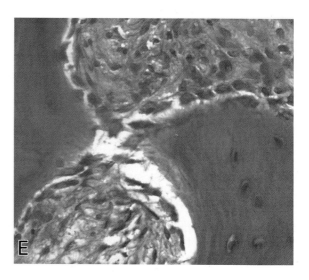

of the mandible (65). Distant metastases were reported in 20 percent of the maxillary lesions and 53 percent of the mandibular lesions in this series of cases. Metastases in jaw osteosarcomas have been reported to develop within 20 to 29 months of diagnosis compared to only 6 months for all other osteosarcomas (92). There are several factors that may contribute to the somewhat better overall survival for patients with osteosarcomas located in the jaw as compared to other sites. These include the tendency to local recurrence rather that distant metastasis and a higher incidence of neoplasms of lower histologic grade (44 percent of jaw sarcomas compared to 20 percent for extragnathic lesions in the Mayo Clinic series [67]).

CARTILAGINOUS LESIONS

Osteochondroma

Definition. Osteochondroma is an osteochondromatous exophytic mass arising from the region of the metaphysis and diaphysis. It has limited growth potential and it is uncertain whether the lesion is of a developmental, neoplastic, or reactive nature.

Clinical Features. There are less than 50 reported cases of osteochondroma involving the jaw bones. More than half of the reported cases involve the coronoid process, with the condyle being the second most frequent site (105,106). Occasional lesions have involved the symphysis and other sites. The mean age at diagnosis is about 40 years and unlike osteochondromas in the extragnathic skeleton, these lesions may continue to grow even after skeletal maturity has been achieved. Females are more commonly affected than males.

Osteochondroma involving the coronoid process most commonly causes difficulty in opening the mouth, whereas involvement of the condyle produces symptoms and signs of temporomandibular joint dysfunction, namely, pain, clicking, malocclusion, facial asymmetry, and posterior apertognathia (101,107). There may also be swelling in the region of the temporomandibular joint.

Radiologic Findings. The lesion is a dome- or mushroom-shaped exophytic bony mass. The cortical component of the pedicle blends with the

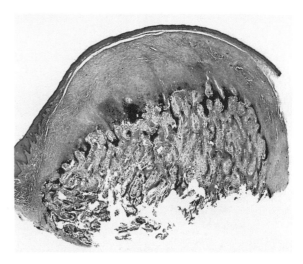

Figure 8-73
OSTEOCHONDROMA OF MANDIBLE

Dome-shaped, exophytic lesion is comprised of a surface cartilaginous cap, a narrow transverse zone of endochondral ossification, and underlying parallel trabeculae of woven and lamellar bone. Oral mucous membrane is stretched over the surface of the lesion. (Figures 8-73 and 8-74 are from the same patient.)

cortex of the underlying bone in the form of a cortical flare and the medullary region of the pedicle is in continuity with the medulla of the host bone. This is best visualized on CT images (103). Osteochondroma of the condyle projects from the anteromedial surface while osteochondroma of the coronoid process arises from the anterior aspect.

Pathologic Findings and Pathogenesis. As in osteochondromas in extragnathic locations, the pedicle of the lesion arises from a metadiaphyseal location. The surface is covered by a cap of fairly well-organized hyaline cartilage with an underlying, well-defined zone of endochondral ossification. This subsequently matures into cortical and medullary bone with marrow that merges with the cortex and medulla of normal bone (figs. 8-73, 8-74). It has been variously postulated that the proliferating cartilage cells of the lesion represent displaced epiphyseal cartilage cells, or cartilage cells derived from stimulated mesenchymal cells at sites of tendinous insertion or from pleuripotential periosteal cells (107). Osteochondromas should not be confused with simple hyperplasia of the condylar process and should also be distinguished from the rarely occurring chondroma of the jaw (102,104).

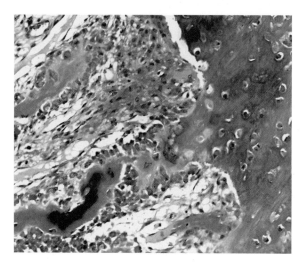

Figure 8-74
OSTEOCHONDROMA OF MANDIBLE
A cartilaginous cap is seen on the right side of photomicrograph and a zone of endochondral ossification on the left.

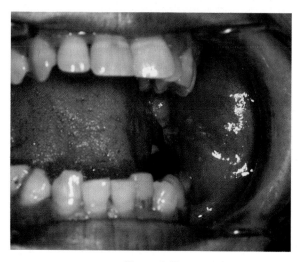

Figure 8-75
CHONDROMYXOID FIBROMA
Swelling of inner aspect of right cheek in a 38-year-old female. (Courtesy of Dr. H. Hashimoto, Kitakyushu, Japan.) (Figures 8-75–8-80 are from the same patient.)

Treatment and Prognosis. Osteochondroma of the jaw is best treated by simple local excision. Unlike osteochondromas occurring elsewhere, there have been no reports of chondrosarcoma or recurrence complicating this lesion (103,107).

Chondroblastoma

Chondroblastoma has been reported so infrequently in a gnathic location that readers are referred to the Fascicle, Tumors of the Bones and Joints (108a) for a detailed description. Three such lesions have been reported in the mandible and one in the maxilla and they exhibit no differences from their extragnathic counterparts (108,109).

Chondromyxoid Fibroma

Definition. Chondromyxoid fibroma is a benign, multilobulated neoplasm arising most commonly in the metaphyseal region of long bones.
Clinical and Radiologic Features. By 1993, 19 well-documented cases had been reported in the jaw bones, all but 4 of which were in the mandible (fig. 8-75) (111). Jaw lesions constitute about 2 percent of all reported chondromyxoid fibromas. All 4 of the maxillary lesions were found between central incisors and canines. The patients ranged in age from 10 to 67 years, with a mean

age of 28 years; over two thirds occurred in patients in the second and third decades. Pain and swelling are the usual clinical manifestations. The radiologic and histologic features are identical to those of such lesions occurring elsewhere in the skeleton. In long bones, the neoplasm is believed to originate from epiphyseal cartilage; in the mandible remnants of Meckel's cartilage may be the nidus of origin.

Radiologically, the lesion produces a well-delineated, radiolucent image with a sclerotic margin and trabeculation. There may be expansion of the bone with thinning or even dissolution of the cortical margin. However, the tumor is always delineated by intact periosteum (figs. 8-76–8-78). Evidence of mineralization is sometimes seen. As a consequence of the high fluid content of the matrix, the signal intensity of the lesion is bright in T2-weighted images (fig. 8-78, right). Loss of lamina dura, root resorption, and displacement of teeth have been reported in association with this tumor (110).

Pathologic Findings. Histologically, the lesion is composed of variable-sized lobules of chondromyxoid tissue, each delineated by cellular fibrovascular bands. Within the lobules, the stellate myxoid cells tend to be more centrally located, whereas toward the periphery, the lobules are more cellular and the cells more polygonal or

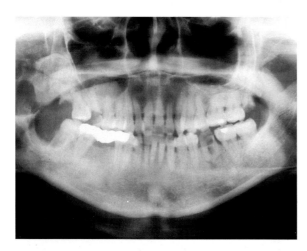

Figure 8-76
CHONDROMYXOID FIBROMA
Expansile, multilocular, lytic lesion of right ramus of mandible. The lesion is well-circumscribed. (Courtesy of Dr. H. Hashimoto, Kitakyushu, Japan.)

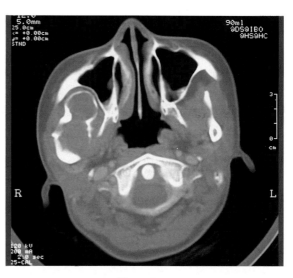

Figure 8-77
CHONDROMYXOID FIBROMA
Axial CT scan shows the lesion expanding the right ramus of the mandible. A thin cortical shell of bone delimits much of the lesion. (Courtesy of Dr. H. Hashimoto, Kitakyushu, Japan.)

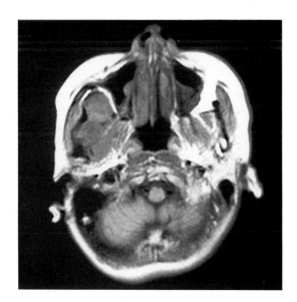

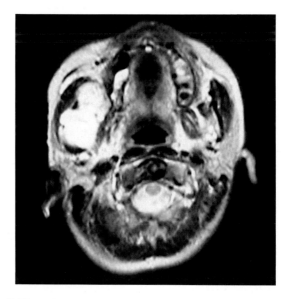

Figure 8-78
CHONDROMYXOID FIBROMA
Left: Axial T1-weighted MRI.
Right: Axial T2-weighted MRI. Note the high signal intensity of the lesion in the T2-weighted image resulting from the high fluid content of the chondromyxoid tissue. (Courtesy of Dr. H. Hashimoto, Kitakyushu, Japan.)

chondroid (figs. 8-79, 8-80). The chondroid cells may show some degree of cytologic atypia. Multinucleate osteoclast type giant cells may be seen at the periphery of the lobules. The pathologist may fail to recognize the distinctive lobulation on small biopsy specimens and erroneously diagnose a myxoma or chondrosarcoma, depending on whether the myxoid or chondroid elements of

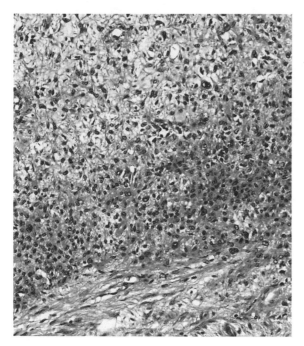

Figure 8-79
CHONDROMYXOID FIBROMA
A portion of the nodule is delimited by a fibrous band (bottom). Polygonal chondroid cells are concentrated toward the periphery of the nodule and the myxoid cells towards the center. (Courtesy of Dr. H. Hashimoto, Kitakyushu, Japan.)

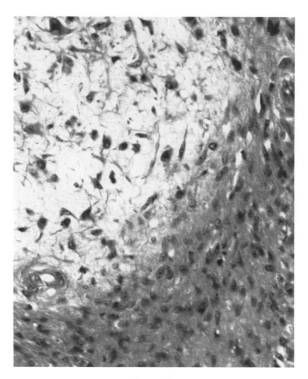

Figure 8-80
CHONDROMYXOID FIBROMA
Stellate myxoid cells are surrounded by polygonal chondroid cells, seen at higher magnification. (Courtesy of Dr. H. Hashimoto, Kitakyushu, Japan.)

the neoplasm are dominant in the specimen. The possibility of misdiagnosis of chondrosarcoma is heightened because of the cytologic atypia alluded to above. The danger of such errors in diagnosis stresses the need for close radiologic-pathologic correlation. Immunohistochemical stains have demonstrated positivity for S-100 protein in the chondroid elements and electron microscopic studies have shown the presence of chondroblastic type cells, suggesting that the neoplasm is primarily of chondroid histogenesis and could be more aptly named fibromyxoid chondroma (111,112).

Treatment and Prognosis. Chondromyxoid fibroma is usually adequately treated by thorough curettage, enucleation, or local resection. In view of the cosmetic deformity which would result from en bloc resection in the jaw bones, a thorough curettage has been advocated as the treatment of choice. Although the recurrence rate in the extragnathic location is about 20 percent, only two recurrences were reported in the 19 documented jaw tumors (111).

Chondrosarcoma

Definition. Chondrosarcoma is a malignant mesenchymal neoplasm associated with the production of cartilaginous matrix directly from neoplastic cells. Any production of osteoid matrix by neoplastic cells, albeit a minor component, precludes a diagnosis of chondrosarcoma and establishes that of an osteosarcoma. Endochondral ossification on the surface of a neoplastic cartilaginous island may, however, be seen in chondrosarcoma and accounts for the ring-like calcification so typical of the roentgenographic appearance of cartilaginous neoplasms.

Incidence. Chondrosarcoma of the craniofacial bones constitutes between 1 and 10 percent of all chondrosarcomas (117). The maxilla is involved slightly more frequently than the mandible. In a recent review of 56 cases from the Mayo Clinic, the maxilla was the most commonly involved region, followed by the central facial bones (nasal septum, ethmoid, and sphenoid), with only few cases involving the mandible (124).

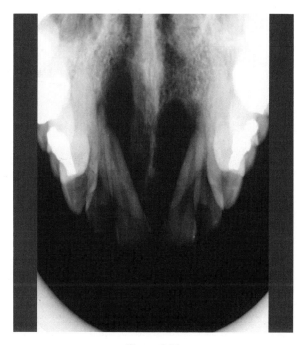

Figure 8-81
CHONDROSARCOMA
A radiolucent lesion with a fairly well-circumscribed margin extends on both sides of the midline and anteriorly in a 29-year-old man. (Figures 8-81–8-88 are from the same patient.)

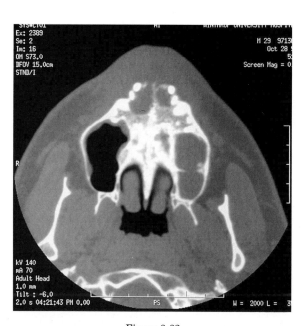

Figure 8-82
CHONDROSARCOMA
The extent of the lesion is illustrated in this axial CT scan.

The mandibular lesions usually occur in the region of the angle and adjacent body and ramus (119). A few cases have involved the mandibular condyle (122). The neoplasm affects patients of a wide age spectrum but is most common in the third decade. The mean age of patients in the Mayo Clinic series was 41.6 years. The sex incidence is about equal.

Clinical Features. The usual presentation is that of swelling and deformity of the involved region. In some cases this may be associated with pain or trismus. Maxillary chondrosarcoma may produce nasal obstruction, epistaxis, proptosis, blurred vision, and diplopia. Odontogenic symptoms include malocclusion, progressive diastema, and loosening and exfoliation of teeth. Chondrosarcoma may, on rare occasions, complicate fibrous dysplasia, especially in cases treated by irradiation, although osteosarcoma is the more usual histologic type of malignant degeneration (116).

Radiologic Findings. While the radiologic features are frequently nonspecific, they are usually those of an aggressive lesion (figs. 8-81–8-83) (117). The lesion is usually radiolucent and poorly

marginated, destroying normal bony contours and extending into adjacent soft tissue. A peripheral sunburst appearance similar to that of osteosarcoma is seen in a minority of cases. A pattern of spotty or ring-like mineralization is a more specific radiologic finding. Chondrosarcoma may widen the periodontal ligament space as may occur in osteosarcoma (123). CT scans are particularly helpful in evaluating the extent of the lesion, especially in maxillary lesions where plain radiographs are difficult to evaluate because the complicated anatomy produces overlapping shadows (figs. 8-82, 8-83). MRI is a potentially valuable imaging modality because cartilaginous lesions have a low signal intensity in T1-weighted images but are very bright in T2-weighted images.

Pathologic Findings. The histogenesis of the neoplasm is still uncertain. It has been postulated to arise from embryonic cartilaginous rests such as occur in the nasopalatine duct region, from remnants of Meckel's cartilage in the mandible, or from uncommitted stem cells (120).

Grossly, the tumor has the usually translucent, grayish, lobulated appearance seen in its extragnathic counterpart. Histologically, it is composed of islands and lobules of cartilage in

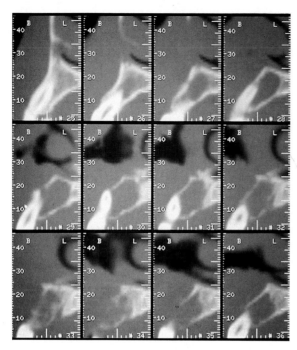

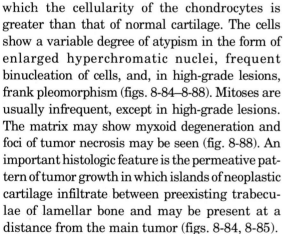

Figure 8-83
CHONDROSARCOMA
A series of sagittal CT images demonstrates the expansile and lytic nature of the lesion. In some of the cuts, the cortical plate has been violated by the neoplasm.

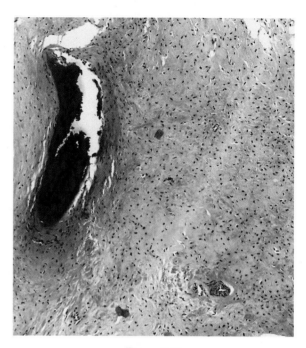

Figure 8-84
CHONDROSARCOMA
The neoplasm has entrapped an island of residual cortical bone.

which the cellularity of the chondrocytes is greater than that of normal cartilage. The cells show a variable degree of atypism in the form of enlarged hyperchromatic nuclei, frequent binucleation of cells, and, in high-grade lesions, frank pleomorphism (figs. 8-84–8-88). Mitoses are usually infrequent, except in high-grade lesions. The matrix may show myxoid degeneration and foci of tumor necrosis may be seen (fig. 8-88). An important histologic feature is the permeative pattern of tumor growth in which islands of neoplastic cartilage infiltrate between preexisting trabeculae of lamellar bone and may be present at a distance from the main tumor (figs. 8-84, 8-85).

Chondrosarcomas have been graded from 1 to 3, with the grade 1 lesions showing only minor histologic deviation from their benign counterpart and the grades 2 and 3 lesions showing readily identifiable malignant features (117). The majority of craniofacial chondrosarcomas are well differentiated and constituted 77 percent of the Mayo Clinic series (124). These low-grade lesions are notoriously difficult to differentiate on

histologic grounds from benign chondroma. The diagnosis frequently requires thorough clinico-radiologic-pathologic correlation. Factors such as the age of the patient, the presence or absence of pain, and the size and radiologic appearance of the lesion are important in this evaluation. However, benign cartilaginous lesions are so infrequent in the craniofacial bones that any cartilaginous neoplasm occurring in such a location should be considered malignant and resected in its entirety (113,118,121,124).

Differential Diagnosis. The lesion most likely to be confused with chondrosarcoma is an osteosarcoma with a prominent chondrocytic component (chondroblastic osteosarcoma) (124). Since the two lesions behave differently and have been shown to have a different prognoses, their distinction has clinical relevancy. Chondrosarcoma of the jaws tends to be more slowly growing than osteosarcoma and, unlike osteosarcoma of the jaw, seldom metastasizes. In cases treated at the Mayo Clinic, the overall 5-year survival rate for patients with gnathic osteosarcoma was 45

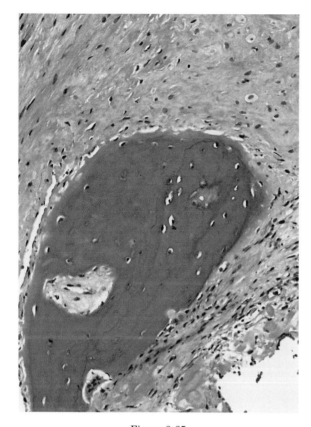

Figure 8-85
CHONDROSARCOMA
Entrapment of another island of cortical bone is seen at higher magnification.

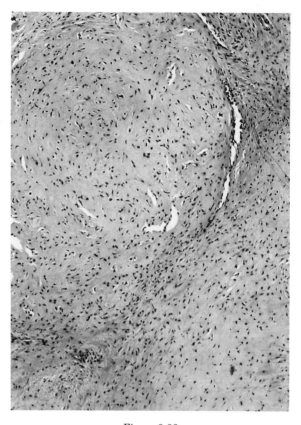

Figure 8-86
CHONDROSARCOMA
Low-power view shows the ill-defined nodular growth pattern.

percent and for chondrosarcoma, 68 percent (124). Since the osteoid component of a chondroblastic osteosarcoma may constitute a minor component of the lesion, it is important to thoroughly examine the tumor histologically and to submit at least one tissue block for each centimeter of the maximum diameter of the tumor in cases in which the osteoid component may be sparse.

Myxoma of the jaw is more uniformly myxoid in appearance and more uniform in cellularity and cytology than chondrosarcoma. A benign mixed salivary gland tumor with a prominent cartilaginous component may mimic a cartilaginous neoplasm but other elements of the neoplasm are invariably present. A chordoma may also resemble a chondrosarcoma, particularly a chondroid chondroma, but knowledge of its relation to the clivus and its midline location should point to the correct diagnosis (117).

Treatment and Prognosis. Chondrosarcoma of jaw bones tends to be slow growing and locally invasive, with little tendency to nodal or blood-borne metastasis. As a consequence of the difficulty in completely excising the lesion, there is a significant incidence of local recurrence, and death usually results from invasion of local vital structures. Although most tumors are of low histologic grade, the recurrent lesion may progress to a higher grade. Factors that have been described to influence prognosis include histologic differentiation, the location of the lesion, and the size of the lesion although none of these factors was of statistical significance in the large Mayo Clinic series (117,124).

The only effective therapy to date has been radical surgical ablation. In the mandible, this requires removal of the grossly visible tumor with a 2 to 3 cm margin, and in the maxilla, a radical maxillectomy. Radiotherapy and chemotherapy have proven to be of little value.

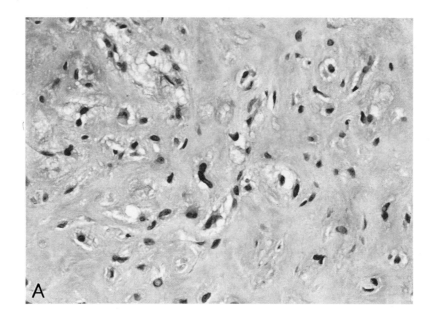

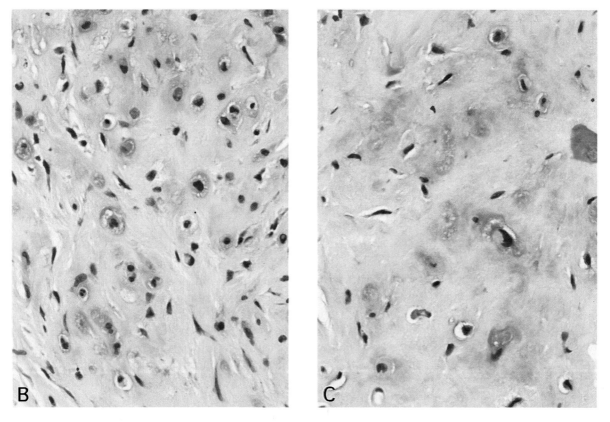

Figure 8-87
CHONDROSARCOMA

The chondrosarcoma exhibits a moderate degree of cellularity and a moderate degree of cellular pleomorphism. Nuclear hyperchromasia, multilobulation, and scattered binucleate cells are readily identifiable. Mitotic figures were not observed. This would constitute a moderately differentiated (grade 2) chondrosarcoma.

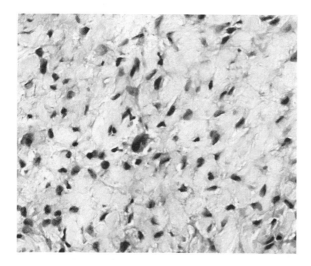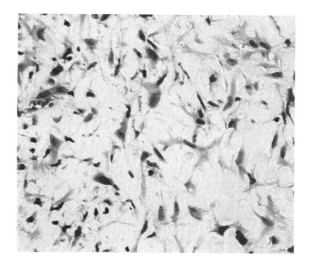

Figure 8-88
CHONDROSARCOMA
Areas of the neoplasm have a myxoid appearance. The stellate chondrocytes exhibit distinct nuclear hyperchromasia and atypism.

The overall 5-year survival rate varies from 40 to 60 percent (117). In a subset of patients treated at the Mayo Clinic, the 5-, 10-, and 15-year survival rates were 68, 54, and 44 percent, respectively (124).

Special Variants of Chondrosarcoma. Some chondrosarcoma variants such as *clear cell chondrosarcoma* and *dedifferentiated chondrosarcoma* in the jaw are so rare as to be medical curiosities (125). However, *mesenchymal chondrosarcoma* is a highly distinctive histologic variant that has a predilection for involving the jaw bones and ribs (115). By 1993, over 40 cases had been documented (126). Most patients are in the second and third decades of life, with a mean age of 27 years; the sex incidence is equal. The maxilla and mandible are nearly equally affected. The clinical and radiologic features are similar to those for chondrosarcoma of the usual type. Histologically, the tumor is composed of monotonous cells with spindle-shaped to ovoid nuclei arranged around endothelial-lined vascular spaces in a hemangiopericytomatous pattern. In fact, if the diagnostic element of the lesion is inconspicuous or even absent, as it may be in a biopsy specimen, a misdiagnosis of hemangiopericytoma may be rendered. The diagnostic feature of mesenchymal chondrosarcoma is the presence of multiple small foci of chondroid differentiation within the cellular lesion. There is usually a fairly abrupt transition from the cellular component to the cartilaginous islands.

As discussed, differential diagnosis includes hemangiopericytoma as well as monophasic synovial sarcoma. However, the multiple foci of chondroid differentiation are so distinctive that the lesion is usually instantly recognized.

The neoplasm is much more aggressive than chondrosarcoma of the standard variety. One third to half of reported cases exhibit both local recurrence and distant metastases (114,115). These adverse outcomes may be long delayed so that long-term follow-up is required.

The mainstay of therapy is radical surgical ablation. In contrast to chondrosarcoma, there has been a response to radiation and chemotherapy in mesenchymal chondrosarcoma.

FIBROUS LESIONS

Desmoplastic Fibroma

Definition. Desmoplastic fibroma is the osseous counterpart of soft tissue fibromatosis (desmoid) (134). It is composed of bland fibrocytic type cells and a collagenous matrix, grows in an infiltrative fashion, and has a significant propensity for local recurrence but no metastatic potential.

Historical Features. The entity was first reported by Jaffe in 1958 (132). Griffith and Irby (131) described the first case involving jaw bones in 1965. To date, only about 60 cases involving the jaw have been documented. The rarity of this lesion is illustrated by Dahlin and Unni (129), who have only 9 documented cases of desmoplastic fibroma among the 8,542 primary bone tumors in the files of the Mayo Clinic; 2 of these 9 cases involved the mandible. Nine cases were reported by Vally et al. (137) from the University of Witwatersrand.

Clinical Features. Except for a few cases of maxillary involvement, the gnathic lesions have occurred in the mandible. The right side is involved twice as often as the left. The tumor most frequently occurs in the posterior region of the body, at the angle and adjacent ramus (130). There is an almost equal sex incidence and most cases manifest during the first three decades of life; the mean age at presentation is about 15 years (130). The usual presentation is that of swelling and facial deformity in the affected region without pain (fig. 8-89). Extension beyond the confines of the bone into adjacent skeletal muscle is seen in 42 percent of cases at the time of surgery and may induce trismus (130).

Radiologic Findings. The affected bone shows a fairly well-circumscribed, radiolucent defect with a unilocular or multilocular configuration (fig. 8-90) (128). Less commonly, the lesion is poorly marginated. There may be expansion of the bone. The cortical plate frequently shows foci of disruption as a result of extension of the process beyond the confines of the bone: at the time of surgery, as many as 77 percent of lesions had eroded the cortical plate (130). The roots of the teeth may be eroded (fig. 8-90). Early lesions may present as a periapical radiolucency which mimics periapical osteitis (136). The above described radiologic

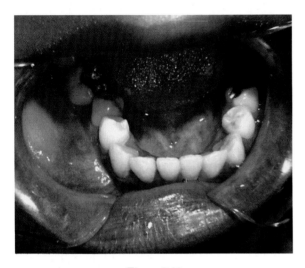

Figure 8-89
DESMOPLASTIC FIBROMA
The lesion expands the buccal plate of the left mandible in the region of canine and premolar teeth. (Figure 1 from Freedman PD, Cardo VA, Kerpel SM, Lumerman H. Desmoplastic fibroma (fibromatosis) of the jawbones. Oral Surg Oral Med Oral Path 1978;46:386-95.)

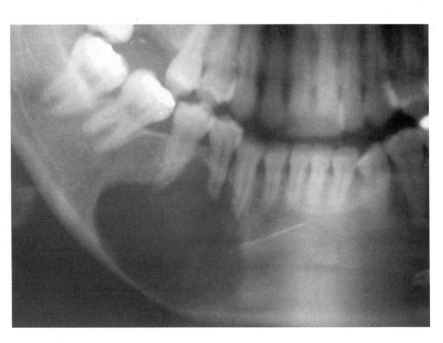

Figure 8-90
DESMOPLASTIC FIBROMA
A well-defined radiolucent lesion in the body of the mandible has caused root resorption of canine and premolar teeth. (Fig. 2 from Freedman PD, Cardo VA, Kerpel SM, Lumerman H. Desmoplastic fibroma (fibromatosis) of the jawbones. Oral Surg Oral Med Oral Path 1978;46:386-95.)

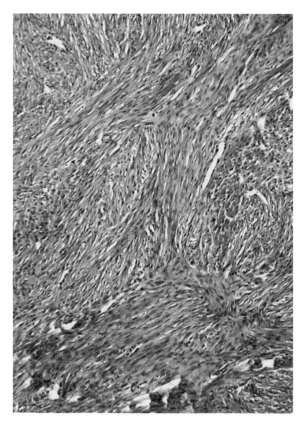

Figure 8-91
DESMOPLASTIC FIBROMA
The neoplasm is composed of fascicles of spindle-shaped fibroblasts and collagen fibers. (Fig. 3 from Freedman PD, Cardo VA, Kerpel SM, Lumerman H. Desmoplastic fibroma (fibromatosis) of the jawbones. Oral Surg Oral Med Oral Path 1978;46:386-95.)

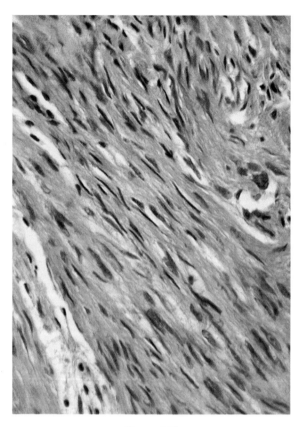

Figure 8-92
DESMOPLASTIC FIBROMA
Detail of uniformly distributed, elongated and spindle-shaped bland nuclei of fibroblastic cells separated by abundant collagen fibers. (Courtesy of Dr. S. Kerpel, New York, NY.)

features are not specific and a similar pattern could result from an ameloblastoma, odontogenic cyst, eosinophilic granuloma, fibro-osseous lesion, aneurysmal bone cyst, odontogenic myxoma, chondromyxoid fibroma, and hemangioma (135).

Pathologic Findings. The gross appearance is that of a rubbery, firm, whitish mass that appears to be well circumscribed. Histologically, the lesion is composed of extremely uniform fibrocytic cells evenly distributed in a collagen-rich matrix (fig. 8-91); the nuclei are ovoid to spindle shaped. Mitoses are absent or sparse and are never abnormal. The degree of cellularity may vary from one lesion to another and even within the same lesion but is generally minimal (figs. 8-92, 8-93).

Although the lesion appears grossly to be well circumscribed, histologically it is not encapsu-

lated. Tongues of tumor extend into surrounding bone and marrow tissue. Lesions that have penetrated cortical bone grow in a prong-like manner into adjacent soft tissue, including skeletal muscle, entrapping atrophic fibers. This appearance is identical to that seen in extragnathic fibromatosis and accounts for the view that desmoplastic fibroma represents the skeletal counterpart of that lesion. Ultrastructurally, the fibrocytic cells show features of myofibroblasts, namely, peripherally located cytoplasmic filament bundles with zones of condensation as seen in smooth muscle cells and a centrally located racemose network of rough endoplasmic reticulum.

Differential Diagnosis. The most difficult entity in the differential diagnosis is low-grade fibrosarcoma. Low-grade fibrosarcoma is somewhat more cellular, shows less uniformity of the fibrocytic nuclei, has more frequent mitoses, and

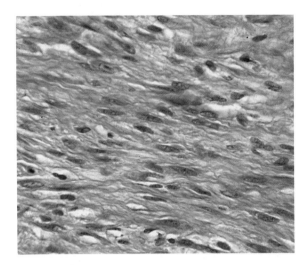

Figure 8-93
DESMOPLASTIC FIBROMA
The fibroblast nuclei contain finely granular and evenly distributed chromatin and a small single nucleolus. The nuclei are evenly dispersed between the collagenous matrix. (Fig. 6 from Freedman PD, Cardo VA, Kerpel SM, Lumerman H. Desmoplastic fibroma (fibromatosis) of the jawbones. Oral Surg Oral Med Oral Path 1978;46:386-95.)

tends to have a pushing border rather than the stellate infiltrating pattern seen in desmoplastic fibroma. The difficulty is compounded in infants and young children since fibromatosis tends to be more cellular and more mitotically active in this group than in adult patients. Infantile myofibromatosis is more cellular and also more mitotically active than desmoplastic fibroma.

There is usually no histologic problem in distinguishing desmoplastic fibroma from other gnathic lesions with a prominent fibrocytic component. The intimate admixture of woven bone spicules clearly identifies the fibro-osseous lesions, fibrous dysplasia and ossifying fibroma. In low-grade central osteosarcoma, as in low-grade fibrosarcoma, the fibrocytic component may closely resemble desmoplastic fibroma. However, the production of neoplastic woven bone, especially if laid down in apposition to preexisting, partially resorbed or necrotic fragments of invaded lamellar bone, helps establish a diagnosis of osteosarcoma. The heterogenous appearance of giant cell granuloma, with clustering of osteoclast type giant cells and deposition of hemosiderin, should readily distinguish it from desmoplastic fibroma. As the radiologic appearance is nonspecific, diagnostic problems may be

encountered when the biopsy is so small that it is difficult to conclude that the fibrocytic process resembling a desmoplastic fibroma is indeed representative of the entire lesion. In such cases, it is prudent to recommend a more liberal biopsy before embarking on definitive therapy.

Treatment and Prognosis. The rate of local recurrence has variously been reported as between 24 and 30 percent (133,135). No case of metastatic disease has been documented. The recurrence rate is higher when the lesion has been simply curetted and when it extended into soft tissue. It has also been suggested that there is a higher recurrence rate in more cellular lesions (133). A variety of therapeutic modalities have been proposed. There is universal agreement that complete resection of the lesion with a margin of normal bone achieves the highest cure rate (135). Such therapy often requires a hemimandibulectomy. However, for smaller and better circumscribed lesions, a more conservative approach seems justified. A thorough curettage or curettage with cryotherapy or marginal osteotomy using a bone burr achieves a high cure rate (127). A more extensive resection can be reserved for cases which recur following curettage. When the lesion has already extended into soft tissue, a radical resection is required. It is recommended that the surgeon attempt to obtain a 2 cm clear margin of resection within the soft tissue. The adequacy of the resection margin can be monitored by multiple frozen sections (133). As the lesion is slow growing, no patient should be considered cured unless they are recurrence free for a minimum of 3 years.

Fibrosarcoma

Definition. This malignant mesenchymal neoplasm of jaw bones resembles its soft tissue counterpart and is composed of malignant fibrocytic cells growing in a fascicular or "herringbone" pattern. It is an extremely rare neoplasm and can be broadly categorized into *ameloblastic* and *nonameloblastic types.*

Incidence. Fibrosarcoma of the jaws occurs over a wide age spectrum but is most common in the third decade (148). Rare cases have been reported in children (138,140). The sex incidence has been reported to be equal or to exhibit a male predominance (144,148). In the few reported series

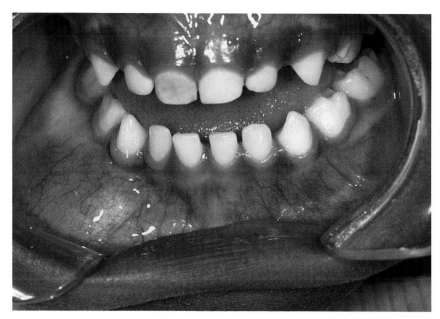

Figure 8-94
FIBROSARCOMA
The fibrosarcoma caused swelling of body of the right side of mandible. (Figures 8-94 and 8-95 are from the same patient.)

of cases, 8 to 14 percent of all osseous fibrosarcomas have involved the jaw bones (141,144, 148). The mandible is involved more frequently than the maxilla.

Clinical Features. Patients present most often with pain, swelling, or a combination of both in the affected jaw bone (fig. 8-94). Other symptoms and signs include paresthesias, trismus, facial deformity, pathologic fracture, loosening of teeth, and orbital displacement with proptosis. Although most fibrosarcomas arise ab-initio, there are reports of development of fibrosarcoma in association with ameloblastic fibroma, myxoma, and Paget's disease, and following radiation therapy for fibrous dysplasia and retinoblastoma (142,145,147,149).

Radiologic Findings. The radiologic features are generally those of an ill-defined radiolucent process, with a "moth-eaten" appearance; the cortical margins may or may not be violated. In later stages, there may be an associated soft tissue component, in which case it may be impossible to determine whether the neoplasm is of osseous or soft tissue origin (fig. 8-95). There may be erosion of the roots of teeth. Less commonly, the lesion appears as a more circumscribed lytic process and mimics a benign lesion. The lytic features described above are nonspecific and can be produced by any number of malignant lesions affecting the jaw bones.

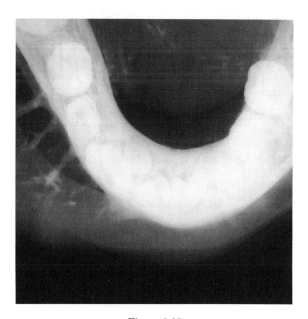

Figure 8-95
FIBROSARCOMA
This fibrosarcoma caused a soft tissue swelling in a juxta-cortical location. There is an associated periosteal reaction.

Pathologic Findings. The precise cell of origin of fibrosarcoma within jaw bones is obscure. In cases of ameloblastic fibrosarcoma, the histogenesis is related to odontogenic mesenchyme. In such lesions, cords or islands of odontogenic epithelium are embedded within the fibrosarcomatous

213

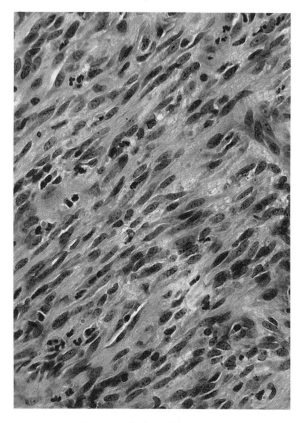

Figure 8-96
FIBROSARCOMA
The cellular neoplasm is composed of uniform spindle-shaped fibroblasts in a fascicular arrangement.

element. The ameloblastic fibrosarcoma may arise de novo or evolve from a preexisting ameloblastic fibroma or an ameloblastic fibro-odontoma (146).

Histologically, fibrosarcoma of the jaw is identical to its soft tissue counterpart and is usually comprised of a uniformly cellular population of spindle-shaped cells arranged in a fascicular or "herringbone" pattern, with a variable amount of collagen production (fig. 8-96). Parts or all of the lesion may be more myxoid in appearance and such lesions have been labeled *myxofibrosarcomas*. Lesions with greater cytologic pleomorphism and a storiform pattern resemble soft tissue malignant fibrous histiocytomas but have been included within the fibrosarcoma group because of their small number and identical behavior to fibrosarcoma.

Fibrosarcoma is distinguished from osseous fibromatosis (desmoplastic fibroma) by the presence of readily identifiable mitoses in the former and their extreme paucity or absence in the latter. Minimal cellularity and a uniform cellular distribution, associated with an abundant collagenous matrix, favors a diagnosis of desmoplastic fibroma. In some instances it may be difficult to distinguish desmoplastic fibroma from low-grade fibrosarcoma, in which case it is advisable to aim for complete eradication of the lesion.

Figure 8-97
MYOFIBROMA
OF MANDIBLE

A mass in the right medial retromolar region in a young girl displaced the tongue. (Figures 8-97, 8-98, and 8-100–8-104 are from the same patient.)

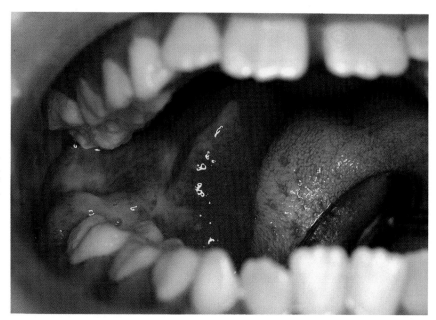

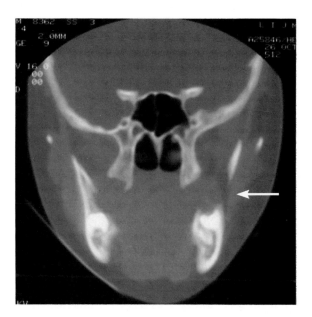

Figure 8-98
MYOFIBROMA OF MANDIBLE
The mass has eroded the medial plate of the left body of the mandible.

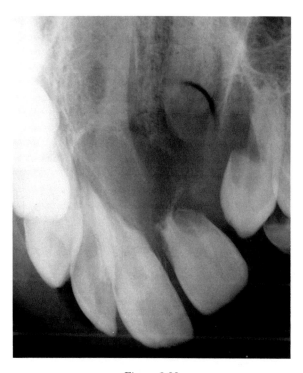

Figure 8-99
MYOFIBROMA OF MAXILLA
The lesion has produced a defect in the anterior maxilla and eroded the roots of incisor teeth.

Treatment and Prognosis. The only effective therapy for fibrosarcoma is radical surgery. There is a high incidence of local recurrence and blood-borne metastases to the lungs; lymph node dissemination is not a feature. For this reason, a cervical lymph node dissection is not part of the standard therapeutic regimen. Radiotherapy and chemotherapy have not proven to be effective measures. The 5-year survival rate in three reported series of patients with gnathic fibrosarcoma was 71 percent, 40 percent, and 27 percent (138,139,148); these figures are higher than the reported 5-year survival rate of 25 to 34 percent for extragnathic fibrosarcomas in bone (148). In a series from Memorial Sloan Kettering Hospital, this improved survival rate for patients with fibrosarcoma of jaw bones was not observed at the 5-year follow-up but was noted at 10 years (27 versus 17 percent survival rate) (143). The better survival rate for patients with gnathic fibrosarcoma has been attributed to histologically lower grade lesions. Ameloblastic fibrosarcomas have a much better prognosis; although local recurrence is common, metastases are rare (146).

Myofibroma (Infantile Myofibromatosis)

Definition. Myofibroma is a benign tumor composed of fibroblasts and myofibroblasts, occurring most commonly as a solitary lesion of soft tissue, skin, or bone in infancy. A less frequent multicentric form involving viscera and skeleton has a more guarded prognosis.

Clinical Features. Nearly 80 percent occur in children of less than 2 years of age (150). In a review of over 900 soft tissue tumors occurring before the age of 20 years, Coffin and Dehner (151) found that myofibroma constituted the largest group (22 percent). The tumor occurs with greatest frequency in the head and neck region, followed by the skin of the trunk. The mandible is the bone most commonly involved. In a series of 24 myofibromas involving the head and neck region in a pediatric age group, Sugatani et al. (152) documented involvement of the mandible in 15 of these cases (62.5 percent) (fig. 8-97). Radiologically, the lesions are well circumscribed (figs. 8-98, 8-99).

215

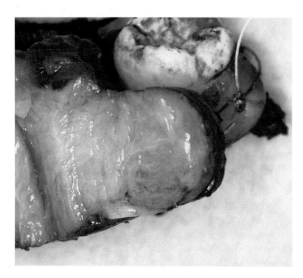

Figure 8-100
MYOFIBROMA OF MANDIBLE
Gross specimen shows a whorled, pale, cut surface and resected molar tooth.

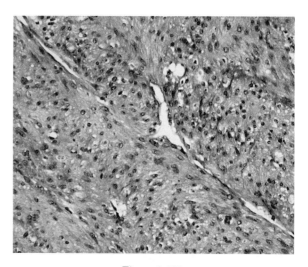

Figure 8-102
MYOFIBROMA OF MANDIBLE
The fascicular pattern, uniformity, and moderate degree of cellularity are shown at higher magnification.

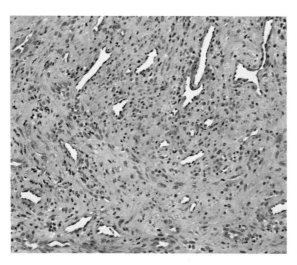

Figure 8-101
MYOFIBROMA OF MANDIBLE
Uniformly distributed spindle-shaped cells. The lesion is of moderate cellularity and contains branching endothelial-lined vascular channels imparting a hemangiopericytomatous appearance.

Pathologic Findings. The lesion presents as a circumscribed nodule composed of fascicles of spindle-shaped cells with fibroblastic and myofibroblastic features (figs. 8-100–8-102). Focally, a hemangiopericytomatous pattern may be present as well as foci of necrosis (figs. 8-101, 8-102). Mitotic figures may be seen but there is no

cellular pleomorphism (fig. 8-103). Immunohistochemically, the cells are decorated by antibodies to vimentin and alpha-smooth muscle actin; their fibroblastic and myofibroblastic features can also be demonstrated ultrastructurally (fig. 8-104).

Treatment and Prognosis. The solitary lesions always behave in a benign fashion and are cured by curettage or simple excision. If the lesion is a component of systemic multifocal disease with visceral involvement, the prognosis is guarded.

HEMATOPOIETIC, LYMPHOID, AND HISTIOCYTIC LESIONS

Langerhans' Cell Histiocytosis

Definition. Langerhans' cell histiocytosis is an idiopathic disorder considered to be reactive in type and involving the skeletal system and visceral organs. Lesions within bone are monostotic or polyostotic. Although the entities separately described as *eosinophilic granuloma, Hand-Schuller-Christian disease,* and *Letterer-Siwe disease* are histologically similar and hence grouped together under the rubric "histiocytosis X," they are clinically distinctive with no evidence of progression from one to another. Eosinophilic granuloma and Hand-Schuller-Christian disease exhibit an indolent course whereas Letterer-Siwe disease is disseminated and may pursue an aggressive fatal

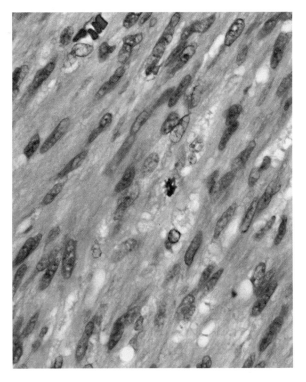

Figure 8-103
MYOFIBROMA OF MANDIBLE
Myofibroblasts have lightly basophilic cytoplasmic cell processes and are separated by collagenous matrix. Note the occasional mitotic figures.

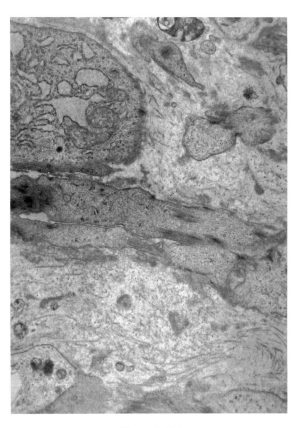

Figure 8-104
MYOFIBROMA OF MANDIBLE
Electron photomicrograph demonstrates racemose profiles of rough endoplasmic reticulum and filament bundles with zones of condensation in a subplasmalemmal location.

course in infancy. The above tumors are used as synonyms for Langerhans' cell histiocytosis.

Jaw Involvement. The jaw bones are a common site of involvement, with mandibular lesions being more common than maxillary ones (figs. 8-105–8-107). Only a few cases have been reported with condylar involvement. Hartman (154) documented oral involvement in 114 of 1,120 cases of Langerhans' cell histiocytosis (10.2 percent): the mandible was involved in 73 percent, with the posterior region the predominant site. Other frequent sites of bony involvement include ribs, shoulder girdle, and skull. Males are affected twice as frequently as females and most patients are in the second and third decades of life (153).

Clinically, the patients present with pain, swelling, or loosening of teeth. Radiologically, the features are fairly nonspecific although the lytic lesions may affect alveolar supporting tissue resulting in the appearance of "floating teeth" (153,155).

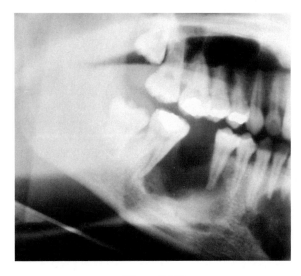

Figure 8-105
LANGERHANS' CELL HISTIOCYTOSIS
Two fairly well-marginated radiolucent lesions in the body of the mandible of a 16-year-old boy.

217

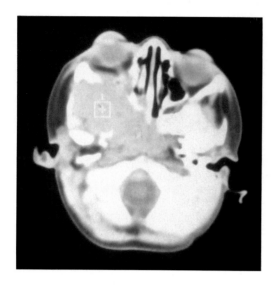

Figure 8-106
LANGERHANS' CELL HISTIOCYTOSIS
This 1-year-old boy presented with swelling of the infratemporal fossa. The axial CT scan shows involvement of the right maxilla with extension into the posterior orbit, posterior nasal cavity, and prevertebral space. (Figures 8-106–8-113 are from the same patient.)

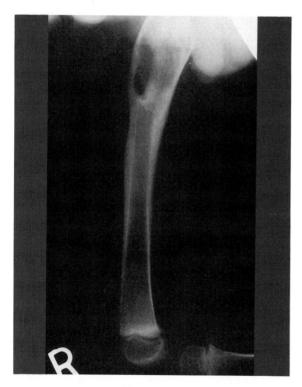

Figure 8-107
LANGERHANS' CELL HISTIOCYTOSIS
About 1 year later the child depicted in figure 8-106 developed this well-defined radiolucent lesion in the metaphysis of the right femur.

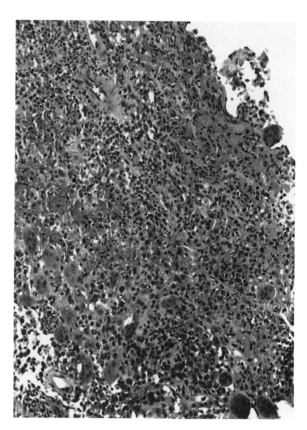

Figure 8-108
LANGERHANS' CELL HISTIOCYTOSIS
Biopsy from the maxillary lesion shows a mixed "inflammatory" cell infiltrate including numerous osteoclast type giant cells.

Pathologic Findings. Histologically, the appearance is usually distinctive. There are sheets of uniform, uninucleate and some multinucleate, benign-looking histiocytic cells (figs. 8-108–8-111). A helpful diagnostic feature is the presence of nuclear indentation producing a reniform or "coffee bean" appearance (figs. 8-110, 8-111). The cells are usually accompanied by numerous eosinophils and smaller numbers of other inflammatory cell types. Secondary infection following ulceration may result in the appearance of a nonspecific inflammatory process with necrosis which may mask and render difficult the diagnosis of the underlying lesion (figs. 8-108, 8-109).

A number of special procedures are helpful in firmly establishing a diagnosis. Immunohistochemistry shows the histiocytic cells to be decorated by antibody to S-100 protein. If fresh tissue is available and frozen sections prepared, the

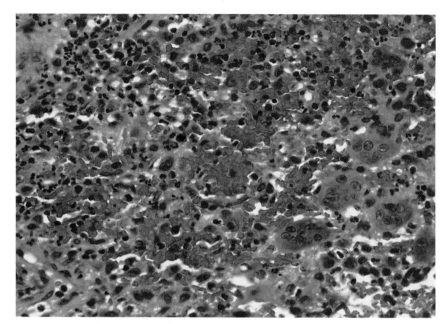

Figure 8-109
LANGERHANS' CELL
HISTIOCYTOSIS
This higher magnification of figure 8-108 shows a mixed inflammatory cell infiltrate including numerous neutrophils, histiocytes, and osteoclast type giant cells. The infiltrate might suggest an acute inflammatory lesion.

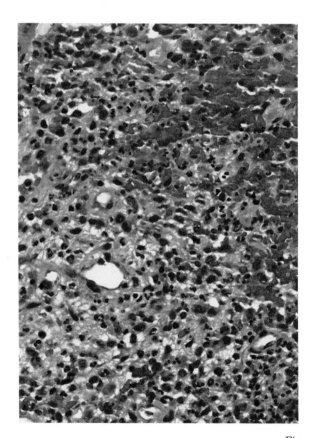

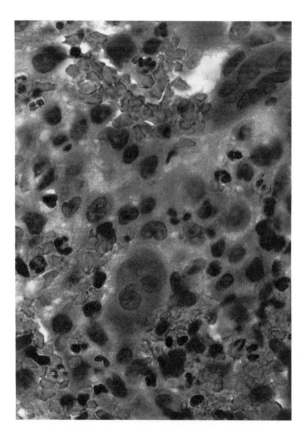

Figure 8-110
LANGERHANS' CELL HISTIOCYTOSIS
Left: In this field mononuclear histiocytes predominate and some of the nuclei have a reniform configuration. In addition to neutrophils, a few eosinophils are seen.
Right: High-power view demonstrates a deep nuclear cleft in the mononuclear histiocytes, producing the reniform shape.

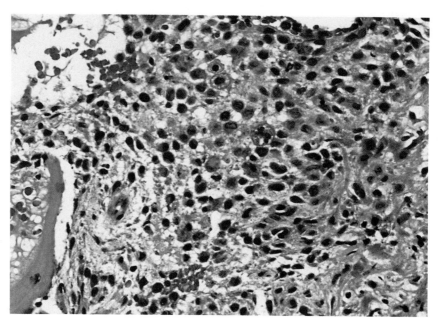

Figure 8-111
LANGERHANS' CELL
HISTIOCYTOSIS
Lesional tissue from the femoral lesion shown in figure 8-107. Sheets of mononuclear histiocytic cells with reniform nuclei are shown.

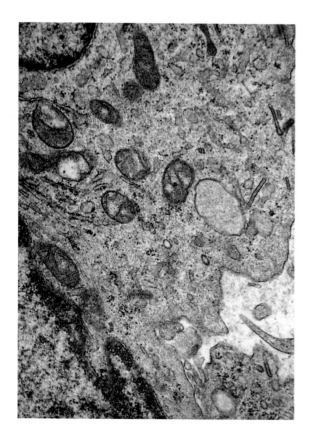

Figure 8-112
LANGERHANS' CELL HISTIOCYTOSIS
Electron photomicrograph of cells from the maxillary lesion shows numerous intracytoplasmic Birbeck granules.

histiocytes can be stained for the antigen CD1a (T6). Electron microscopy remains a helpful diagnostic tool. The histiocytic cells contain distinctive granules, Birbeck granules, seen in no other condition. They have a trilaminate structure with one bulbous end, resembling a racket, and can be seen to originate from the plasma membrane (figs. 8-112, 8-113).

Treatment. Langerhans' cell histiocytosis is best treated by simple curettage, although low-dose radiotherapy can be utilized for lesions in surgically inaccessible regions. Chemotherapy should be reserved for the aggressive disseminated lesions of infantile Letterer-Siwe disease (153).

Myeloma

Definition. Myeloma is a neoplastic proliferation of plasma cells usually involving the red bone marrow of the axial skeleton and frequently associated with the production of a monoclonal paraprotein (fig. 8-114). Involvement of the jaw bones may be a primary manifestation of the disease but more commonly is part of systemic skeletal involvement. For a more detailed discussion of plasma cell dyscrasias and related disorders, the reader is referred to the third series, Atlas of Tumor Pathology text, Tumors of the Bone Marrow, by Brunning and McKenna (156).

Clinical Features. The jaw bones are involved in 5 to 30 percent of cases of multiple

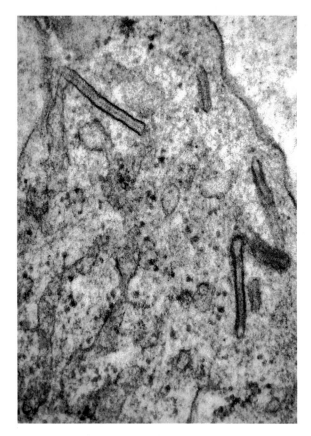

Figure 8-113
LANGERHANS' CELL HISTIOCYTOSIS
Detail of a Birbeck granule shows a trilaminar structure
and drumstick-shaped extremity.

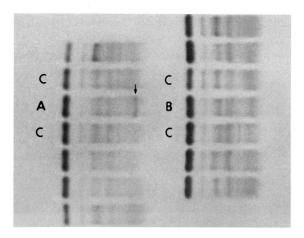

Figure 8-114
SOLITARY MYELOMA
Serum electrophoretogram shows a monoclonal band
(arrow) in patient's serum preoperatively (A) which disap-
peared following excision of the lesion (B). Control sera (C).
(Fig. 2 from Lipper S, Kahn LB, Heselson NG. Localized
myeloma with osteogenesis and Russell body formation. S
Afr Med J 1975;49:2041-5.) (Figures 8-114, 8-117, 8-118,
8-120, and 8-121 are from the same patient.)

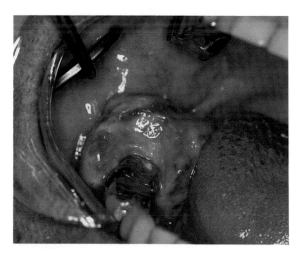

Figure 8-115
MULTIPLE MYELOMA INVOLVING MANDIBLE
A mucosal-covered mass involves left retromolar trigone
region.

myeloma as compared to 45 percent for skull
bones (159). Nearly all jaw lesions involve the
mandible, with only isolated cases reported in
the maxilla (157,164). The jaw bones have been
documented as the presenting location of the
disease in 12 to 15 percent of cases. In a review
of 18 cases of oral and maxillofacial manifestations of myeloma from three hospitals in Barce-
lona, jaw involvement was the first sign of the
disease in 13 (72 percent), with the mandible
involved in 10 cases and the maxilla in 8 (160).
Myelomatous involvement of jaw bones was the
first manifestation of the disease in 6 of 13 patients reported by Pisano et al. (162). Solitary
myeloma of the skeletal system occurs in 3 to 7
percent of all cases of myeloma but is exceedingly
rare in the jaw (166): 1 of 46 cases of myeloma of
the jaw bones from the Mayo Clinic was of solitary type (158).

Myeloma usually manifests between the ages
of 50 and 70 years. In the jaw symptoms and
signs include swelling, toothache, loosening or
loss of vitality of teeth, pain, paresthesia of lips,
excessive postextraction hemorrhage, and
rarely, pathologic fracture (fig. 8-115) (160).

Radiologic Findings. Radiologically, the typical feature is that of single or multiple, lytic "punched-out" lesions, occurring most frequently in the angle and molar-premolar region where the bulk of the red bone marrow resides (fig. 8-116) (161). However, any part of the mandible may be involved including the condylar process (160). Punched-out lesions occurring in the apical regions may be misconstrued as periapical inflammatory disease. Other radiologic features include generalized rarefaction and, rarely, an osteoblastic appearance with surface "sun-ray" spiculation (figs. 8-117, 8-118) (163).

Pathologic Findings. The histopathologic features are identical to those seen in the extragnathic skeleton and include the presence of sheets of plasma cells showing mild to severe cytologic atypism, with some binucleate forms (figs. 8-119–8-121). Well-differentiated lesions in which the degree of cellular atypia is minimal need to be differentiated from inflammatory lesions with a predominant plasma cell population. In the oral cavity, gingivitis, periodontitis, and periapical "granulomas" may contain sheets of plasma cells. The intensity of the inflammation may even induce some reactive atypia, including binucleate forms, within the plasma cell infiltrate. However, the lesional tissue always includes other inflammatory cell types, notably lymphocytes, macrophages, and neutrophils. Intracytoplasmic Russell bodies are usually readily identifiable

within the reactive plasma cells although they may occasionally be seen within neoplastic plasma cells (fig. 8-121). In cases in which histologic distinction between these entities is difficult, correlation with clinical and radiologic features is helpful. The immunohistochemical demonstration of clonal light chain restriction in

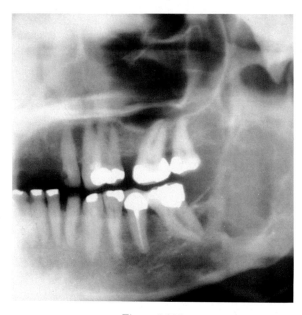

Figure 8-116
MULTIPLE MYELOMA INVOLVING MANDIBLE
Extensive osteolytic destruction of both body and ramus of mandible.

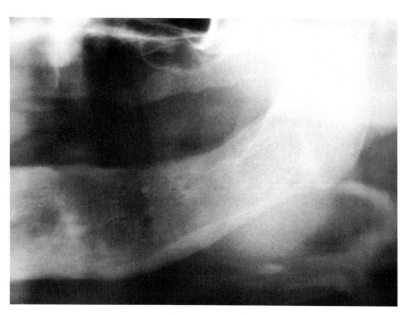

Figure 8-117
SOLITARY MYELOMA
Unusual osteoblastic "sun-ray" surface spiculation of myeloma involving angle of mandible. (Fig. 1 from Lipper S, Kahn LB, Heselson NG. Localized myeloma with osteogenesis and Russell body formation. S Afr Med J 1975;49:2041-5.)

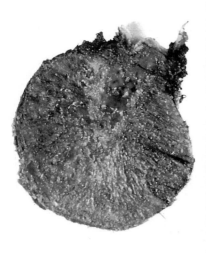

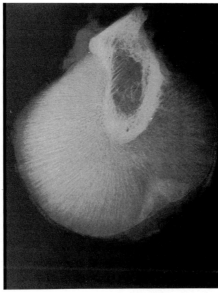

Figure 8-118
SOLITARY MYELOMA
Gross (left) and specimen radiograph (right) of cut surface of specimen demonstrating prominent "sunray" spiculation radiating from the surface of the bone. (Fig. 4 from Lipper S, Kahn LB, Heselson NG. Localized myeloma with osteogenesis and Russell body formation. S Afr Med J 1975;49:2041-5.)

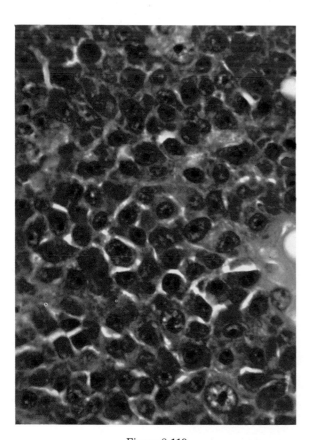

Figure 8-119
MULTIPLE MYELOMA INVOLVING MANDIBLE
These immature plasmablasts have prominent nucleoli, eccentric nuclei, paranuclear Golgi "hof," and lilac-colored cytoplasm.

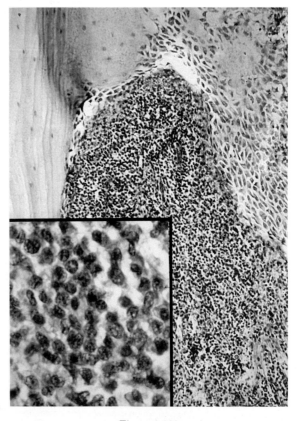

Figure 8-120
SOLITARY MYELOMA
Sheets of neoplastic cells are surrounded by lamellar bone and osteoblasts (top). Inset shows detail of neoplastic plasma cells. (Fig. 5 from Lipper S, Kahn LB, Heselson NG. Localized myeloma with osteogenesis and Russell body formation. S Afr Med J 1975;49:2041-5.)

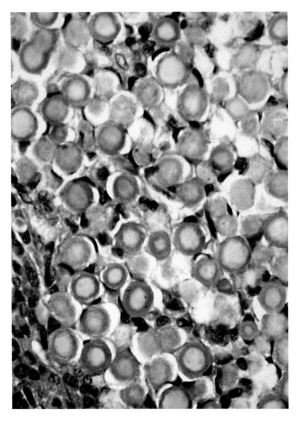

Figure 8-121
SOLITARY MYELOMA
Profusion of intracytoplasmic Russell bodies. (Fig. 6 from Lipper S, Kahn LB, Heselson NG. Localized myeloma with osteogenesis and Russell body formation. S Afr Med J 1975;49:2041-5.)

paraffin-embedded tissue can be used to establish a diagnosis of myeloma.

Deposition of amyloid may be seen in association with the myelomatous infiltrate. Amyloid deposition may also occur in the absence of any overt evidence of myeloma (165). In the oral and maxillofacial regions, amyloid deposition occurs most frequently in the tongue (macroglossia), the buccal mucosa and gingiva (nodules and plaques), and the salivary gland (xerostomia) (167).

Treatment and Prognosis. The prognosis and therapy for jaw myeloma as a manifestation of multiple myeloma is identical to that of myeloma elsewhere in the skeleton. Solitary myeloma has a more indolent course although most patients eventually progress to the systemic form of the disease.

Leukemia and Lymphoma

Leukemia. Apart from gingival hypertrophy (fig. 8-122), involvement of the jaw bones as a manifestation of leukemia is uncommon. There are reports of relapse manifesting as isolated jaw involvement (180,185). Radiologically, jaw involvement by leukemia causes osteolysis. The lesion is poorly circumscribed and there may be associated loss of lamina dura and widening of the periodontal ligament space (172,173). Leukemias that involve the jaw include acute lymphoblastic and myeloblastic types. Jaw involvement in acute or

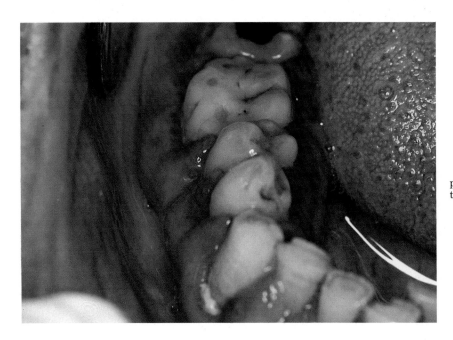

Figure 8-122
LEUKEMIC INFILTRATION OF GINGIVA
Prominent gingival hypertrophy is produced by leukemic infiltration of the soft tissue.

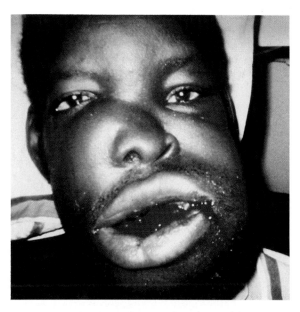

Figure 8-123
BURKITT'S LYMPHOMA
Involvement of all four quadrants of the jaw in a 28-year-old black male. (Courtesy of Dr. H. Coleman, Johannesburg, South Africa.)

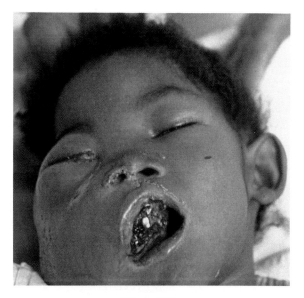

Figure 8-124
BURKITT'S LYMPHOMA
Involvement of right maxilla and mandible in a black child. (Courtesy of Dr. J. Posen, Johannesburg, South Africa.)

chronic myeloid leukemia (chloroma) may precede the diagnosis of bone marrow and peripheral blood involvement or these sites of involvement may be diagnosed synchronously (168,171).

Diagnosing acute myeloid leukemia involving a jaw bone may be difficult since the infiltrate closely resembles other large cell malignant lymphoproliferative disorders. Leukemia should be suspected if any eosinophil precursor leukocytes can be identified within the lesion, or when the cells in a suspected neoplastic lymphoproliferative process fail to stain immunohistochemically for the usual battery of pan-B and pan-T cell markers. A useful confirmatory histochemical stain is the identification of chloroacetate esterase (Leder stain) although primitive myeloid cells may not contain the enzyme. A Leder stain is considered positive even if only a small number of the immature cells are reactive. The presence of stained mature non-neoplastic neutrophils within the infiltrate should not be misconstrued as a positive test and this finding serves as a useful internal control for the Leder stain. Electron microscopy may demonstrate leukocytic granules. If lesional tissue is available for flow cytometry, antigen CD43 positivity is an invaluable confirmatory finding.

Non-Hodgkin's Lymphoma. With the exception of Burkitt's lymphoma, jaw involvement by non-Hodgkin's lymphoma is uncommon. Non-Hodgkin's lymphoma of bone comprised 3.4 to 5.0 percent of all primary bone neoplasms; about 100 cases have been reported in jaw bones (178). Burkitt's lymphoma is endemic in tropical and East Africa and frequently manifests in children before the age of 10 years. All four quadrants of the jaw are involved. The jaw bones are reported to be involved in up to 60 percent of endemic cases (figs. 8-123–8-129) and 20 percent of sporadic nonendemic cases (American type), which occur in a slightly older age (185). Ninety-two of 98 children with lymphoma diagnosed over a recent 7-year period in northeastern Brazil had Burkitt's lymphoma but only 3 presented with a jaw mass (181).

Other non-Hodgkin lymphomas that involve the jaw are usually of diffuse large cell type (figs. 8-130–8-133). They involve the maxilla more frequently than the mandible possibly because of origin from lymphoid tissue of the mucosal lining of the maxillary sinus (169). In the largest series of mandibular lymphomas published, 15 of 17 were of B cell immunophenotype (177).

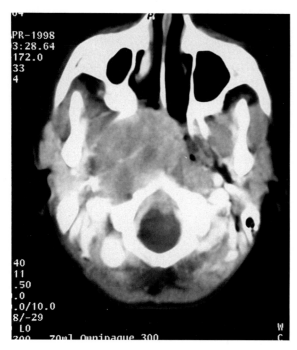

Figure 8-125
BURKITT'S LYMPHOMA

An axial CT scan shows a large prevertebral and naso-pharyngeal mass causing destruction of the pterygoid plate. (Courtesy of Dr. J. Posen, Johannesburg, South Africa.) (Figures 8-125 and 8-126 are from the same patient.)

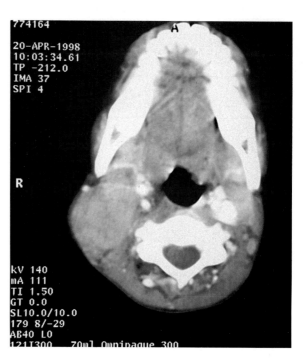

Figure 8-126
BURKITT'S LYMPHOMA

Axial CT scan shows a large right posterior cervical node. (Courtesy of Dr. J. Posen, Johannesburg, South Africa.)

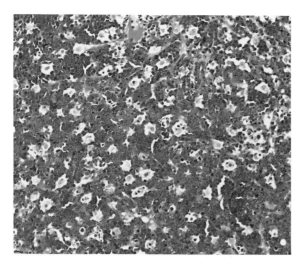

Figure 8-127
BURKITT'S LYMPHOMA

The typical "starry-sky" pattern results from isolated and uniformly distributed tingible body macrophages scattered throughout the neoplasm. (Courtesy of Dr. H. Coleman, Johannesburg, South Africa.) (Figures 8-127–8-129 are from the same patient.)

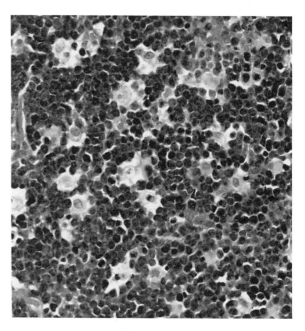

Figure 8-128
BURKITT'S LYMPHOMA

Sheets of uniform, intermediate-sized (15 μm), rounded nuclei with inconspicuous nucleoli, fine chromatin, and scant cytoplasm. The nuclei of the tingible body macrophages are slightly larger than the neoplastic cells. Mitoses are frequent. (Courtesy of Dr. H. Coleman, Johannesburg, South Africa.)

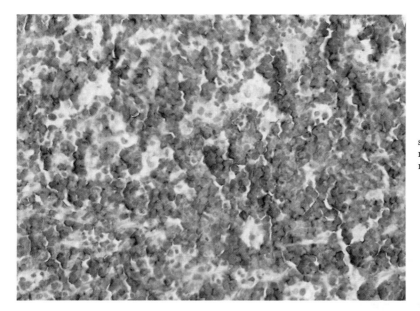

Figure 8-129
BURKITT'S LYMPHOMA
Uniform cytoplasmic membrane staining of neoplastic cells by pan B-cell marker, CD20. (Courtesy of Dr. H. Coleman, Johannesburg, South Africa.)

As occasionally occurs with lymphoma involving visceral organs, the presence of collagenous fibers may impart a sarcomatous appearance to the jaw lymphoma and result in an erroneous diagnosis (fig. 8-130). Immunohistochemical studies establish the true nature of the neoplasm when the possibility of a lymphoma is considered in the differential diagnosis (fig. 8-131) (178). A variety of other lymphoma types may involve the jaw bones but much less frequently than the diffuse large cell type (figs. 8-133–8-137). Extranodal lymphomas are a well-recognized complication of human immunodeficiency virus (HIV) infection, most commonly involving the digestive tract and central nervous system. In a review of 465 patients with HIV infection, 5 developed lymphoma of the jaw bones, 3 in the maxilla and 2 in the mandible (174). A primary anaplastic large cell (Ki-1) lymphoma of the jaw has been reported as the initial manifestation of acquired immunodeficiency syndrome (AIDS) in a pediatric patient (184). An AIDS-related, small, noncleaved cell lymphoma of non-Burkitt's type in the mandible has also been documented as the initial presentation of the disease (183).

Radiologically, non-Hodgkin's lymphomas produce an ill-defined osteolytic lesion with loss of lamina dura, depression of the alveolar margin, widened periodontal ligament space, and destruction of the cortical plate (fig. 8-138) (182). The bone destruction may result in the appear-

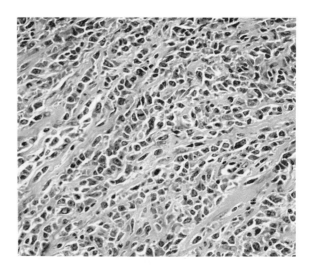

Figure 8-130
DIFFUSE LARGE CELL LYMPHOMA
OF MAXILLARY SINUS
Sheets of large lymphoma cells with irregular nuclear outlines and scanty cytoplasm. The presence of fibrous bands may complicate the diagnosis. (Figures 8-130 and 8-131 are from the same patient.)

ance of "floating teeth" (176). There are too few cases with jaw involvement to assess whether this feature has any prognostic significance. In a review of 17 patients, Soderholm et al. (182) found that 11 had involvement at other sites as a result of staging procedures; 9 died of the disease after a mean period of 19 months.

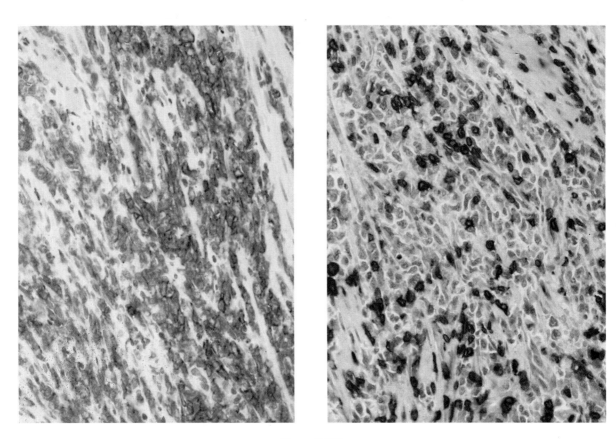

Figure 8-131
DIFFUSE LARGE CELL LYMPHOMA OF MAXILLARY SINUS
Uniform membrane staining of neoplastic cells for pan B-cell marker (left) and negative staining for pan T-cell marker CD3 (right) confirms the diagnosis of a B-cell lymphoma. The stained cells on the right are scattered reactive T cells.

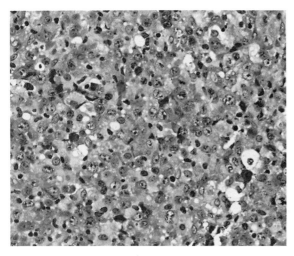

Figure 8-132
DIFFUSE LARGE CELL LYMPHOMA OF MAXILLA
The neoplastic cells have large vesicular nuclei with multiple nucleoli.

Hodgkin's Disease. Although bone involvement in Hodgkin's disease has been reported to occur in from 7 to 34 percent of cases, the jaw bones are uncommon as a primary or clinically significant secondary site; less than 10 such cases had been documented by 1988 (170,175,179). Histologically, the lesion is frequently of the lymphocytic depleted type, clinically is widely disseminated, and the prognosis has been poor (179). The histologic diagnosis has been complicated in a few of the reported cases by the presence of an associated fracture and osteomyelitis (170). Hodgkin's disease in such an extranodal setting may be difficult to differentiate from other non-Hodgkin lymphomas, in particular anaplastic or Ki-1 lymphomas as well as from other nonlymphomatous metastatic malignancies. Immunohistochemical demonstration of the antigens CD15 (Leu-M1) and CD30 (Ki-1) in at least some of the neoplastic cells is of significant diagnostic value, especially

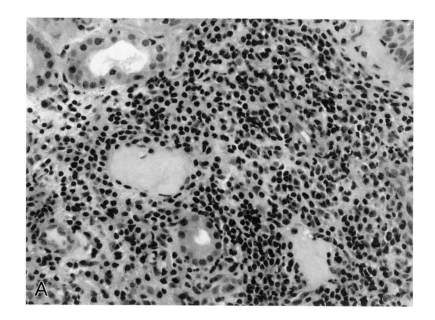

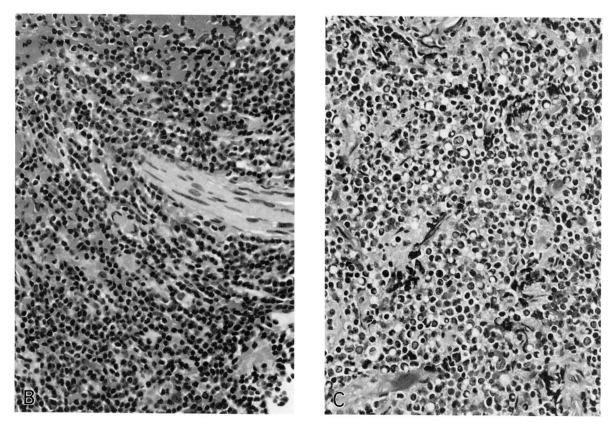

Figure 8-133
PATTERNS OF SMALL CELL LYMPHOMA, ALL FROM MAXILLARY LESIONS
A: There is infiltration of maxillary mucosa by chronic lymphocytic leukemia. Note the absence of other inflammatory cell types.
B: Waldenstrom macroglobulinemia.
C: Small cell lymphocytic lymphoma with signet ring cell features.

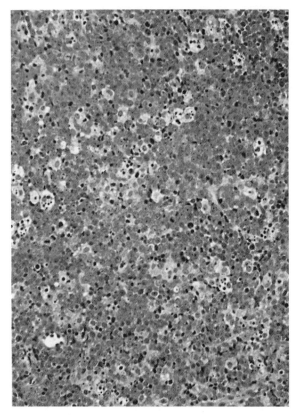

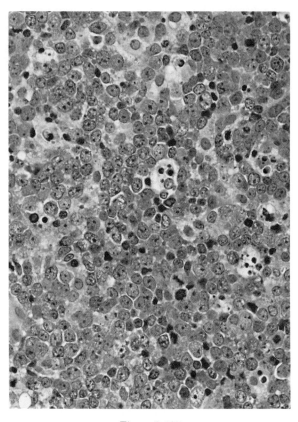

Figure 8-134
UNDIFFERENTIATED NON-BURKITT'S
TYPE LYMPHOMA

Unilateral involvement of maxilla and mandible by lymphoma of high grade in a 23-year-old man. The "starry-sky" pattern mimics Burkitt's lymphoma. (Figures 8-134 and 8-135 are from the same patient.)

Figure 8-135
UNDIFFERENTIATED
NON-BURKITT'S LYMPHOMA

The nuclei of the neoplastic cells are larger than in Burkitt's lymphoma (20 to 25 μm), more vesicular, and more variable in size.

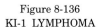

Figure 8-136
KI-1 LYMPHOMA

Lesion from the mandible of a 50-year-old man. The lymphoma cells show severe anaplasia and are large (anaplastic large cell lymphoma). The light microscopic appearance closely resembles a poorly differentiated carcinoma.

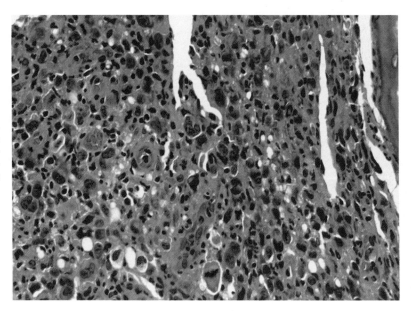

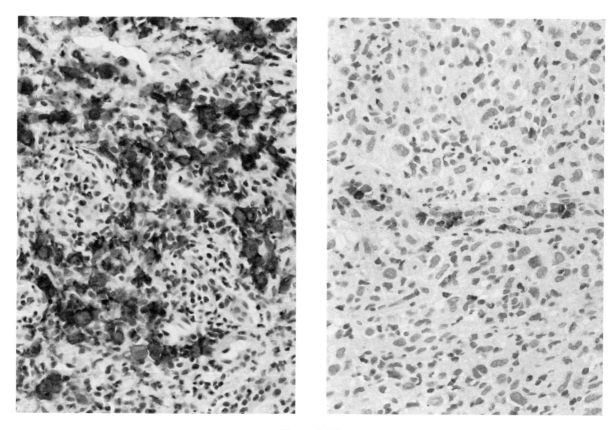

Figure 8-137
KI-1 LYMPHOMA
The neoplastic cells stain intensely with Ki-1 antibody (left) but fail to stain with Leu-M1 (CD15) antibody (right). Leukocytes within a capillary provides a useful internal control.

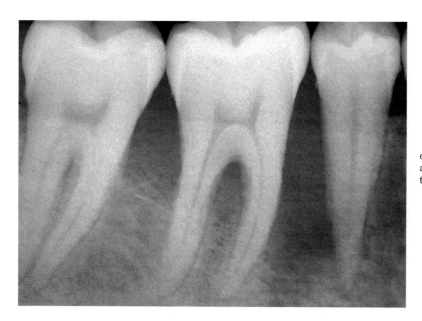

Figure 8-138
LYMPHOMA OF JAW
Ill-defined radiolucent lesion with loss of normal trabecular markings involves alveolar bone around canine and premolar teeth. The alveolar margin is lost.

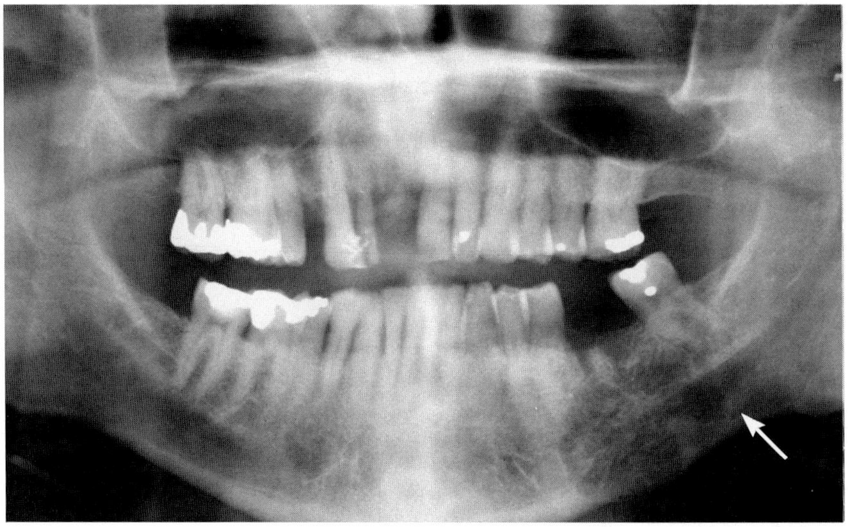

Figure 8-139
HEMANGIOMA
OF MANDIBLE
A large, ovoid, well-circumscribed lytic lesion is within the body of the left mandible.

in the absence of staining for leukocyte common antigen within these cells.

VASCULAR LESIONS

Angioma

Definition. This is a benign vascular neoplasm or hamartoma involving the jaw bones. It encompasses both the slow flow capillary and cavernous type hemangiomas as well as the rapid flow venous hemangioma (arteriovenous malformations).

Incidence. Hemangiomas in the orofacial region occur most commonly in the lips, tongue, palate, and buccal mucosa. They are rare in bones, constituting less than 0.7 percent of all bony neoplasms. Within the skeleton they occur with greatest frequency in the skull and vertebrae (187). Mandibular and maxillary involvement has been documented in more than 100 cases (191), usually in patients in the second decade of life; females outnumber males 2 to 1. Venous angiomatous lesions have been documented in the maxillary bones of a patient with Sturge-Weber syndrome (192).

Clinical Features. The lesion may be found incidentally on radiographic examination. Expansion of the affected bone may cause nonpainful swelling or deformity. There may be oozing of blood from the gingival crevice or severe hemorrhage following a biopsy or dental extraction. The lesion may present as a compressible bluish swelling submucosally if it erodes through cortical bone. Mobility of teeth may be noted. In the rapid flow arteriovenous type lesion, the patient may be aware of a pulsatile or throbbing sensation and a bruit may even be heard. Of particular concern is the danger of catastrophic hemorrhage following biopsy or surgical intervention (186,191).

Radiologic Findings. The radiologic features may be nonspecific, consisting of a radiolucent lesion with or without expansion of the bone and thinning of the cortex (fig. 8-139). There may be resorption of the roots of teeth or displacement of teeth. In some cases, radiating spicules of bone separating vascular channels within the lesion produce patterns variously described as soap bubble, honeycomb, spokewheel, sunray, or sunburst (191). There are several other imaging modalities that provide important information about the lesion. A CT scan is of value in demonstrating the extent of the lesion, in particular the presence of bony erosion and soft tissue extension. MRI helps identify rapid flow feeder vessels as well as vessels with rapid flow within arteriovenous type lesions, as these appear as signal flow void areas in both T1- and T2-weighted images. Foci of bright signal intensity in T2-weighted images indicate areas of slow flow or stagnation of blood, cysts, or necrosis within the lesion (fig. 8-140). Due to the vascularity of the lesion, there is prominent signal enhancement with gadolinium (190). Angiography is of particular value in demonstrating the vascular nature of the lesion and in identifying feeding vessels which may require

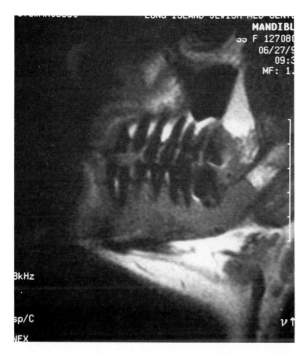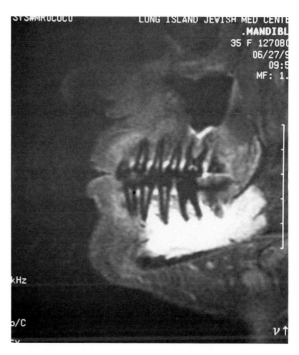

Figure 8-140
CAVERNOUS HEMANGIOMA OF MANDIBLE
Comparison of T1- (left) and T2-weighted (right) images demonstrates high intensity signal in the latter image related to stagnation of blood within the tumor. (Figures 8-140–8-143 are from the same patient.)

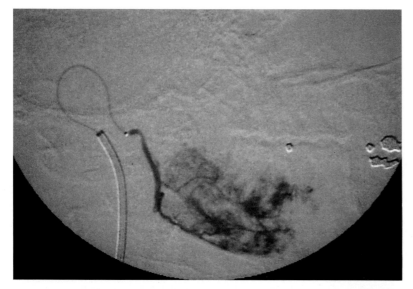

Figure 8-141
CAVERNOUS HEMANGIOMA
OF MANDIBLE
Angiogram demonstrates feeding vessels and tumor blush resulting from the presence of numerous cavernous type vascular channels.

ligation preoperatively to obviate severe bleeding (fig. 8-141) (189). The radiologic differential diagnosis includes aneurysmal bone cyst, telangiectatic osteosarcoma, ameloblastoma, odontogenic keratocyst, central giant cell reparative granuloma, and hyperparathyroidism (187).

Pathologic Findings. Capillary and cavernous hemangiomas resemble their counterparts at other sites in the body (figs. 8-142, 8-143). Rapid flow venous type angiomas consist of endothelial-lined vascular channels that contain variable amounts of smooth muscle in their walls

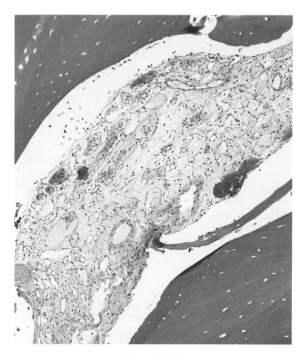

Figure 8-142
CAVERNOUS HEMANGIOMA OF MANDIBLE
Distended, endothelial-lined vascular channels fill the intertrabecular spaces.

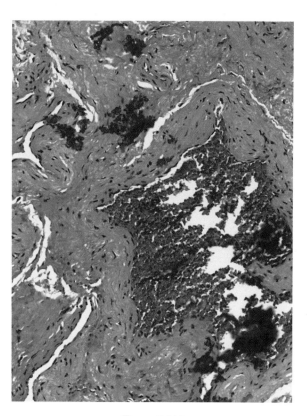

Figure 8-144
VENOUS HEMANGIOMA OF MANDIBLE
The distended and tortuous vascular channels have convoluted thick walls containing smooth muscle.

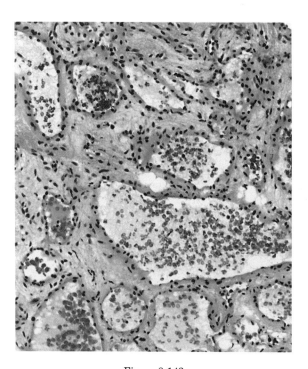

Figure 8-143
CAVERNOUS HEMANGIOMA OF MANDIBLE
Endothelial-lined vascular channels are shown at higher magnification.

and resemble venous structures (fig. 8-144). These are separated from one another by variable amounts of stromal connective tissue.

Treatment and Prognosis. If hemangioma is suspected based on the clinical or radiologic features, a needle aspiration should be performed rather than an open biopsy because of the danger of severe hemorrhage. Brisk bleeding at the time of needle biopsy suggests the possibility of a high flow vascular neoplasm. Under such circumstances, curettage should be avoided and an en bloc resection performed, preceded by embolization or ligation of feeding afferent vessels (186). A variety of other therapeutic modalities have been utilized including curettage and packing with hemostatic agents for low flow lesions, sclerosing agents, embolization, radiotherapy, and carbon dioxide and argon laser therapy (189). Unfortunately, recurrence is frequent with these alternative forms of therapy because of a rich collateral vascular supply.

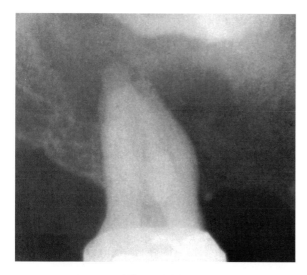

Figure 8-145
ANGIOSARCOMA
A large radiolucent lesion surrounds the roots of the maxillary left second molar and extends to the distal second premolar. (Courtesy of Dr. Paul Freedman, New York, NY.) (Figures 8-145–8-151 are from the same patient.)

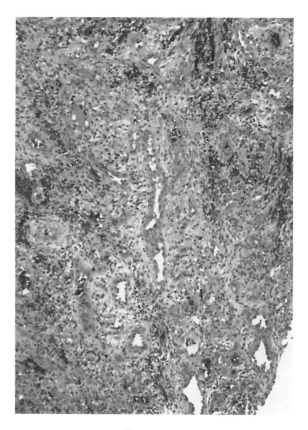

Figure 8-146
ANGIOSARCOMA
Low-power photomicrograph shows a neoplasm composed of a network of luminated and nonluminated endothelial-lined vascular channels. (Courtesy of Dr. Paul Freedman, New York, NY.)

In addition to benign hemangioma of the jaws, a sporadic case of *lymphangioma of the jaw* has been described (188).

Angiosarcoma

Definition. Angiosarcoma is a malignant mesenchymal neoplasm of endothelial derivation.

Clinical Features. Angiosarcoma occurs infrequently within jaw bones. By 1989, only 13 cases had been documented within the maxilla (195). In an extensive literature review in 1980, Zachariades et al. (197) documented mandibular involvement in 17 cases. Ellis and Kratochvil (193) documented 12 cases from the head and neck region but none of these involved the mandible or maxilla. The symptoms vary and depend on the local tissue elements involved by the neoplasm. As with benign vascular neoplasms, there is a tendency to significant hemorrhage following minor traumatic events (198). Radiologically, the lesion is purely osteolytic and, if the tooth-bearing region is involved, the appearance may be that of "teeth floating in space" (fig. 8-145).

Pathologic Findings. Histologically, the neoplasm is a sarcoma with vasoformative features. In low-grade, well-differentiated lesions this takes the form of anastomosing channels lined by mildly atypical, hyperchromatic endothelial cells. There may be endovascular papillary formations. These channels can be seen to infiltrate or dissect surrounding native stromal tissue. Mitoses are infrequent. High-grade or poorly differentiated angiosarcomas show primitive neovascularization in which slit-like vascular spaces containing red blood cells are lined by plump, atypical endothelial cells which may have a hobnail configuration (figs. 8-146–8-148). These cells have prominent eosinophilic nucleoli and frequent mitoses (figs. 8-149, 8-150). More compact cord-like or sheet-like patterns may be present in which the only evidence of an angiomatous histogenesis is intracytoplasmic vacuolation, representing an abortive attempt at vascularization (fig. 8-151). Areas of the tumor may be hemorrhagic and necrotic.

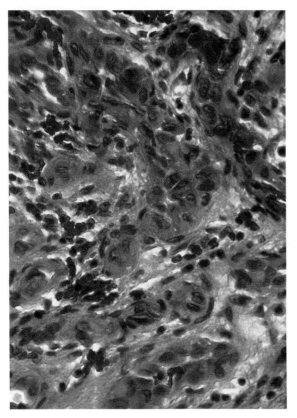

Figure 8-147
ANGIOSARCOMA

Luminated and nonluminated vascular channels are lined by plump polygonal epithelioid type endothelial cells showing moderate nuclear atypism. (Courtesy of Dr. Paul Freedman, New York, NY.)

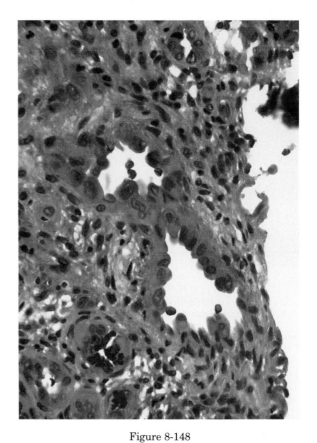

Figure 8-148
ANGIOSARCOMA

The epithelioid endothelial cells show a distinctly hobnail configuration. (Courtesy of Dr. Paul Freedman, New York, NY.)

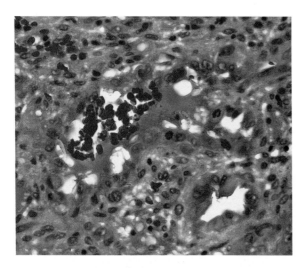

Figure 8-149
ANGIOSARCOMA

Numerous mitotic figures are present within the endothelial cells. (Courtesy of Dr. Paul Freedman, New York, NY.)

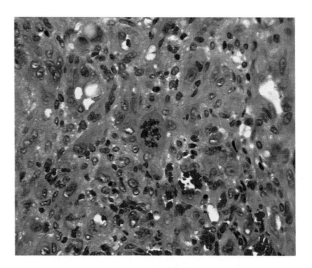

Figure 8-150
ANGIOSARCOMA

Abnormal mitotic figure in a neoplastic cell (center). (Courtesy of Dr. Paul Freedman, New York, NY.)

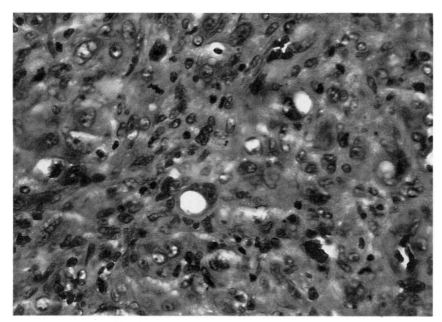

Figure 8-151
ANGIOSARCOMA
Intracytoplasmic vacuoles represent an attempt at neolumen formation in several malignant endothelial cells. Note the mitotic figures and significant nuclear pleomorphism. (Fig. 6 from Freedman PD, Kerpel SM. Epithelioid angiosarcoma of the maxilla. A case report and review of the literature. Oral Surg Oral Med Oral Pathol 1992;74:319-25.)

A variant of angiosarcoma in which the endothelial cells are large and polygonal, resembling epithelial cells, has been termed *epithelioid hemangioendothelioma (low-grade epithelioid angiosarcoma)* and *epithelioid angiosarcoma (high-grade epithelioid angiosarcoma)*. Freedman and Kerpel (194) have described this variant in the maxilla. Epithelioid hemangioma is a circumscribed lesion in which vascular differentiation is well developed, with formation of multicellular, canalized channels rather than the abortive structures present in epithelioid hemangioendothelioma.

It is important to distinguish low-grade angiosarcoma from a non-neoplastic reparative lesion, namely, Masson's intravascular papillary hemangioendothelioma. The pattern of anastomosing slit-like vascular channels with endovascular papillary formations lined by plump active endothelial cells closely resembles low-grade angiosarcoma. Two important distinguishing features are the confinement of the Masson's lesion to the lumen of a large vascular channel and its development in relation to a thrombus.

Treatment and Prognosis. Angiosarcomas are aggressive sarcomas that disseminate widely, particularly the high-grade lesions. Of 46 cases of low-grade epithelioid hemangioendothelioma, the local recurrence rate was 13 percent and the metastatic rate, 31 percent (196). Care should be taken when biopsying a suspected lesion because of the danger of severe hemorrhage. Radical surgery is the treatment of choice. Embolization prior to surgery may reduce the incidence of hemorrhage. Radiotherapy may be used as an adjunct either preoperatively or postoperatively.

SYNOVIAL AND TEMPOROMANDIBULAR JOINT LESIONS

Synovial Chondromatosis

Definition. This is a monoarticular, idiopathic, metaplastic disorder of synovial tissue, which results in the formation of multiple osteocartilaginous nodules in continuity with synovial membrane as well as lying free as loose bodies within the joint space. The joints most frequently involved include knee, hip, and elbow, followed by wrist and ankle.

Historical Features. This condition was first mentioned by Ambroise Pare in 1558, while Laennec was the first to suggest a metaplastic pathogenesis in 1813. In 1764, Baron Albrecht von Haller described loose bodies in the temporomandibular joint (TMJ). The first case of synovial chondromatosis involving the TMJ was reported by Axhausen in 1933 (206). To date, over 60 cases have been documented.

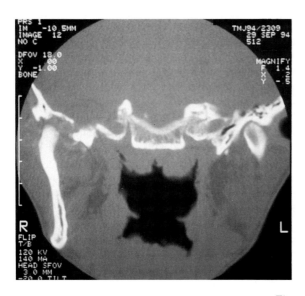 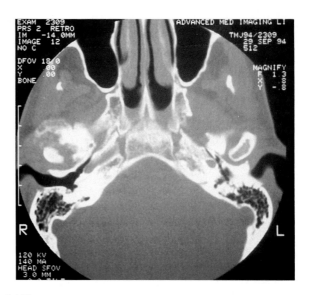

Figure 8-152
SYNOVIAL CHONDROMATOSIS
Coronal (left) and axial (right) CT scans show destruction of right mandibular condyle and nodular densities within the joint space. (Figures 8-152–8-157 are from the same patient.)

Clinical Features. There is a wide age range of 18 to 75 years, with a mean in the mid-forties and a majority of cases occurring in the fourth and fifth decades. Females outnumber males by a ratio of 1.5 to 1. About 70 percent of patients present with swelling or pain in the region of the TMJ or in the parotid region; about 45 percent present with both swelling and pain. Limitation of motion of the TMJ is the next most frequent complaint and occurs in 24 percent of patients. Less common clinical features include clicking, crepitus, locking of the joint, and displacement of the mandible (203). The lesion may erode through the external auditory canal and the floor of the middle cranial fossa causing auditory symptoms (207).

Radiologic Findings. In about 40 percent of cases the plain radiographs are within normal limits, so that other imaging modalities may be necessary to demonstrate the lesion (204). Any abnormal findings on plain radiographs frequently cannot be distinguished from those seen in degenerative joint disease, including sclerosis and erosion of the mandibular condyle and glenoid fossa. The joint space may be widened and the condyle displaced. Mineralization of metaplastic nodules and loose bodies would render them visible and facilitate the correct diagnosis

(203). As mentioned previously, the lesion may, on rare occasions, erode the external auditory canal and middle cranial fossa (207).

CT and MRI studies may identify the lesion when plain radiographs appear normal (figs. 8-152, 8-153). The CT scan is particularly helpful in distinguishing synovial chondromatosis from lesions arising in the parotid gland. The T2-weighted MRI image demonstrates the high signal intensity of cartilaginous nodules and loose bodies.

Pathologic Findings. The etiology of synovial chondromatosis is unknown although a few patients have had a well-substantiated history of prior trauma (200). Macroscopically, multiple cartilaginous nodules, ranging in size from less than 1 mm to 1 cm or more, stud the synovial surfaces of the joint space and also lie free as rounded loose bodies within the joint space. Some of these may be heavily mineralized or ossified so that they can only be sectioned following decalcification.

Histologically, the lesion develops as a metaplasia of mesenchymal cells immediately beneath the lining surface synovial cells. Rounded islands and nodules of cartilage of varying size are surrounded by subsynovial connective tissue, with the synovial surface layer encompassing the lesion (figs. 8-154–8-156). As the nodules

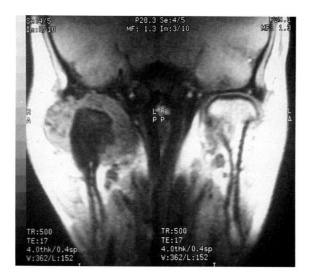 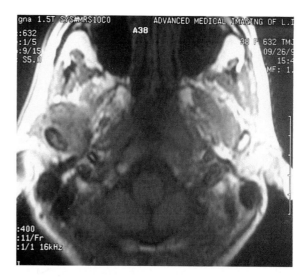

Figure 8-153
SYNOVIAL CHONDROMATOSIS
Coronal (left) and axial (right) T1-weighted MRIs show destruction of right mandibular condyle and nodular densities within the joint space.

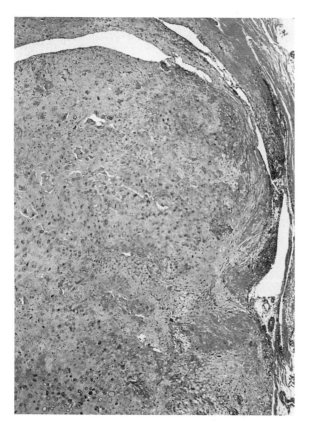 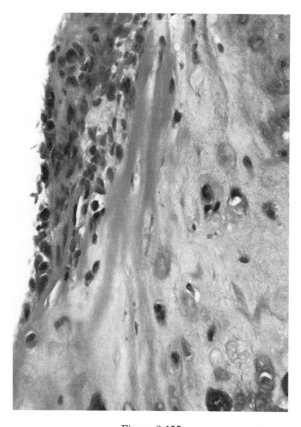

Figure 8-154
SYNOVIAL CHONDROMATOSIS
Cartilaginous nodules within joint space.

Figure 8-155
SYNOVIAL CHONDROMATOSIS
Layer of cuboidal synovial cells contiguous to and merging with nodule of cartilaginous tissue.

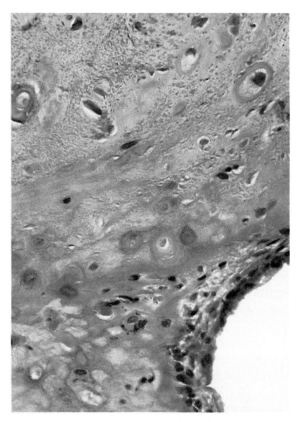

Figure 8-156
SYNOVIAL CHONDROMATOSIS
Surface synovial cells, mild nuclear atypism, and early speckled mineralization of matrix are seen.

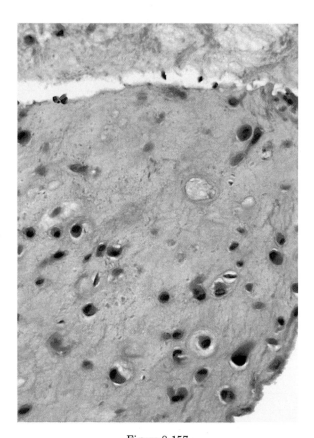

Figure 8-157
SYNOVIAL CHONDROMATOSIS
There is a moderate degree of nuclear atypism and hyperchromasia.

expand, they bulge into the joint space and eventually detach from their synovial moorings and form loose bodies. These loose bodies are bathed in and nourished by synovial fluid and continue to grow as a result of the proliferation of the chondrocytes. As the lesion ages, the loose bodies become mineralized and exhibit varying degrees of endochondral ossification. Of particular importance is the fact that the chondrocytes may show cytologic atypia, usually of a mild degree, but on occasion, fairly severe (fig. 8-157) (199, 201,204,205). There may be double nucleated chondrocytes and clustering of chondrocytes producing hypercellularity. These histologic features may result in an erroneous diagnosis of chondrosarcoma. Such histologic features fall within the spectrum of those seen in synovial chondromatosis and should not be misconstrued as evidence of malignancy, even though identical histologic features observed in a large cartilagi-

nous neoplasm arising in the long or flat bones would certainly be indicative of a chondrosarcoma. Myxoid change and necrosis are features seen in chondrosarcoma but not in synovial chondromatosis. Merrill et al. (202) recently diagnosed a synovial chondrosarcoma of the temporomandibular joint based on the presence of pleomorphic chondrocytes, myxoid degeneration, and foci of necrosis. However, at surgery the lesion resembled synovial chondromatosis and the patient was without evidence of recurrence 8 months after a high condylectomy.

Differential Diagnosis. Synovial osteochondromatosis clinically may mimic a parotid gland lesion and a biopsy showing islands of cartilage may be misconstrued as a component of a benign mixed tumor of the parotid gland. However, no myxoid or epithelial elements are seen and the continuity of the cartilaginous nodules with synovial tissue establishes the diagnosis.

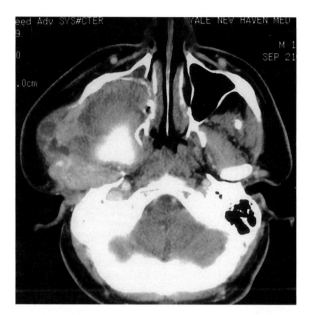

Figure 8-158
PIGMENTED VILLONODULAR SYNOVITIS
CT scan demonstrates destruction of mandibular condyle and an associated large mass extending into right maxillary sinus and infratemporal space. (Courtesy of Dr. H. D. Dorfman, Bronx, NY.) (Figures 8-158–8-162 are from the same patient.)

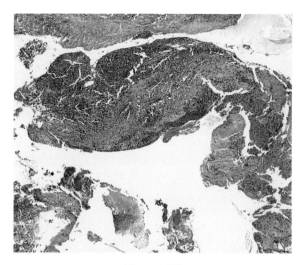

Figure 8-159
PIGMENTED VILLONODULAR SYNOVITIS
At low magnification, a villonodular configuration of the process is evident. (Courtesy of Dr. H. D. Dorfman, Bronx, NY.)

Loose bodies within the joint may also be seen in several other diseases, namely, osteoarthritis with detachment of osteocartilaginous fragments, neuropathic joint disease, osteochondritis dissecans, traumatic avulsion of osteochondral tissue, and pigmented villonodular synovitis (199,203).

Treatment and Prognosis. Surgical intervention is required to remove the loose bodies and resect the affected regions of synovium. This can usually be accomplished by a partial synovectomy although more extensive joint involvement may necessitate a complete synovectomy or even a discectomy if the disc is involved. The recurrence rate is extremely low (204).

Pigmented Villonodular Synovitis

Definition. This is a proliferative lesion of unknown etiology that produces villonodular or multilobulated masses arising from the synovium of joints and tendon sheaths, respectively. It is usually monoarticular and more commonly affects knee, hip, wrist, shoulder, or ankle. By 1992, only 12 cases involving the TMJ had been reported (208).

Clinical Features. Patients with temporomandibular involvement have ranged in age from 22 to 62 years, with an equal sex distribution. The symptoms and signs are similar to those of synovial chondromatosis, namely, swelling, pain, decreased range of motion, and clicking. Radiologically, the lesion may cause pressure erosion of adjacent bone including the articular surface (fig. 8-158). Eisig et al. (208) and O'Sullivan et al. (209) reported cases in which the lesion had eroded into the middle cranial fossa and into the external auditory canal.

Pathologic Findings. Controversy exists as to whether the lesion represents a neoplastic or reactive process, although most authorities consider pigmented villonodular synovitis and the related giant cell tumor of tendon sheath to be reactive or inflammatory in nature. Grossly, the lesion in the joint has a villous or villonodular configuration and the affected synovium is usually brown due to prominent hemosiderin deposition. Histologically, the synovial villi are expanded by a proliferation of uniform, polygonal to ovoid cells of histiocytic derivation (figs. 8-159–8-162). They frequently manifest their histiocytic potential by showing evidence of lipid accumulation ("foamy histiocytes") and intracytoplasmic hemosiderin deposition (fig. 8-162). Multinucleate giant cells are distributed throughout the lesion fairly uniformly or in an irregular pattern. The giant cells may be of

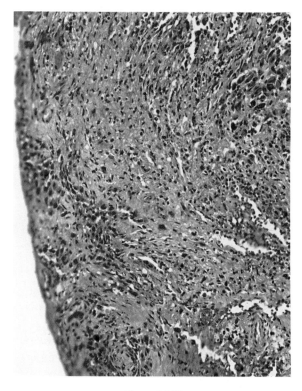

Figure 8-160
PIGMENTED VILLONODULAR SYNOVITIS
A nodule is partly lined by synovium. Aggregates of hemosiderin-laden phagocytic cells are separated by a broad fibrous band. (Courtesy of Dr. H. D. Dorfman, Bronx, NY.)

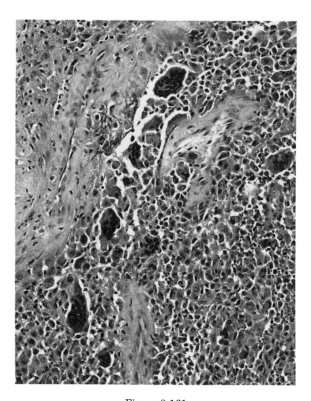

Figure 8-161
PIGMENTED VILLONODULAR SYNOVITIS
Sheets of polygonal mononuclear histiocytic cells with scattered osteoclast type giant cells and fibrovascular bands. (Courtesy of Dr. H. D. Dorfman, Bronx, NY.)

osteoclast or Touton type (fig. 8-162). There may be a variable degree of fibrosis, with transformation of polygonal histiocytic cells to facultative type fibroblasts (figs. 8-160, 8-161). Mitoses may be identified in actively proliferative lesions.

Three examples of *synovial sarcoma* involving the TMJ have been described (210).

Treatment and Prognosis. The affected synovial tissue requires surgical excision. The surgery may be complicated when the lesion involves the TMJ and especially if the lesion has eroded into adjacent structures such as the floor of the cranial cavity or the middle ear. Recurrences have been described in some patients (209).

Tophaceous Pseudogout

Definition. Tophaceous pseudogout is a juxta-articular mass resulting from deposition of calcium pyrophosphate and the associated histiocytic and foreign body giant cell reaction and metaplastic cartilaginous change.

Clinical Features. Deposition of crystals of calcium pyrophosphate within or adjacent to joints (calcium pyrophosphate deposition disease: CPPD) usually does not result in symptoms and is an incidental histologic finding. However, it may cause a painful arthropathy (pseudogout) and, least commonly, may produce a tophus (tophaceous pseudogout). By 1995, there were only about 30 documented cases of tophaceous pseudogout (211). Most occurred in middle-aged or elderly individuals who presented with a juxta-articular, painless or painful soft tissue mass. The TMJ region was involved in 10 cases.

Radiologic Findings. Radiologically, the lesion presents as a calcified soft tissue mass in the region of the TMJ (figs. 8-163, 8-164). The calcification is of a granular or fluffy texture and there may be pressure erosion of the adjacent bone. The lesion is frequently misdiagnosed preoperatively as a malignant tumor, usually as a chondrosarcoma.

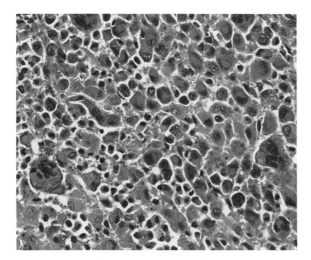

Figure 8-162
PIGMENTED
VILLONODULAR SYNOVITIS
Sheets of polygonal, mononuclear histiocytic cells with abundant eosinophilic cytoplasm and occasional multinucleate cells. Many of the cells contain hemosiderin pigment. (Courtesy of Dr. H. D. Dorfman, Bronx, NY.)

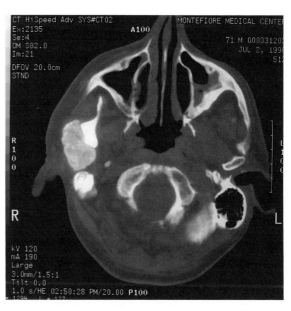

Figure 8-163
TOPHACEOUS PSEUDOGOUT
Axial CT scan demonstrates a well-circumscribed mineralized mass involving the temporomandibular joint. (Courtesy of Dr. H. Dorfman, Bronx, NY.) (Figures 8-163–8-167 are from the same patient.)

Pathologic Findings. The mass may measure up to 4 cm in greatest dimension and has a gray-white chalky appearance. Microscopically, the most distinctive feature is the presence of islands of basophilic crystalline material in which individual crystals have a needle-like or rhomboid configuration (figs. 8-164–8-166). The crystals are birefringent (fig. 8-166, inset). They induce a histiocytic and foreign body giant cell reaction and, in about half of the cases, a chondrometaplastic reaction. The chondrocytes may exhibit significant cytologic atypia (fig. 8-167). As a consequence of the presence of this metaplastic change, the lesion has been histologically misdiagnosed as soft tissue chondroma, synovial chondromatosis, and most seriously, chondrosarcoma. Such a misdiagnosis may be abetted when the crystalline structures are lost as a consequence of decalcification procedures. The presence of the granulomatous reaction should alert the pathologist to the possibility of the correct diagnosis and a careful examination by polarized microscopy undertaken.

Treatment and Prognosis. The lesion should be locally excised. A recurrence rate of about 20 percent has been reported (211).

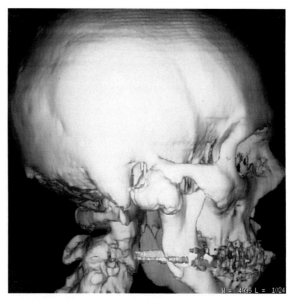

Figure 8-164
TOPHACEOUS PSEUDOGOUT
Three-dimensional reconstruction shows a circumscribed mineralized mass in the region of the temporomandibular joint. (Courtesy of Dr. H. Dorfman, Bronx, NY.)

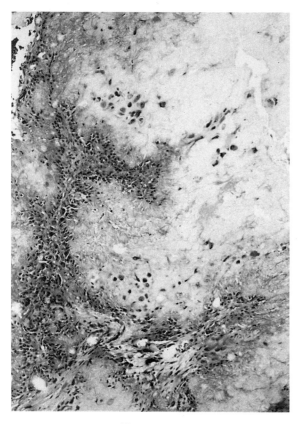

Figure 8-165
TOPHACEOUS PSEUDOGOUT
Nodular aggregates of crystalline material are surrounded by histiocytic cells. (Courtesy of Dr H. Dorfman, Bronx, NY.)

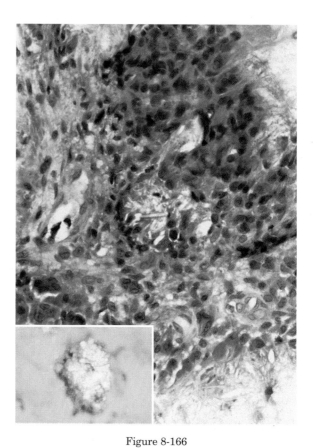

Figure 8-166
TOPHACEOUS PSEUDOGOUT
Aggregates of crystals are surrounded by sheets of histiocytic cells. Individual crystals have a rhomboid configuration. Inset shows birefringence of crystals with polarized light. (Courtesy of Dr. H. Dorfman, Bronx, NY.)

Figure 8-167
TOPHACEOUS PSEUDOGOUT
Chondroid metaplasia with cytologic atypia. (Courtesy of Dr. H. Dorfman, Bronx, NY.)

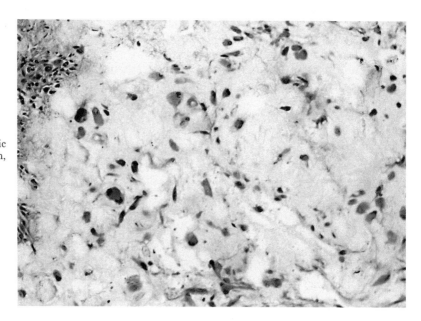

REFERENCES

Giant Cell Granuloma

1. Abrams B, Shear M. A histological comparison of the giant cells in the central giant cell granuloma of the jaws and the giant cell tumors of long bone. J Oral Pathol 1974;3:217–23.
2. Auclair FL, Cuenin P, Kratochvil FJ, Slater LJ, Ellis GL. A clinical and histomorphologic comparison of the central giant cell granuloma and the giant cell tumor. Oral Surg Oral Med Oral Pathol 1988;66:197–208.
3. Bhambhani M, Lamberty BG, Clements MR, Skingle SJ, Crisp AJ. Giant cell tumours in mandible and spine: a rare complication of Paget's disease of bone. Ann Rheum Dis 1992;51:1335–7.
4. Chuong R, Kaban LB, Kozakewich H, Perez-Atayde A. Central giant cell lesions of the jaws: a clinicopathologic study. J Oral Maxillofac Surg 1986;44:708–13.
5. El-Labban NG. Ultrastructural study of intranuclear tubulo-filaments in a giant cell tumour of bone in a patient with Paget's disease. J Oral Pathol 1984;13:650–60.
6. Ficcarra G, Kaban LB, Hansen LS. Giant cell lesions of the jaws: a clinicopathologic and cytometric study. Oral Surg Oral Med Oral Pathol 1987;64:44–9.
7. Flanagan AM, Tinkler SM, Horton MA, Williams DM, Chambers TJ. The multinucleate giant cells in giant cell granulomas of the jaw are osteoclasts. Cancer 1988;62:1139–45.
8. Jackson CE, Norum RA, Boyd SB, et al. Hereditary hyperparathyroidism and multiple ossifying jaw fibromas: a clinically and genetically distinct syndrome. Surgery 1990;108:1006–13.
9. Jacobs TP, Michelsen J, Polay JS, D'Adamo AC, Canfield RE. Giant cell tumor in Paget's disease of bone: familial and geographic clustering. Cancer 1979;44:742–7.
10. Jaffe HL. Giant cell reparative granuloma, traumatic bone cyst and fibrous (fibro-osseous) dysplasia of the jaw bones. Oral Surg Oral Med Oral Pathol 1953;6:159–75.
11. Kaffe I, Ardekian L, Taicher S, Littner MM, Buchner A. Radiologic features of central giant cell granuloma of the jaws. Oral Surg Oral Med Oral Pathol Radiol Endod 1996;81:720–6.
12. Mills BG. Comparison of the ultrastructure of a malignant tumor of the mandible containing giant cells with Paget's disease of bone. J Oral Pathol 1981;10:203–15.
13. Minic A, Stajcic Z. Prognostic significance of cortical perforation in the recurrence of central giant cell granulomas of the jaws. J Craniomaxillofac Surg 1996;24:104–8.
14. Mintz GA, Abrams AM, Carlsen GD, Melrose RJ, Fister HW. Primary malignant giant cell tumor of the mandible. Report of a case and review of the literature. Oral Surg Oral Med Oral Pathol 1981;51:164–71.
15. O'Malley M, Pogrel MA, Stewart JC, Silva RG, Regezi JA. Central giant cell granulomas of the jaws: phenotype and proliferation-associated markers. J Oral Pathol Med 1997;26:159–63.
16. Quick CA, Anderson R, Stool S. Giant cell tumors of the maxilla in children. Laryngoscope 1980;90:784–91.
17. Stolovitzky JP, Waldron CA, McConnel FM. Giant cell lesions of the maxilla and paranasal sinuses. Head Neck 1994;16:143–8.
18. Waldron CA, Shafer WG. The central giant cell reparative granuloma of the jaws. An analysis of 38 cases. Am J Clin Pathol 1966;45:437–47.
19. Whitaker SB, Vigneswaran N, Budnick SD, Waldron CA. Giant cell lesions of the jaws: evaluation of nucleolar organizer regions in lesions of varying behavior. J Oral Pathol Med 1993;22:402–5.
20. Whitaker SB, Waldron CA. Central giant cell lesions of the jaws. A clinical, radiologic, and histopathologic study. Oral Surg Oral Med Oral Pathol 1993;75:199–208.

Cherubism

21. Arnott DG. Cherubism: an initial unilateral presentation. Br J Oral Surg 1978;16:38–46.
22. Betts NJ, Stewart JC, Fonseca RJ, Scott RF. Multiple central giant cell lesions with a Noonan-like phenotype. Oral Surg Oral Med Oral Pathol 1993;76:601–7.
23. Cannon ML, Spiegel RE, Cooley RO. Hereditary fibrous dysplasia of the jaws (cherubism): report of a case. J Dent Child 1983;50:292–5.
24. Dunlap C, Neville B, Vickers RA, O'Neil D, Barker B. The Noonan syndrome/cherubism association. Oral Surg Oral Med Oral Pathol 1989;67:698–705.
25. Hille JJ, Buch B, Evans WG, Shakenovsky B, Butz S. Cherubism: two case reports and a review of the literature. J Dent Assoc S Afr 1986;41:461–6.
26. Jones WA. Familial multilocular cystic disease of the jaws. Am J Cancer 1933;17:946–50.
26a. Jones WA. Further observations regarding familial multilocular cystic disease of the jaw. Br J Radiol 1938;11:227–40.
27. Koury ME, Stella JP, Epker BN. Vascular transformation in cherubism. Oral Surg Oral Med Oral Pathol 1993;76:20–7.
28. Peters WJ. Cherubism: a study of twenty cases from one family. Oral Surg Oral Med Oral Pathol 1979;47:307–11.
29. Ramon Y, Engelberg IS. An unusually extensive case of cherubism. J Oral Maxillofac Surg 1986;44:325–8.

Aneurysmal Bone Cyst

30. Bataineh AB. Aneurysmal bone cysts of the maxilla: a clinicopathologic review. J Oral Maxillofac Surg 1997;55:1212–6.
31. Matt BH. Aneurysmal bone cyst of the maxilla; case report and review of the literature. Int J Pediatr Otorhinolaryngol 1993;25:217–26.
32. Revel MP, Vanel D, Sigal R, et al. Aneurysmal bone cysts of the jaws. CT and MR findings. J Comput Assist Tomogr 1992;16:84–6.
33. Toljanic JA, Lechewski E, Huvos AG, Strong EW, Schweiger AW. Aneurysmal bone cysts of the jaws: a case study and review of the literature. Oral Surg Oral Med Oral Pathol 1987;64:72–7.

Osteoma

34. Bessho K, Murakami KI, Iizuka T, Ono T. Osteoma in mandibular condyle. Int J Oral Maxillofac Surg 1987;16:372–5.

35. Cutilli BJ, Quinn PD. Traumatically induced peripheral osteoma. Report of a case. Oral Surg Oral Med Oral Pathol 1992:73:667–9.

36. Gordon NC, Swann NP, Hansen LS. Median palatine cyst and maxillary antral osteoma: report of an unusual case. J Oral Surg 1980;38:361–5.

37. Kurita K, Kawai T, Ikeda N, Kameyama Y. Cancellous osteoma of the mandibular coronoid process: report of a case. J Oral Maxillofac Surg 1991;49:753–6.

38. Rajayogeswarau V, Eveson JW. Endosteal (central) osteoma of the maxilla. Br Dent J 1981;150:162–3.

39. Richards HE, Strider JW, Short SG, Theisen FC, Larson WJ. Large peripheral osteoma arising from the genial tubercle area. Oral Surg Oral Pathol Oral Med 1986;61:268–71.

40. Schneider LC, Dolinsky HB, Grodjesk JE. Solitary peripheral osteoma of the jaws: report of case and review of literature. J Oral Surg 1980;38:452–5.

41. Williams SC, Peller PJ. Gardner's syndrome. Case report and discussion of the manifestations of the disorder. Clin Nucl Med 1994;19:668–70.

42. Wolf J, Jarvinen HJ, Hietanen J. Gardner's dento-maxillary stigmas in patients with familial adenomatous coli. Br J Oral Maxillofac Surg 1986;24:410–16.

Osteoblastoma/Osteoid Osteoma

43. Ataoglu 0, Oygur T, Yamalik K, Yucel E. Recurrent osteoblastoma of the mandible. A case report. J Oral Maxillofac Surg 1994;52:86–90.

44. Dorfman HD, Weiss SW. Borderline osteoblastic tumors: problems in the differential diagnosis of aggressive osteoblastoma and low grade osteosarcoma. Sem Diag Pathol 1984;1:215–34.

45. Eisenbud L, Kahn LB, Friedman E. Benign osteoblastoma of the mandible: fifteen year follow-up showing spontaneous regression after biopsy. J Oral Maxillofac Surg 1987;45:53–7.

46. Farman AG, Nortje CJ, Grotepass F. Periosteal benign osteoblastoma of the mandible. Report of a case and review of the literature pertaining to benign osteoblastic neoplasms of the jaws. Br J Oral Surg 1976;14:12–22.

47. Kramer HS. Benign osteoblastoma of the mandible. Report of a case. Oral Surg Oral Med Oral Pathol 1967;24:842–51.

48. Ohkubo T, Hernandez JC, Ooya K, Kratchhoff DJ. "Aggressive" osteoblastoma of the maxilla. Oral Surg Oral Med Oral Pathol 1989;68:69–73.

49. Schajowicz F, Lemos C. Malignant osteoblastoma. J Bone Joint Surg (Br) 1976;58:202–11.

50. Slootweg PJ. Cementoblastoma and osteoblastoma: a comparison of histologic features. J Oral Pathol Med 1992;21:385–9.

51. Svensson B, Isacsson G. Benign osteoblastoma associated with an aneurysmal bone cyst of the mandibular ramus and condyle. Oral Surg Oral Med Oral Pathol 1993;76:433–6.

52. Ueno H, Ariji E, Tanaka T, et al. Imaging features of maxillary osteoblastoma and its malignant transformation. Skeletal Radiol 1994;23:509–12.

53. van der Waal I, Greebe RB, Elias EA. Benign osteoblastoma or osteoid osteoma of the maxilla. Report of a case. Int J Oral Surg 1983;12:355–8.

54. Weinberg S, Katsikeris N, Pharoah M. Osteoblastoma of the mandibular condyle: review of the literature and report of a case. J Oral Maxillofac Surg 1987;45:350–5.

55. Zulian MA, Vincent SK, Hiatt WR. Osteoid osteoma of the mandibular ramus. J Oral Maxillofac Surg 1987;45:712–4.

Osteosarcoma

56. Adekeye EO, Chau KK, Edwards MB, Williams HK. Osteosarcomas of the jaws—a series from Kaduna, Nigeria. Int J Oral Maxillofac Surg 1987;16:205–13.

57. Ajagbe HA, Junaid TA, Daramola JO. Osteogenic sarcoma of the jaw in an African community: report of twenty-one cases. J Oral Maxillofac Surg 1986;44:104–6.

58. Arlen M, Shah IC, Higinbotham N, Huvos AJ. Osteogenic sarcoma of head and neck induced by radiation therapy. NY State J Med 1972;72:929–34.

59. Ashman S, Lever S, Weiss M. Osteogenic sarcoma and Paget's disease of the mandible. Review of the literature and case report. J MD State Dent Assoc 1986;29:53–5.

60. Baker CG, Tishler JM. Malignant disease of the jaws. J Can Assoc Radiol 1977;28:129–41.

61. Batsakis JG. Pathology consultation. Osteogenic and chondrogenic sarcoma of the jaws. Ann Otol Rhinol Laryngol 1987;96:474–5.

62. Bertoni F, Dallera P, Bacchini P, Marchetti C, Campobassi A. The Instituto Rizzoli-Baretta experience of osteosarcoma of the jaw. Cancer 1991;68:1555–63.

63. Bohay RN, Daley T. Osteosarcoma and fibrous dysplasia. Radiologic features in the differential diagnosis: a case report. J Can Dent Assoc 1993;59:931–4.

64. Bras JM, Donner R, van der Kwast WA, Snow GB, van der Waal I. Juxtacortical osteogenic sarcoma of the jaws. Review of the literature and report of a case. Oral Surg Oral Med Oral Pathol 1980;50:535–44.

65. Caron AS, Hajdu SI, Strong EW. Osteogenic sarcoma of the facial and cranial bones. A review of forty-three cases. Am J Surg 1971;122:719–25.

66. Chan CW, Kung TM, Ma L. Telangiectatic osteosarcomas of the mandible. Cancer 1986;58:2110–5.

67. Clark JL, Unni KK, Dahlin DC, Devine KD. Osteosarcoma of the jaw. Cancer 1983;51:2311–16.

68. Colmenero C, Rodejas EG, Colmenero B, Lopez-Barea F. Osteogenic sarcoma of the jaws: malignant fibrous histiocytoma subtype. J Oral Maxillofac Surg 1990;48:1323–8.

69. Dahlin DC, Unni KK. Bone tumors: general aspects and data on 8,542 cases, Springfield, Il: Charles C Thomas, 1986:271.

70. Delgado R, Maafs E, Alfeiran A, et al. Osteosarcoma of the jaw. Head Neck 1994;16:246–52.

71. Dickens P, Wei WI, Sham JS. Osteosarcoma of the maxilla in Hong Kong Chinese post-irradiation for nasopharyngeal carcinoma. A report of four cases. Cancer 1990;66:1924–6.

72. Ebata K, Takeshi U, Tohnai I, Kaneda T. Chondrosarcoma and osteosarcoma arising in polyostotic fibrous dysplasia. J Oral Maxillofac Surg 1992;50:761–4.

73. Fechner RE, Mills SE. Tumors of the bones and joints. Atlas of Tumor Pathology, 3rd Series, Fascicle 8. Washington, DC: Armed Forces Institute of Pathology, 1993:38–9.

74. Finkelstein JB. Osteosarcoma of the jaw bones. Radiol Clin North Am 1970;8:425–43.

75. Forteza G, Colmenero B, Lopez-Barea F. Osteogenic sarcoma of the maxilla and mandible. Oral Surg Oral Med Oral Pathol 1986;62:179–84.

76. Gardner DG, Mills DM. The widened periodontal ligament of osteosarcoma of the jaws. Oral Surg Oral Med Oral Pathol 1976;41:652–6.

77. Gardner GM, Steiniger JR. Family cancer syndrome: a study of the kindred of a man with osteogenic sarcoma of the mandible. Laryngoscope 1990;100:1259–63.

78. Garrington GE, Scofield HH, Cornyn J, Hooker SP. Osteosarcoma of the jaws. Analysis of 56 cases. Cancer 1967;20:377–91.

79. Giangaspero F, Stracca V, Visona A, Eusebi V. Small cell osteosarcomas of the mandible. Case report. Appl Pathol 1984;2:28–31.

80. Hoffman S, Jacoway JR, Krolls SO. Intraosseous and parosteal tumors of the jaws. Atlas of Tumor Pathology, 2nd Series, Fascicle 24. Washington, DC: Armed Forces Institute of Pathology, 1987:170–80.

81. Hutchison IL, Hopper C, Coonar HS. Neoplasia masquerading as periapical infection. Br Dent J 1990;168:288–94.

82. James PL, O'Reagan MB, Speight PM. Well differentiated intraosseous osteosarcoma in the mandible of a six-year-old child. J Laryngol Otol 1990;104:335–40.

83. Kim J, Ellis GL, Mounsdon TA. Usefulness of antikeratin immunoreactivity in osteosarcoma of the jaw. Oral Surg Oral Med Oral Pathol 1991;72:213–7.

84. Lee YY, Van Tassel P, Nauert C, Raymond AK, Edeiken J. Craniofacial osteosarcomas: plain film, CT, and MR findings in 46 cases. Am J Roentgenol 1988;150:1397–402.

85. Lindqvist C, Teppo L, Sane J, Holmstrom T, Wolf J. Osteosarcoma of the mandible. Analysis of nine cases. J Oral Maxillofac Surg 1986;44:459–64.

86. Liu SK. Neoplasms of bone. In: Whittick WG, ed. Canine orthopedics. Philadelphia: Lea and Febiger, 1990:867–9.

87. Millar BG, Browne RM, Flood TR. Juxtacortical osteosarcoma of the jaws. Br J Oral Maxillofac Surg 1990;28:73–9.

88. Patterson A, Greer RO Jr, Howard D. Periosteal osteosarcoma of the mandible. A case report and review of the literature. J Oral Maxillofac Surg 1990;48:522–6.

89. Potdar GG. Osteogenic sarcoma of the jaws. Oral Surg Oral Med Oral Pathol 1970;30:381–9.

90. Regezi JA, Zarbo RJ, McClatchey KD, Courtney RM, Crissman JD. Osteosarcomas and chondrosarcomas of the jaws: immunohistochemical correlations. Oral Surg Oral Med Oral Pathol 1987;64:302–7.

91. Russ JE, Jesse RH. Management of osteosarcoma of the maxilla and mandible. Am J Surg 1980;140:572–6.

92. Slootweg PJ, Muller H. Osteosarcoma of the jaw bones. Analysis of eighteen cases. J Maxillofac Surg 1985;13:158–66.

93. Smith J, Botet JF, Yeh SD. Bone sarcomas in Paget's disease: a study of 85 patients. Radiology 1984;152:583–90.

94. Struthers PJ, Shear M. Aneurysmal bone cysts of the jaws. (II). Pathogenesis. Int J Oral Surg 1984;13:92–100.

95. Tanzawa H, Uchiyama S, Sato K. Statistical observation of osteosarcoma of the maxillofacial region in Japan. Analysis of 114 Japanese cases reported between 1930 and 1989. Oral Surg Oral Med Oral Pathol 1991;72:444–8.

96. Tillman HH. Paget's disease of bone. A clinical radiographic and histopathologic study of twenty-four cases involving the jaws. Oral Surg Oral Med Oral Pathol 1962;15:1225–34.

97. Vener J, Rice DH, Newman AN. Osteosarcoma and chondrosarcoma of the head and neck. Laryngoscope 1984;94:240–2.

98. Vincent SD, Lilly GE, Ruskin JD. Recurrent enlargement of the left maxillary alveolus. J Oral Maxillofac Surg 1993;51:671–5.

99. Yabut SM, Kenan S, Sissons HA, Lewis MM. Malignant transformation of fibrous dysplasia. A case report and review of the literature. Clin Orthop 1988;228:281–9.

100. Zarbo RJ, Regezi JA, Baker SR. Periosteal osteogenic sarcoma of the mandible. Oral Surg Oral Med Oral Pathol 1984;57:643–7.

Osteochondroma

101. Asanami S, Kasazaki Y, Uchida I. Large exostosis of the mandibular coronoid process. Report of a case. Oral Surg Oral Med Oral Pathol 1990;69:559–62.

102. Forssell H, Happonen RP, Forssell K, Virolainen E. Osteochondroma of the mandibular condyle. Report of a case and review of the literature. Br J Oral Maxillofac Surg 1985;23:183–9.

103. Gaines RE Jr, Lee MB, Crocker DJ. Osteochondroma of the mandibular condyle: case report and review of literature. J Oral Maxillofac Surg 1992;50:899–903.

104. Goyal M, Sidhu SS. A massive osteochondroma of the mandibular condyle. Br J Oral Maxillofac Surg 1992;30:66–8.

105. Henry CH, Granite EL, Rafetto LK. Osteochondroma of the mandibular condyle: report of a case and review of the literature. J Oral Maxillofac Surg 1992;50:1102–8.

106. Kerscher A, Piette E, Tideman H, Wu PC. Osteochondroma of the coronoid process of the mandible. Report of a case and review of the literature. Oral Surg Oral Med Oral Pathol 1993;75:559–64.

107. Loftus MJ, Bennett JA, Fantasia JE. Osteochondroma of the mandibular condyles. Report of three cases and review of the literature. Oral Surg Oral Med Oral Pathol 1986;61:221–6.

Chondroblastoma

108. Al-Deurachi HS, Al-Naib N, Sangal BC. Benign chondroblastoma of the maxilla: a case report and review of chondroblastomas in facial bones. Br J Oral Surg 1980;18:150–6.

108a. Fechner RE, Mills SE. Tumors of the bones and joints. Atlas of Tumor Pathology. 3rd Series, Fascicle 8. Washington, D.C.: Armed Forces Institute of Pathology, 1993.

109. Payne M, Yusuf H. Benign chondroblastoma involving the mandibular condyle. Br J Oral Maxillofac Surg 1982;25:250–5.

Chondromyxoid Fibroma

110. Danielsen B, Ritsau M, Wenzel A. Recurrence of chondromyxoid fibroma: a case report. Dentomaxillofac Radiol 1991;20:65–7.

111. Lingen MW, Solt DB, Polverini PJ. Unusual presentation of a chondromyxoid fibroma of the mandible. Report of a case and a review of the literature. Oral Surg Oral Med Oral Pathol 1993;75:615–21.

112. Muller S, Whitaker SB, Weathers DR. Chondromyxoid fibroma of the mandible. Diagnostic image cytometry findings and review of the literature. Oral Med Oral Surg Oral Pathol 1992;73:465–8.

Chondrosarcoma

113. Berktold R, Krespi YP, Bytell DE, Ossoff RH. Chondrosarcoma of the maxilla. Otolayngol Head Neck Surg 1984;92:484–6.

114. Bottrill ID, Wood S, Barrett-Lee P, Howard DJ. Mesenchymal chondrosarcoma of the maxilla. J Laryngol Otol 1994;180:785–7.

115. Christensen RE Jr. Mesenchymal chondrosarcoma of the jaws. Oral Surg Oral Med Oral Pathol 1982;54:197–206.

116. Ebata K, Usami T, Tohnai I, Kaneda T. Chondrosarcoma and osteosarcoma arising in polyostotic fibrous dysplasia. J Oral Maxillofac Surg 1992;50:761–4.

117. Garrington GE, Collett WK. Chondrosarcoma. I. A selected review of the literature. J Oral Pathol 1988;17:1–11.

118. Hackney FL, Aragon SB, Aufdemorte TB, Holt GR, van Sickels JE. Chondrosarcoma of the jaws: clinical findings, histopathology and treatment. Oral Surg Oral Med Oral Pathol 1991;71:139–43.

119. Happonen RP, Heikinheimo K, Aitasalo K, Ekfors TO, Calonius PE. Chondrosarcoma of the jaws. Review of the literature and report of two cases. Proc Finn Dent Soc 1985;81:135–41.

120. Krolls SO, Schaffer RC, O'Rear JW. Chondrosarcoma and osteosarcoma of the jaws in the same patient. Oral Surg Oral Med Oral Pathol 1980;50:146–50.

121. Lurie R. Solitary enchondroma of the mandibular condyle: a review and case report. J Dent Assoc S Afr 1975;30:589–93.

122. Nortje GJ, Farman AG, Grotepass FW, van Zyl A. Chondrosarcoma of the mandibular condyle. Report of a case with special reference to radiographic features. Br J Oral Surg 1976;14:101–11.

123. Ormiston IW, Piette E, Tideman H, Wu PC. Chondrosarcoma of the mandible presenting as periodontal lesions: report of two cases. J Craniomaxillofac Surg 1994;22:231–5.

124. Saito K, Unni KK, Wollan PC, Lund BA. Chondrosarcoma of the jaw and facial bones. Cancer 1995;76:1550–8.

125. Slootweg PJ. Clear-cell chondrosarcoma of the maxilla. Report of a case. Oral Surg Oral Med Oral Pathol 1980;50:233–7.

126. Takahashi K, Sato K, Kanazawa H, Wang XL, Kimura T. Mesenchymal chondrosarcoma of the jaw—report of a case and review of 41 cases in the literature. Head Neck 1993;15:459–64.

Desmoplastic Fibroma

127. Bertoni F, Present D, Marchetti C, Bacchini P, Stea G. Desmoplastic fibroma of the jaw: the experience of the Institute Beretto. Oral Surg Oral Med Oral Pathol 1986;61:179–84.

128. Crim JR, Gold RH, Mirra JM, Eckardt JJ, Bassett LW. Desmoplastic fibroma of bone: radiographic analysis. Radiology 189;172:827–32.

129. Dahlin DC, Unni KK. Bone tumors: general aspects and data on 8,542 cases, 4th ed. Springfield, Ill: Charles C. Thomas, 1986:3–17, 209–307, 366–78.

130. Freedman PD, Cardo VA, Kerpel SM, Lumerman H. Desmoplastic fibroma (fibromatosis) of the jawbones. Report of a case and review of the literature. Oral Surg Oral Med Oral Pathol 1978;46:386–95.

131. Griffith JG, Irby WB. Desmoplastic fibroma: report of a rare tumor of the oral structures. Oral Surg Oral Med Oral Pathol 1965;20:269–75.

132. Jaffe HL. Tumors and tumorous conditions of the bones and joints. Philadelphia: Lea & Febiger, 1958:298–303.

133. Kwon PH, Horswell BB, Gatto DJ. Desmoplastic fibroma of the jaws: surgical management and review of the literature. Head Neck 1989;11:67–75.

134. Rabhan WN, Rosai J. Desmoplastic fibroma. Report of ten cases and review of the literature. J Bone Surg 1968;50:487–502.

135. Sugiura I. Desmoplastic fibroma. Case report and review of the literature. J Bone Joint Surg 1976;58:126–30.

136. Valente G, Migliario N, Bianchi SD, Vercellino V. Desmoplastic fibroma of the mandible: a case with an unusual clinical presentation. J Oral Maxillofac Surg 1989;47:1087–9.

137. Vally IM, Altini N. Fibromatoses of the oral and paraoral soft tissues and jaws. Review of the literature and report of 12 new cases. Oral Med Oral Surg Oral Pathol 1990;69:191–8.

Fibrosarcoma

138. Bang G, Baardsen R, Gilhaus-Moe 0. Infantile fibrosarcoma in the mandible: case report. J Oral Pathol Med 1989;18:339–43.

139. Dahlin DC, Ivins JC. Fibrosarcoma of bone. A study of 114 cases. Cancer 1969;23:35–41.

140. Dehner LP. Tumors of the mandible and maxilla in children. II. A study of 14 primary and secondary malignant tumors. Cancer 1973;32:112–20.

141. Eyre-Brook AL, Price CH. Fibrosarcoma of bone. Review of fifty consecutive cases from the Bristol Bone Tumour Registry. J Bone Joint Surg 1969;51B:20–37.

142. Ferlito A, Recher G, Tomazzoli L. Radiation-induced fibrosarcoma of the mandible following treatment for bilateral retinoblastoma. J Laryngol Otol 1979;93:1015–20.

143. Huvos AG, Higinbotham NL. Primary fibrosarcoma of bone. A clinicopathologic study of 130 patients. Cancer 1975;35:837–47.

144. Jeffree GM, Price CH. Metastatic spread of fibrosarcoma of bone. A report on forty-nine cases and a comparison with osteosarcoma. J Bone Joint Surg 1976;58B:418–25.

145. Moloy PJ, Kowal KA, Siegel WM. Fibrosarcoma of the mandible following supravoltage irradiation. Report of a case. Arch Otolaryngol Head Neck Surg 1989;115:1250–2.

146. Reichart PA, Zobl H. Transformation of ameloblastic fibroma to fibrosarcoma. Int J Oral Surg 1978;7:503–7.

147. Slootweg PJ, Muller H. Fibrosarcoma of the jaws. A study of 7 cases. J Maxillofac Surg 1984;12:157–62.

148. Taconis WK, van Ryssel TG. Fibrosarcoma of the jaws. Skeletal Radiol 1986;15:10–3.

149. Van Blarcom CW, Masson JK, Dahlin DC. Fibrosarcoma of the mandible. A clinicopathologic study. Oral Surg Oral Med Oral Pathol 1971;32:428–39.

Myofibroma (Infantile Myofibromatosis)

150. Chung E, Enzinger FM. Infantile myofibromatosis. Cancer 1981;48:1807–18.

151. Coffin CM, Dehner LP. Fibroblastic-myofibroblastic tumors in children and adolescents: a clinicopathologic study of 108 examples in 103 patients. Pediatr Pathol 1991;11:569–88.

152. Sugatani T, Inui N, Tagawa T, Seki Y, Mori A, Yoneda J. Myofibroma of the mandible. Clinicopathologic study and review of the literature. Oral Surg Oral Med Oral Pathol Oral Radiol Endod 1995;80:303–9.

Langerhans' Cell Histiocytosis

153. Bhaskar PB, White CS, Baughman RA. Eosinophilic granuloma of the mandibular condyle. A case report and management discussion. Oral Surg Oral Med Oral Pathol 1993;76:557–60.

154. Hartman KS. Histiocytosis X: a review of 114 cases with oral involvement. Oral Surg Oral Med Oral Pathol 1980;49:38–54.

155. Ragab RR, Rake 0. Eosinophilic granuloma with bilateral involvement of both jaws. Int J Oral Surg 1975;4:73–9.

Myeloma

156. Brunning RD, McKenna RW. Tumors of the bone marrow. Atlas of Tumor Pathology, 3rd Series, Fascicle 9. Washington, D.C.: Armed Forces Institute of Pathology 1994:323–67.

157. Epstein JB, Voss NJ, Stevenson-Moore P. Maxillofacial manifestations of multiple myeloma. An usual case and review of the literature. Oral Surg Oral Med Oral Pathol 1984;57:267–71.

158. Frassica FJ, Schray MF, Sim FH, Kyle RA. Solitary plasmacytoma of bone: Mayo Clinic experience. Int J Radiat Oncol Biol Phys 1989;16:43–8.

159. Furutani M, Ohnishi M, Tanaka Y. Mandibular involvement in patients with multiple myeloma. J Oral Maxillofac Surg 1994;52:23–5.

160. Gonzales J, Elizondo J, Trull M, De Torres I. Plasma cell tumours of the condyle. Br J Oral Maxillofac Surg 1991;29:274–6.

161. Monje F, Gil-Diez JL, Campano FJ, Alonso del Hoyo JR. Mandibular lesion as the first evidence of multiple myeloma. Case report. J Craniomaxfac Surg 1989;17:315–7.

162. Pisano JJ, Coupland R, Chew SY, Miller AS. Plasmacytoma of the oral cavity and jaws. Oral Surg Oral Med Oral Pathol Oral Radiol Endod 1997;83:265–71.

163. Ramon Y, Oberman M, Horowitz I, Freedman A, Tadmor R. A large mandibular tumor with a distinct radiological "sun-ray" effect as the primary manifestation of multiple myeloma. J Oral Surg 1978;36:52–4.

164. Raubenheimer EJ, Lello GI, Dauth J, Fayman MS, Dvornak N, Senekal JC. Multiple myeloma presenting as localized expansile jaw tumour. Int J Oral Maxillofac Surg 1988;17:382–5.

165. Rennie JS, Critchlow HA. Solitary oral amyloid. A report of two cases. Int J Oral Surg 1982;11:73–6.

166. Tamir R, Pick AI, Calderone S. Plasmacytoma of the mandible: a primary presentation of multiple myeloma. J Oral Maxillofac Surg 1992;50:408–13.

167. Zachariades N, Papanicolaou S, Papavassiliou D, Vairaktaris E, Triantafyllou D, Mezitis M. Plasma cell myeloma of the jaws. Int J Oral Maxillofac Surg 1987;16:510–5.

Leukemia and Lymphoma

168. Castella A, Davey FR, Elbadawi A, Gordon GB. Granulocytic sarcoma of the hard palate: report of the first case. Hum Pathol 1984;15:1190–2.
169. Choukas NC. Lymphosarcoma of the maxilla. Oral Surg Oral Med Oral Pathol 1967;23:567–72.
170. Cohen MA, Bender S, Struthers PJ. Hodgkin's disease of the jaws. Review of the literature and report of a case. Oral Surg Oral Med Oral Pathol 1984;57:413–7.
171. Conran MJ, Keohane C, Kearney PJ. Chloroma of the mandible: a problem of diagnosis and management. Acta Paediatr Scand 1982;71:1041–3.
172. Hiraki A, Nakamura S, Abe K, et al. Numb chin syndrome as an initial symptom of acute lymphocytic leukemia: report of three cases. Oral Surg Oral Med Oral Pathol Oral Radiol Endod 1997;83:555–61.
173. Huffman GG. Mandibular involvement in acute lymphocytic leukemia: report of a case. J Oral Surg 1976;34:842–3.
174. Langford A, Dienemann D, Schurman D, et al. Oral manifestations of AIDS–associated non-Hodgkin's lymphomas. Int J Oral Maxillofac Surg 1991;20:136–41.
175. Lello GE, Raubenheimer E. Hodgkin's disease presenting in the maxilla. A case report. Int J Oral Maxillofac Surg 1989;18:7–9.
176. Li TK, MacDonald-Janowski DS. An unusual presentation of a high-grade non-Hodgkin's lymphoma in the maxilla. Dentomaxillofac Radiol 1991;19:224–6.
177. Pileri SA, Montanari M, Falini B, et al. Malignant lymphoma involving the mandible: clinical, morphologic and immunohistochemical study of 17 cases. Am J Surg Pathol 1990;14:652–9.
178. Rios-Martin JJ, Villar-Rodriguez JL, Vasquez-Ramirez FJ, et al. Mandibular lymphomas with sclerosis. Oral Surg Oral Med Oral Pathol Oral Radiol Endod 1996;81:321–7.
179. Ronchi P, Epifani C, Lunetta PH. Hodgkin's disease of the jaw: report of a case. J Oral Maxillofac Surg 1988;46:155–8.
180. Rush M, Toth BB, Pinkel D. Clinically isolated mandibular relapse in childhood acute leukemia. Cancer 1990;66:369–72.
181. Sandlund JT, Fonseca T, Leimig T, et al. Predominance and characteristics of Burkitt lymphoma among children with non-Hodgkin lymphoma in northeastern Brazil. Leukemia 1997;11:743–6.
182. Soderholm AL, Lindqvist C, Heikinheimo K, Forssell K, Happonen RP. Non-Hodgkin's lymphoma presenting through oral symptoms. Int J Oral Maxillofac Surg 1990;19:131–4.
183. Stolarski CR, Boguslaw BI, Hoffman CH, Gates PE. Small-cell noncleaved non-Hodgkin's lymphoma of the mandible in previously unrecognized human immunodeficiency virus infection: report of a case. J Oral Maxillofac Surg 1997;55:853–6.
184. Willard CC, Foss RD, Hobbs TJ, Audair PL. Primary anaplastic large cell (Ki-1 positive) lymphoma of the mandible as the initial manifestation of acquired immunodeficiency syndrome in a pediatric patient. Oral Surg Oral Med Oral Pathol Oral Radiol Endod 1995;80:67–70.
185. Williams SA, Duggan MB, Bailey CC. Jaw involvement in acute lymphoblastic leukemia. Br Dent J 1983;155:164–6.

Hemangioma

186. Bunel K, Sindet-Pedersen S. Central hemangioma of the mandible. Oral Surg Oral Med Oral Pathol 1993;75:565–70.
187. DelBalso AM, Banyas JB, Wild LM. Hemangioma of the mandibular condyle and ramus. Am J Neuroradiol 1994;15:1703–5.
188. Ellis GL, Brannon RB. Intraosseous lymphangiomas of the mandible. Skeletal Radiol 1950;5:253–6.
189. Greene LA, Freedman PD, Friedman JM, Wolf M. Capillary hemangioma of the maxilla. A report of two cases in which angiography and embolization were used. Oral Surg Oral Med Oral Pathol 1990;70:268–73.
190. van Rensburg LJ, Nortje CJ, Wood RE. Advanced imaging in evaluation of a central mandibular haemangioma. Dentomaxillofac Radiol 1994;23:111–6.
191. Wei-Yung Y, Guang-Sheng M, Merrill RG, Sperry DW. Central hemangioma of the jaws. J Oral Maxillofac Surg 1989;47:1154–60.
192. Yukna RA, Cassingham RJ, Carr RF. Periodontal manifestations and treatment in a case of Sturge-Weber syndrome. Oral Surg Oral Med Oral Pathol 1979;47:408–15.

Angiosarcoma

193. Ellis GL, Kratochvil FJ III. Epithelioid hemangioendothelioma of the head and neck: a clinicopathologic report of twelve cases. Oral Surg Oral Med Oral Pathol 1986;61:61–8.
194. Freedman PD, Kerpel SM. Epithelioid angiosarcoma of the maxilla. A case report and review of the literature. Oral Surg Oral Med Oral Pathol 1992;74:319–25.
195. Lanigan DT, Hey JH, Lee L. Angiosarcoma of the maxilla and maxillary sinus: report of a case and review of the literature. J Oral Maxillofac Surg 1989;47:747–53.
196. Weiss SW, Enzinger FM. Epithelioid hemangioendothelioma. A vascular tumor often mistaken for a carcinoma. Cancer 1982;50:970–81.
197. Zachariades N, Papadakou A, Koundouris J, Constantinidis J, Angelopoulos AP. Primary hemangioendotheliosarcoma of the mandible: review of the literature and report of a case. J Oral Surg 1980;38:288–96.
198. Zakrzewska J. Angiosarcoma of the maxilla. A case report and review of the literature including angiosarcoma of the maxillary sinus. Br J Oral Maxillofac Surg 1986;24:286–92.

Synovial Chondromatosis of the Temporomandibular Joint

199. Ballard R, Weiland LH. Synovial chondromatosis of the temporomandibular joint. Cancer 1972;30:791–5.

200. Deboise A, Roche Y. Synovial chondromatosis of the temporomandibular joint possibly secondary to trauma. A case report. Int J Oral Maxillofac Surg 1991;20:90–2.

201. Fujita S, Iizuka T, Tuboi Y, Hyou Y. Synovial chondromatosis of the temporomandibular joint with immunohistochemical findings. Report of a case. J Oral Maxillofac Surg 1991;49:880–3.

202. Merrill RG, Wei-Yung Y, Shamloo J. Synovial chondrosarcoma of the temporomandibular joint: a case report. J Oral Maxillofac Surg 1997;55:1312–6.

203. Moses JJ, Hosaka H. Arthoscopic punch for definitive diagnosis of synovial chondromatosis of the temporomandibular joint. Case report and pathology review. Oral Surg Oral Med Oral Pathol 1993;75:12–7.

204. Musgrove BT, Moody GH. Synovial chondromatosis of the temporomandibular joint. Int J Oral Maxillofac Surg 1991;20:93–5.

205. Nomoto M, Nagao K, Numata T, Konno A, Kaneko T. Synovial osteochondromatosis of the temporomandibular joint. J Layngol Otol 1993;107:742–5.

206. Quinn PD, Stanton DC, Foote JW. Synovial chondromatosis with cranial extension. Oral Surg Oral Med Oral Pathol 1992;73:398–402.

207. Sun S, Helmy E, Bays R. Synovial chondromatosis with intracranial extension. A case report. Oral Surg Oral Med Oral Pathol 1990;70:5–9.

Pigmented Villonodular Synovitis of the Temporomandibular Joint

208. Eisig S, Dorfman HD, Cusamano RJ, Kantrowitz AB. Pigmented villonodular synovitis of the temporo-mandibular joint. Case report and review of the literature. Oral Surg Oral Med Oral Pathol 1992;73:328–33.

209. O'Sullivan TJ, Alport EC, Whiston HG. Pigmented villonodular synovitis of the temporomandibular joint. J Otolaryngol 1984;13:123–6.

210. White RD, Makar Jr J, Steckler RM. Synovial sarcoma of the temporomandibular joint. J Oral Maxillofac Surg 1992;50:1227–30.

Tophaceous Pseudogout

211. Ishida T, Dorfman MD, Bullough PG. Tophaceous pseudogout (tumoral calcium pyrophosphate dihydrate crystal deposition disease). Human Pathol 1995;26:587–93.

9
MISCELLANEOUS LESIONS

NEUROECTODERMAL TUMORS

Melanotic Neuroectodermal Tumor of Infancy

Definition. This is a dysembryogenetic neoplasm of neural crest origin affecting predominantly the craniofacial region of infants; it is comprised of two main elements, melanocytic and neuroblastic.

Historical Features. The lesion was first described by Krompecher in 1918 (4) and since that time there have been over 200 reported cases (2). One of the largest series is a review of

20 cases from the Armed Forces Institute of Pathology (3). The disputed histogenesis has a spawned a plethora of synonyms including *melanotic progonoma, retinal anlage tumor, melanotic ameloblastoma,* and the currently used terminology proposed by Borello and Gorlin (1), *melanotic neuroectodermal tumor of infancy.*

Clinical Features. Most of the lesions occur before the age of 1 year, with an equal sex distribution. The craniofacial region is involved in 87 percent of cases. About 70 percent of tumors occur in the maxilla, in the region of the anterior alveolar ridge (2). This frequently causes protrusion of the superior lip and, hence, problems with feeding (fig. 9-1). Other craniofacial sites of involvement, in decreasing order of frequency, are skull, dura and brain, mandible, and orbit; infrequent sites include other bones, skin, mediastinum, uterus, and epididymis. The neoplasm is usually not functional but catecholamine secretion has been documented (2). Radiologically, the neoplasm causes expansion and osteolytic destruction of the affected bone (fig. 9-2).

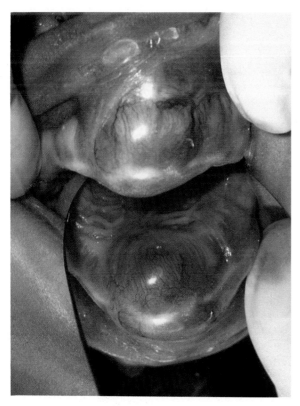

Figure 9-1
MELANOTIC NEUROECTODERMAL TUMOR
OF INFANCY

A dome-shaped swelling with purple discoloration protrudes from the anterior portion of the hard palate. The lesion above is being reflected in a mirror below. (Courtesy of Dr. Michael Kahn, Memphis, TN.) (Figures 9-1 and 9-2 are from the same patient.)

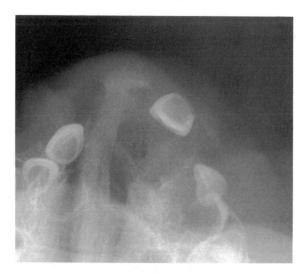

Figure 9-2
MELANOTIC NEUROECTODERMAL TUMOR
OF INFANCY

The radiograph shows a radiolucent lesion in the anterior maxilla causing displacement of teeth. (Courtesy of Dr. Michael Kahn, Memphis, TN.)

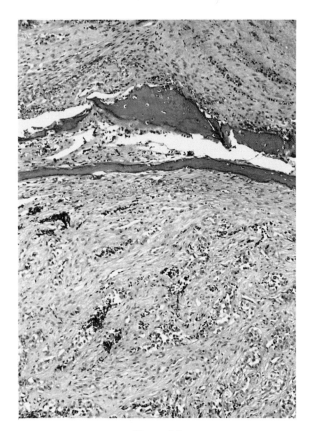

Figure 9-3
MELANOTIC NEUROECTODERMAL
TUMOR OF INFANCY

Nests of tumor cells envelop and have caused partial resorption of maxillary bone. (Courtesy of Dr. Gary Ellis, Washington, D.C.) (Figures 9-3– 9-5 are from the same patient.)

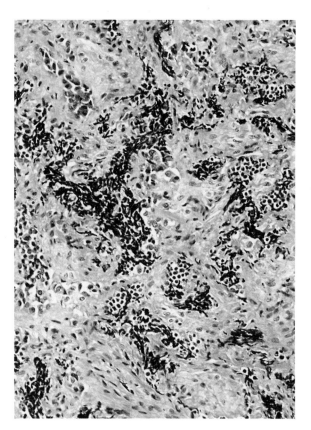

Figure 9-4
MELANOTIC NEUROECTODERMAL
TUMOR OF INFANCY

The tumor is composed of nests and cords, with a biphasic cellular population. More centrally placed are small "blue" cells showing smudging artefact due to nuclear fragility. Surrounding cells are large with abundant cytoplasm. (Courtesy of Dr. Gary Ellis, Washington, D.C.)

Pathologic Findings. The histopathologic features as well as the results of electron microscopic, immunohistochemical, and molecular studies indicate an origin from the neural crest. The presence of cells showing features of both melanocytic and ectodermal type suggested to Pettinato et al. (6) that the neoplasm is attempting to recapitulate retinal development at the 5-week period of gestation.

Histologically, the neoplasm is composed of alveolar nests and tubules separated by a fibrous stroma (figs. 9-3–9-5). The nests and tubules are populated by two distinct cell types: a peripheral layer of melanin-pigmented large cells surrounding groups of small neuroblastic type cells (figs. 9-4, 9-5). A fibrillar network may be seen between the nuclei of the neuroblastic cells. Maturation of neuroblasts to ganglion cells has also been reported (7).

Ultrastructurally, the large melanin-containing cells contain both premelanosomes and melanosomes as well as tonofilament bundles and desmosomes whereas the neuroblastic cells contain dense core neurosecretory type granules, neurotubules, and neurofilaments. These organelles are seen both within the cell body or within cellular cytoplasmic processes.

Immunohistochemically, the neoplasm exhibits a unique multiphenotypic profile of epithelial, melanocytic, and neural markers. The large melanocytic cells stain uniformly for cytokeratin, vimentin, and HMB-45 and may also stain for epithelial membrane antigen and S-100 protein. Both cell types tend to stain for Leu-7 whereas the small neuroblastic cell component may, in addition, stain for synaptophysin, glial fibrillary

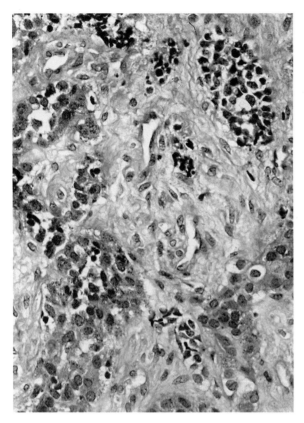

Figure 9-5
MELANOTIC NEUROECTODERMAL
TUMOR OF INFANCY
Nests of neuroblastoma type cells are seen in the upper right and nests of pigmented large melanocytic cells are elsewhere. (Courtesy of Dr. Gary Ellis, Washington, D.C.)

The age of the patient, location of the tumor, and the alveolar histologic pattern may result in a diagnosis of rhabdomyosarcoma. However, the typical biphasic cell population and immunohistochemical profile exclude that possibility.

Treatment and Prognosis. Most of the lesions have behaved in a benign fashion following local resection. A recurrence rate of 10 to 60 percent has been reported (2,6). Kapadia et al. (3) documented a 45 percent recurrence rate (5 of 12 tumors with follow-up) in their series of 20 cases from the Armed Forces Institute of Pathology. In a recent review, metastases were documented in only 13 of 195 reported cases (6.6 percent) (6).

Ewing's Sarcoma

Definition. Ewing's sarcoma is a malignant neoplasm composed of sheets of small round cells. It occurs most commonly in long bones and the flat bones of the pelvis. The histogenesis has remained obscure since its recognition in 1866 but recent evidence suggests a neuroectodermal derivation.

Clinical Features. The jaw bones are infrequently affected by Ewing's sarcoma, with a 1 to 10 percent incidence rate reported in the literature (8). The two largest series involve 19 cases reported by Geschickter and Copeland in 1949 (11) and 17 cases reported by Arafat et al. (8) from the Armed Forces Institute of Pathology in 1983. By the latter date over 80 cases had been reported. As in the extragnathic skeleton, the disease is most common in the second and third decades and males are more frequently affected than females. The mandible is involved more often than the maxilla.

Clinical features include swelling, pain, paresthesia, and loosening and displacement of teeth. Radiologically, there is usually an ill-defined, mottled, radiolucent and sclerotic appearance. An "onion-skin" or "sun-ray" periosteal reaction may be seen but is rare. Due to the lack of specificity of the clinical and radiologic features, the lesion may initially be misdiagnosed as a common dental problem, resulting in a delay in diagnosis and therapy.

Pathologic Findings. Histologically, the lesion is identical to Ewing's sarcoma of other bones and consists of sheets of small dark cells with scant cytoplasm. Foci of necrosis and mitotic activity

acidic protein, and S-100 protein (3). Molecular studies utilizing reverse transcription polymerase chain reaction have demonstrated the presence of melano-transferrin within the neoplastic cells (5). The tumors are either diploid or aneuploid but there have been too few tumors analyzed to attribute any prognostic significance to this finding (3).

Differential Diagnosis. There are three chief differential diagnoses. The lesion may be misinterpreted as a malignant melanoma but the early age at diagnosis, the presence of the neuroblastic cell component, and the unique immunohistochemical profile should exclude that diagnosis. The lesion may resemble a metastatic neuroblastoma; the presence of the melanocytic large cell component and the location of the tumor should trigger the need to perform the battery of immunohistochemical stains mentioned above.

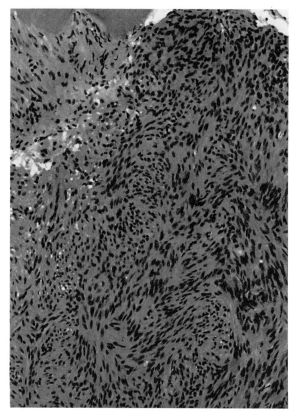

Figure 9-6
LEIOMYOMA OF MANDIBLE
This moderately cellular spindle cell neoplasm has a fascicular cell arrangement. Islands of preexisting bone are seen in left upper corner. (Figures 9-6 and 9-7 are from the same patient.)

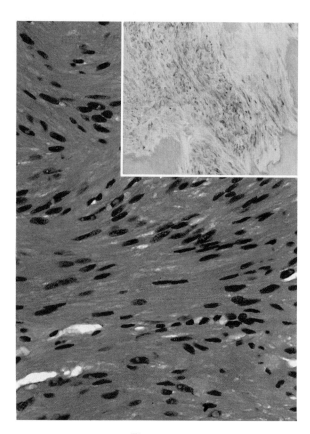

Figure 9-7
LEIOMYOMA OF MANDIBLE
There are elongated, uniform, cigar-shaped nuclei of smooth muscle cells. The elongated cytoplasmic tails of the cells are densely eosinophilic. Inset shows positive staining of the cytoplasm for desmin.

may be conspicuous. Extension of the neoplastic infiltrate into adjacent soft tissue is frequently observed. Glycogen granules can usually be demonstrated within the cytoplasm. Of most diagnostic help is the demonstration of a specific surface glycoprotein which can be demonstrated by the monoclonal antibody HBA-71 (10).

Treatment and Prognosis. The prognosis and therapy do not differ from those of Ewing's sarcoma involving other bones (9).

SMOOTH MUSCLE TUMORS

Definition. Both benign and malignant smooth muscle tumors occur as primary mesenchymal tumors within the jaw bones and are believed to be derived from undifferentiated mesenchymal cells or the smooth muscle of vessels.

Clinical and Radiologic Features. Smooth muscle tumors arising within bone are extremely rare (figs. 9-6, 9-7) and most are malignant. A literature review by Izumi et al. in 1995 (12) produced 60 leiomyosarcomas within the oral cavity of which 41 (28 maxillary and 13 mandibular) involved the jaw bones. A review of leiomyosarcoma of the skeleton by Kratochvil et al. in 1982 (13) demonstrated that the jaw bones comprised 40 percent of all cases. There is a wide age spectrum and males outnumber females. Two maxillary leiomyosarcomas developed in patients who had received radiation therapy for retinoblastoma many years previously (14). Patients usually present with swelling, pain, and loosening of teeth. Radiologically, the lesion is radiolucent, ill-defined, and may cause resorption of the roots of the teeth.

Pathologic Findings. The sarcomas may be poorly differentiated and initially misdiagnosed. A smooth muscle origin should be suspected if the tumor cells have distinctly eosinophilic, elongated, cytoplasmic tails and cigar-shaped nuclei with blunt rounded ends. In the past, simple histochemical stains such as the Masson trichrome stain to demonstrate red coloration of sarcoplasm, phosphotungstic acid hematoxylin to demonstrate longitudinal myofilaments, and periodic acid-Schiff stain with and without subsequent diastase digestion to demonstrate glycogen were useful diagnostic aids. Ultrastructural examination demonstrated cytoplasmic filaments with dense bodies and attachment plaques on the cell membrane. Most laboratories are now able to confirm a smooth muscle origin by immunohistochemical techniques using antibodies against desmin and smooth muscle-specific actin.

The finding of a malignant smooth muscle tumor within bone should always prompt a search for a possible extraskeletal primary site. In female patients particular attention should be paid to the possibility of a primary tumor of the myometrium.

Treatment and Prognosis. The only effective mode of therapy is surgical ablation of the tumor. Radiotherapy and chemotherapy are of limited value and have been used postoperatively or for palliation. Lesions of jaw bones metastasize most commonly to lungs and regional lymph nodes. In a review of intraoral leiomyosarcomas of which 58 percent involved maxilla or mandible, Schenberg et al. (15) reported distant metastases, most commonly to the lung, in 39 percent. Metastases were present in cervical nodes in 15 percent of cases and nearly all of these also had distant spread. The local recurrence rate for surgically treated cases was 35 percent and the 5-year cure rate only 23 percent. These results highlight the aggressive nature of this neoplasm.

PERIPHERAL NERVE SHEATH TUMORS

Definition. Schwannomas, neurofibromas, and malignant peripheral nerve sheath tumors identical to those in extraoral and extragnathic locations occur in the oral cavity and jaws. They are benign or malignant nerve sheath tumors derived from Schwann cells or perineurial fibroblasts.

Clinical and Radiologic Features. About 45 percent of all nerve sheath tumors occur in the head and neck region but less than 10 percent involve the oral cavity, including the jaws (17,19). Within the oral cavity, the sites of involvement in decreasing order of frequency are the anterior portion of the tongue, palate, floor of mouth, oral mucosa, gingiva, lips, and buccal mucosa (26). They constitute less than 1 percent of all benign bone neoplasms. Over 40 cases of peripheral nerve sheath tumors have been documented to involve the jaw bones (26). Nearly all of these have occurred in the posterior body and ramus region of the mandible as they have originated from the inferior dental nerve (16). This nerve courses through a longer bony canal than any other peripheral nerve in the body. Only a few cases have been reported in the anterior portion of the body of the mandible or the maxilla (20,22). These central intraosseous nerve sheath tumors present most frequently in the second and third decades and show a female preponderance in a ratio of 1.6 to 1 (21).

Peripheral nerve sheath tumors usually present with a swelling of the affected jaw. Other less frequently observed symptoms include pain and paresthesia. A few cases have been reported to occur in association with neurofibromatosis. Radiologically, the appearance is that of a nonspecific, radiolucent, unilocular or multilocular lesion (fig. 9-8). The lesion is usually well circumscribed. Teeth may be displaced and occasionally resorbed (24). A nerve sheath tumor should be suspected if there is an expansion of the inferior alveolar canal (fig. 9-9).

Pathologic Findings. Schwannomas are usually well encapsulated and attached to the peripherally displaced nerve from which they originate. Occasionally, the schwannoma may have a plexiform, multinodular configuration. Neurofibromas and malignant peripheral nerve sheath tumors lack such encapsulation. Microscopically, these tumors are identical to their counterparts elsewhere in the body (figs. 9-10–9-12). Most of the well-documented examples of central peripheral nerve sheath tumor appear to represent schwannomas rather than neurofibromas.

Malignant peripheral nerve sheath tumors are difficult to distinguish from sarcomas of other histogenetic types and only a few well-documented examples of such lesions exist in the

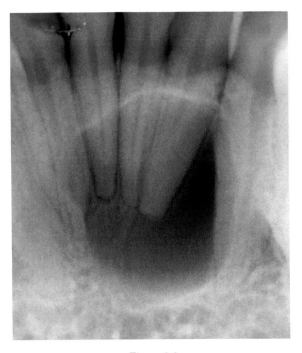

Figure 9-8
NEUROFIBROMA OF MANDIBLE
This neurofibroma has produced a sharply circumscribed lytic lesion in the region of the symphysis.

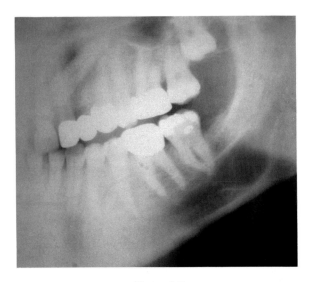

Figure 9-9
NEUROFIBROMA OF INFERIOR DENTAL NERVE
A sharply circumscribed radiolucent lesion in the body of mandible has expanded the dental canal. (Figures 9-9–9-12 are from the same patient.)

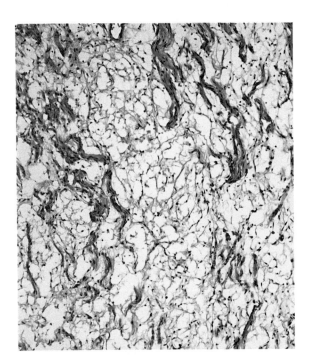

Figure 9-10
NEUROFIBROMA OF INFERIOR ALVEOLAR NERVE
Wavy bundles of nerve sheath cells are separated by nerve sheath elements with a myxoid configuration.

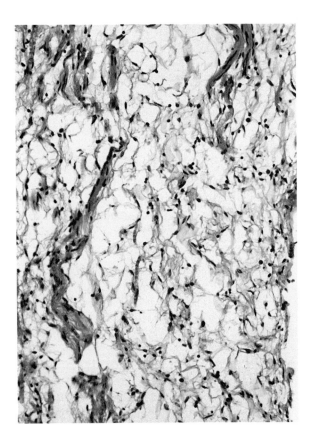

Figure 9-11
NEUROFIBROMA OF INFERIOR ALVEOLAR NERVE
The wavy configuration of the cell processes in both the cell bundles and myxoid component of the lesion is illustrated.

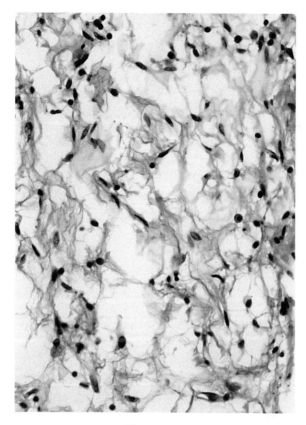

Figure 9-12
NEUROFIBROMA OF INFERIOR ALVEOLAR NERVE
The cells of the neurofibroma are bland and spindle or stellate shaped. A few mast cells are also present.

jaws (18). In order to firmly establish a diagnosis of a sarcoma as being of nerve sheath origin, it should fulfill one or more of the following criteria: develop in a patient with neurofibromatosis; demonstrate attachment to a large peripheral nerve; show histologic evidence of residual foci of neurofibroma; immunoreact with antibody to S-100 protein; or show convincing electron microscopic evidence of derivation from perineurial fibroblasts or Schwann cells.

An interesting histologic finding in a few reported schwannomas has been the presence of nests of epithelial cells within the tumor. The epithelial nests may be solid or show glandular differentiation. In some cases the glandular structures may simply represent an entrapped salivary gland duct within a neurofibroma (23). Solid epithelial nests within a schwannoma have also been shown to be derived from included nests of a vestigial juxtaoral organ of Chievitz (25). This

originates during embryogenesis as a mucosal thickening adjacent to the ridge destined to form the parotid gland. The glandular elements seen within some tumors have been postulated to be derived from displaced ependymal cells, neuroectodermal stem cells, or cells derived from the central canal of the spinal cord (23).

Treatment. Benign peripheral nerve sheath tumors are usually cured by local excision. Every effort should be made to conserve any attached nerve to preserve nerve function.

LIPOMA, LIPOSARCOMA, LIPOBLASTOMA

Intraosseous neoplasms of lipocytic derivation are extremely rare and constitute less than 1 of 1,000 bone neoplasms from the Mayo Clinic (27). By 1992 only eight lipomas involving the jaw had been reported. Oral lipomas are more frequent and involve the following sites in decreasing order of frequency: buccal mucosa, tongue, floor of mouth, buccal sulcus, palate, lips, and gingiva (31). Within bone, mandible and maxilla are affected with no particular site predilection. All patients are adults of equal sex distribution.

Clinically, the lesion may be found as an incidental radiologic abnormality or it may produce swelling, paresthesia, or pain. Radiologically, the lesion produces a well-marginated radiolucent defect which may be unilocular or multilocular and may expand the bone. One case is described as having a radiopaque center resulting from the presence of foci of osseous metaplasia (31). This finding may correspond to the foci of infarction with dystrophic calcification that cause focal radiopacities in lipomas described at other intraosseous sites.

Histologically, the lesion shows the usual pattern of lobules of mature adipose tissue delineated by thin fibrous septa (figs. 9-13–9-15). In a few areas, a prominent vascular component justifies the terminology, *angiolipoma* (28,30). There is some debate in the literature as to whether intraosseous lipomas represent a true neoplasm derived from the marrow fat or a reactive process in which the adipose tissue represents a space-filling defect (27). Treatment consists of simple curettage or enucleation.

To date there are no well-documented examples of liposarcoma within jaw bones. In the rare case

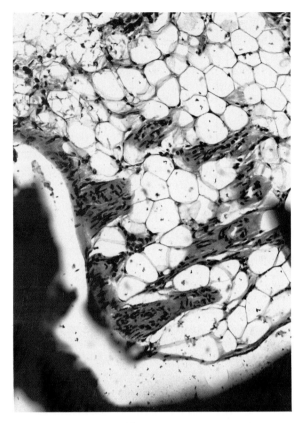

Figure 9-13
LIPOMA OF JAW
A lobule of mature adipose tissue is within bone of the jaw.

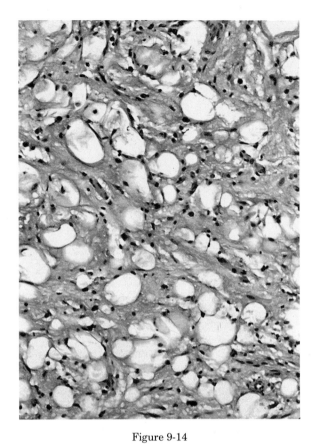

Figure 9-14
MYXOID LIPOMA
Admixture of mature lipocytes and stellate myxoid cells compose this myxoid lipoma of jaw. (Figures 9-14 and 9-15 are from the same patient.)

Figure 9-15
MYXOID LIPOMA
Higher magnification illustrates mature lipocytes and bland stellate myxoma cells.

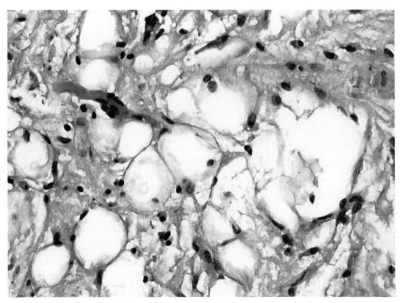

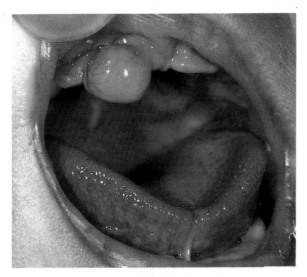

Figure 9-16
CONGENITAL EPULIS OF THE NEWBORN
A pedunculated, smooth-surfaced, nodular mass along the maxillary anterior alveolar crest in a 3-day-old female.

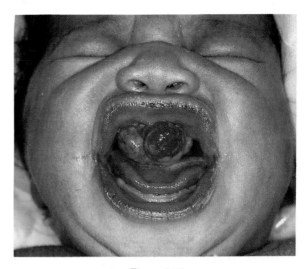

Figure 9-17
CONGENITAL EPULIS OF THE NEWBORN
A bilobed, ulcerated and bulky mass of the anterior maxillary alveolar ridge was obstructing feeding in a female child.

report, the histologic features are either not convincing or it is unclear as to whether the sarcoma arose within bone or adjacent soft tissue.

There is a single case of a well-documented lipoblastoma involving the mandibular ramus of a 26-month-old child (29). The tumor caused marked deformity of the cheek. It was readily enucleated and histologically showed lobules of adipose tissue composed of an admixture of mature adipocytes as well as embryonic multivacuolated fat cells. The child was well without facial deformity 5 years after surgery.

CONGENITAL EPULIS OF THE NEWBORN

Definition. The congenital epulis (*congenital gingival granular cell tumor*) is a rare soft tissue mass of uncertain origin composed of granular cells and located in the anterior segment of the jaws in newborn infants. Sufficient phenotypic and developmental features help separate this lesion from other oral lesions that contain granular cells (35,38). Theories of histogenesis include origin from neural sheath cells (39), myofibroblasts (42), smooth muscle cells (40), macrophages (36), pericytic cells (32), mesenchymal precursors of smooth muscle, or fibroblasts (37,44).

Clinical Features. This benign nonodontogenic tumor is found only in neonates. Up to 90

percent of lesions occur in females, most frequently in the maxillary alveolar ridge (fig. 9-16). The epulis usually presents as a solitary mass, but may be multiple, either in the same region of the affected jaw or within both the maxillary and mandibular arches (43). Patients are asymptomatic and the lesion is usually found incidentally. The mass is often less than 2 cm in diameter but may attain sufficient size to interfere with nutrition by causing oral obstruction (fig. 9-17) (33). Lesions are frequently pedunculated but may be sessile and have a smooth overlying mucosa, although traumatic ulceration may occur in larger lesions.

Pathologic Findings. An attenuated layer of stratified squamous epithelium, often with a flat epithelial-connective tissue junction, covers the mass, which is composed of an unencapsulated aggregate of large, round to polyhedral cells. Individual cells contain moderately basophilic nuclei and abundant, finely granular, eosinophilic cytoplasm (figs. 9-18–9-20). Mitoses are rare and necrosis is absent except in association with surface ulceration. Evenly dispersed, thin-walled vascular spaces are noted and thin fibrous septa may be present (fig. 9-21). Unlike the granular cell tumor (myoblastoma), there is neither overlying pseudoepitheliomatous hyperplasia nor S-100 protein positivity of the granular cell population (41).

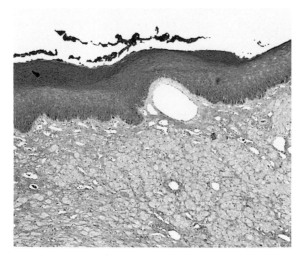

Figure 9-18
CONGENITAL EPULIS OF THE NEWBORN

Attenuated, stratified squamous epithelium covers a cellular mass of polygonal granular cells. A rich network of thin walled blood vessels in a delicate stroma separates the overlying epithelium from the granular cell population.

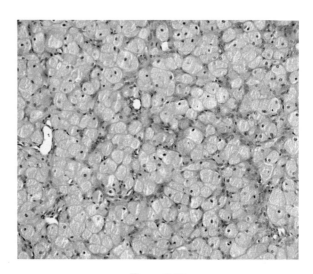

Figure 9-19
CONGENITAL EPULIS OF THE NEWBORN

Round to polygonal cells with laterally placed, evenly stained nuclei and a delicate fibrovascular stromal component are seen.

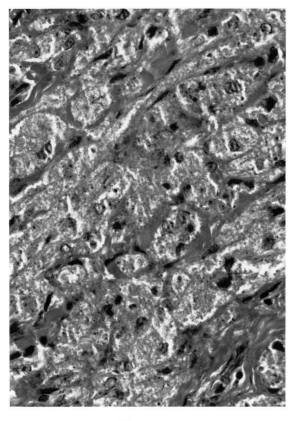

Figure 9-20
CONGENITAL EPULIS OF THE NEWBORN

This trichrome stain allows recognition of the fibrous stroma which delineates small clusters of granular cells.

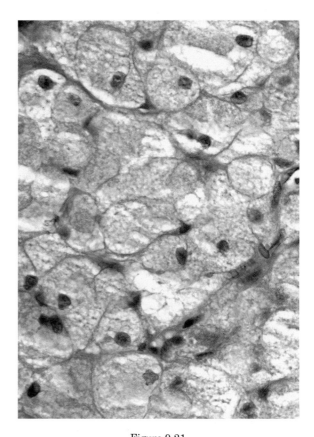

Figure 9-21
CONGENITAL EPULIS OF THE NEWBORN

Uniformly granular cytoplasm fills the large round and polygonal cells. Nuclei are peripherally located.

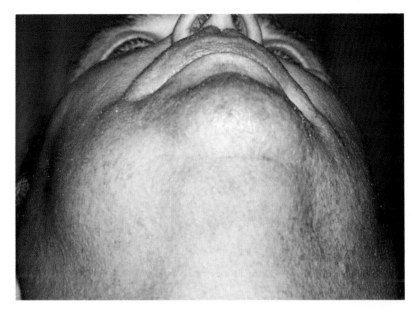

Figure 9-22
MANDIBULAR METASTASIS
This metastatic lesion has caused mandibular swelling in the region of the angle. (Figures 9-22–9-26 are from the same patient.)

Ultrastructurally, tightly aggregated, autophagosome cytoplasmic granules, which are membrane-bound and electron dense, crowd the cytoplasm. Other ultrastructural features within the cytoplasm include the presence of vesicles, banded intracellular collagen fibrils, and thin filaments with focal dense patches (37, 40,44). The cell membrane demonstrates pinocytosis and areas of exocytosis (32). In contrast to the granular cell myoblastoma, however, intracellular, membrane-bound fibrillar bodies (angulate bodies) are absent.

Differential Diagnosis. Clinically, this is a distinct entity, unlikely to be confused with other lesions. Histologically, it closely resembles the more common granular cell tumor (myoblastoma), however, S-100 protein staining is positive in the granular cell tumor and that lesion frequently exhibits pseudoepitheliomatous hyperplasia of the overlying epithelium.

Treatment and Prognosis. Simple excision under local anesthesia is curative. Recurrence is extremely rare, with case reports demonstrating spontaneous regression over a period of a year (34).

METASTATIC TUMORS TO JAW BONES

Metastatic tumors to the oral region are relatively infrequent. A review of cases in the English language literature up to 1991 disclosed 390 cases specifically involving the jaw bones

(45). In this review, the average age of presentation was 45.5 years, with a majority of patients in the fifth to seventh decades. In women, the most frequent primary site was the breast (42 percent), followed by adrenal gland (8.5 percent), colorectum (8 percent), female genital organs (7.5 percent), and thyroid (6 percent); for men it was the lung (22.3 percent), followed by the prostate (12 percent), kidney (10.3 percent), bone (9.2 percent), and adrenal gland (9.2 percent). Isolated case reports of primary lesions from many other sites have been documented.

The mandible alone was involved in 81 percent of cases, the maxilla alone in 13.6 percent, and both jaw bones in 5.4 percent. Within the mandible, the metastases were most frequently located in the molar region (fig. 9-22). Swelling, pain, and paresthesia were the most common symptoms. In 37.2 percent of cases, the jawbone metastasis was the first sign of a metastatic process; in 29.4 percent, the metastatic lesion was the primary manifestation of malignancy. Of note was the presence of a normal radiograph despite the pain and swelling in 5.4 percent of cases. Radiologically, the lesion is usually lytic with ill-defined margins (figs. 9-23, 9-24). The use of technetium-99 m-phosphonate bone scintigraphy, magnetic resonance imaging (MRI), and computed tomography (CT) help evaluate the extent of the metastatic process (fig. 9-25). Histologically, the lesions resemble their counterparts in other bones (fig. 9-26).

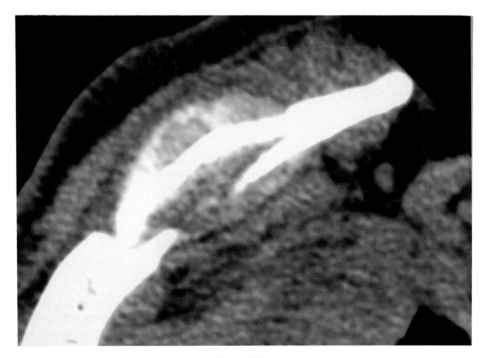

Figure 9-23
MANDIBULAR METASTASIS
Axial CT scan demonstrates a destructive lesion of the mandible that perforates the lingual plate and extends into soft tissue both medially and laterally.

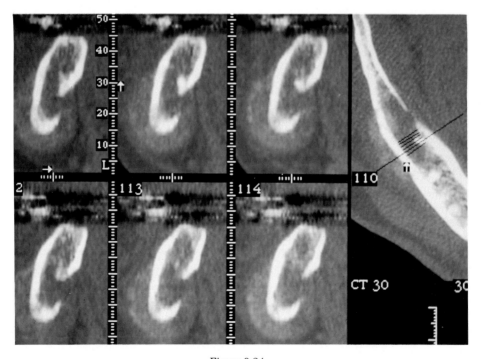

Figure 9-24
MANDIBULAR METASTASIS
Coronal CT sections show perforation of the lingual plate and a soft tissue component wrapping around the inferior aspect of the mandible.

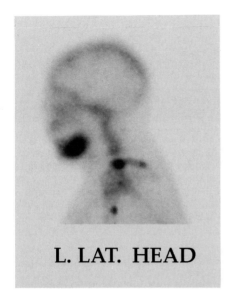 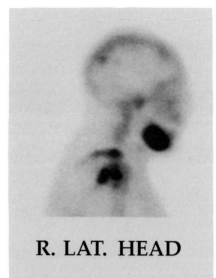

L. LAT. HEAD   **R. LAT. HEAD**

Figure 9-25
MANDIBULAR METASTASIS
Technetium-99 m-phosphon-
ate scintigram demonstrates a
large "hot" lesion within the mandible.

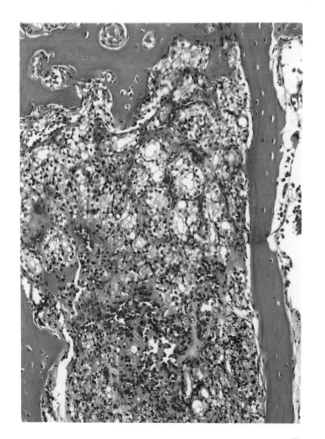 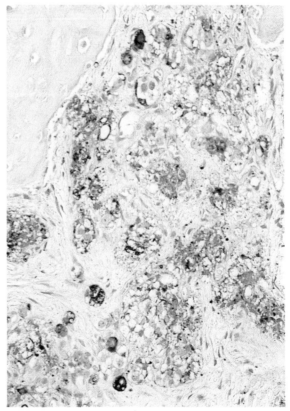

Figure 9-26
MANDIBULAR METASTASIS
Left: Metastatic prostate carcinoma.
Right: Positive staining for prostatic specific antigen by immunohistochemistry.

REFERENCES

Melanotic Neuroectodermal Tumor of Infancy

1. Borello ED, Gorlin RJ. Melanotic neuroectodermal tumor of infancy—a neoplasm of neural crest origin. Report of a case associated with high urinary excretion of vanilmandelic acid. Cancer 1966;19:196–206.
2. Hoshino S, Takahashi H, Shimura T, Nakazawa S, Naito Z, Asano G. Melanotic neuroectodermal tumor of infancy in the skull associated with high serum levels of catecholamine. Case report. J Neurosurg 1994;80:919–24.
3. Kapadia SB, Frisman DM, Hitchcock CL, Ellis GL, Popek EJ. Melanotic neuroectodermal tumor of infancy. Clinicopathological, immunohistochemical, and flow cytometric study. Am J Surg Pathol 1993;17:566–73.
4. Krompecher E. Zur histogenese und morphologie der adamantinome und sonstiger kiefergeschwulste. Beitr Pathol Anat 1918;4:165–97.
5. Nitta T, Endo T, Tsunoda A, Kudota Y, Matsumoto T, Sato K. Melanotic neuroectodermal tumor of infancy: a molecular approach to diagnosis. J Neurosurg 1995;83:145–8.
6. Pettinato G, Manivel C, d'Amore ES, Jaszcz W, Gorlin RJ. Melanotic neuroectodermal tumor of infancy. Am J Surg Pathol 1991;15:233–45.
7. Shah RV, Jambhekar NA, Rana DN, et al. Melanotic neuroectodermal tumor of infancy: report of a case with ganglionic differentiation. J Surg Oncol 1994;55:65–8.

Ewing's Sarcoma

8. Arafat A, Ellis GL, Adrian JC. Ewing's sarcoma of the jaws. Oral Surg Oral Med Oral Pathol 1983;55:589 95.
9. Borghelli RF, Zampieri J. Ewing sarcoma of the mandible, report of case. J Oral Surg 1978;36:473–5.
10. Fechner RE, Mills SE. In: Tumors of the bone and joints. Atlas of Tumor Pathology, 3rd series, Washington, DC: Armed Forces Institute of Pathology 1993:193.
11. Geschickter CF, Copeland M. In: Tumors of bone, 3rd ed. Philadelphia: JB Lippincott 1949:387.

Smooth Muscle Tumors

12. Izumi K, Maeda T, Cheng J, Saku T. Primary leiomyosarcoma of the maxilla with regional node metastases. Report of a case and review of the literature. Oral Surg Oral Med Oral Pathol 1995;80:310–9.
13. Kratochvil FJ, MacGregor SD, Hewan-Lowe K, Allsup HW. Leiomyosarcoma of the maxilla. Report of a case and review of the literature. Oral Surg Oral Med Oral Pathol 1982;54:647–55.
14. Martin-Hirsch DP, Habashi S, Benbow EW, Farrington WT. Post-irradiation leiomyosarcoma of the maxilla. J Laryngol Otol 1991;105:1068–71.
15. Schenberg ME, Slootweg PJ, Koole R. Leiomyosarcomas of the oral cavity. Report of four cases and review of the literature. J Craniomaxillofac Surg 1991;21:342–7.

Peripheral Nerve Sheath Tumors

16. Artzi Z, Taicher S, Nass D. Neurilemmoma of the mental nerve. J Oral Maxillofac Surg 1991;49:196–200.
17. Das Gupta TK, Brasfield RD, Strong EW, Hajdu ST. Benign solitary schwannomas (neurilemmomas). Cancer 1969;24:355–66.
18. David DJ, Speculand B, Vernon-Roberts B, Sach RP. Malignant schwannoma of the inferior dental nerve. Br J Plastic Surg 1978;31:323–33.
19. Ellis GL, Abrams AM, Melrose RJ. Intraosseous benign neural sheath neoplasms of the jaws. Oral Surg Oral Med Oral Pathol 1977;44:731–43.
20. Minic AJ. Central schwannoma of the maxilla. Int J Maxillofac Surg 1992;21:297–8.
21. Murphy J, Giunta JL. Atypical central neurilemmoma of the mandible. Oral Surg Oral Med Oral Pathol 1984;59:275–8.
22. Ord RA, Rennie JS. Central neurilemmoma of the maxilla. Report of a case and review of the literature. Int J Oral Surg 1981;10:137–9.
23. Papanicolaou SJ, Eversole LR. Glandular structures in neural sheath neoplasms. Oral Surg Oral Med Oral Pathol 1982;53:69–72.
24. Rubin MM, Koll TJ. Central neurilemmoma (schwannoma) of the mandible. NY State Dental J 1993;59:43–5.
25. Sciubba JJ, Sachs SA. Schwannoma of the inferior alveolar nerve in association with the organ of Chievitz. J Oral Pathol 1980;9:16–28.
26. Villanueva J, Gigoux C, Sole F. Central neurilemmoma of maxilla. Oral Surg Oral Med Oral Pathol Radiol Endod 1995;79:41–3.

Lipoma, Liposarcoma, Lipoblastoma

27. Barker GR, Sloan P. Intraosseous lipomas: clinical features of a mandibular case with possible aetiology. Br J Oral Maxillofac Surg 1986;24:459–63.
28. Lewis DM, Brannon RB, Isaksson B, Larsson A. Intraosseous angiofibroma of the mandible. Oral Surg Oral Med Oral Pathol 50;2:156–9.
29. Obwegeser HL, Makek MS. Benign lipoblastoma of the mandible. Head Neck Surg 1983;5:251–6.

30. Polte HW, Kolodny SC, Hooker SP. Intra-osseous angiolipoma of the mandible. Oral Surg Oral Med Oral Pathol 1976;41:637–43.

31. To WH, Yeung KH. Intra-oseous lipoma of the maxillary tuberosity. Br J Oral Maxillofac Surg 1992;30:122–4.

Congenital Epulis of the Newborn

32. Damm DD, Cibull ML, Geissler RH, Neville BW, Bowden CM, Lehmann JE. Investigation into the histogenesis of congenital epulis of the newborn. Oral Surg Oral Med Oral Pathol 1993;76:205–12.

33. Eppley BL, Sadore AM, Campbell A. Obstructive congenital epulis in a newborn. Ann Plast Surg 1991;27:152–5.

34. Jenkins HR, Hill CM. Spontaneous regression of congenital epulis of the newborn. Arch Dis Child 1989;64:145–7.

35. Junquera LM, de Vicente JC, Vega JA, Losa JL, Albertos JM, Lopez-Arranz JS. Granular cell tumors: an immunohistochemical study. Br J Oral Maxillofac Surg 1997;35:180–4.

36. Kaiserling E, Ruck P, Xiao JC. Congenital epulis and granular cell tumor: a histologic and immunohistochemical study. Oral Surg Oral Med Oral Pathol 1995; 80:687–97.

37. Kameyama Y, Mizohata M, Takehana S, Murata H, Manabe H, Mukai Y. Ultrastructure of the congenital epulis. Virchows Arch [A] 1983;401:251–60.

38. Mirchandani R, Sciubba JJ, Mir R. Granular cell lesions of the jaws and oral cavity: a clinicopathologic, immunohistochemical and ultrastructural study. J Oral Maxillofac Surg 1989;47:1248–55.

39. Regezi JA, Zarbo RJ, Courtney RM, Crissman JD. Immunoreactivity of granular cell lesions of skin, mucosa and jaw. Cancer 1989;64:1455–60.

40. Semba I, Kitano M, Mimura T. Gingival leiomyomatous hamartoma: immunohistochemical and ultrastructural observations. J Oral Pathol Med 1993;22:468–70.

41. Takahashi H, Fujita S, Satoh H, Okabe H. Immunohistochemical study of congenital gingival granular cell tumor (congenital epulis). J Oral Pathol Med 1990;19:492–6.

42. Tucker MC, Rusnock EJ, Azumi N, Hoy GR, Lack EE. Gingival granular cell tumors of the newborn. An ultrastructural and immunohistochemical study. Arch Pathol Lab Med 1990;114:895–8.

43. Ugras S, Demirtas I, Bekerecioglu M, Kutluhan A, Karakok M, Peker O. Immunohistochemical study on histogenesis of congenital epulis and review of the literature. Pathol Int 1997;47:627–32.

44. Zarbo RJ, Lloyd RV, Beals TF, McClatchey KD. Congenital gingival granular cell tumor with smooth muscle cytodifferentiation. Oral Surg Oral Med Oral Pathol 1983;56:512–20.

Metastatic Tumors to Jawbones

45. Hirshberg A, Leibovich P, Buchner A. Metastatic tumors to the jawbones: analysis of 390 cases. J Oral Pathol Med 1994;23:337–41.

Index*

---

*Numbers in boldface indicate table and figure pages.

✧✧✧